AGING PHENOMENA

Relationships among Different Levels of Organization

ADVANCES IN EXPERIMENTAL MEDICINE AND BIOLOGY

Recent Volumes in this Series

AGING PHENOMENA

Relationships among Different Levels of Organization

Edited by

Kunio Oota
Tokyo Metropolitan Institute of Gerontology
Tokyo, Japan

Takashi Makinodan
Veterans Administration
Wadsworth Medical Center
Los Angeles, California

Masami Iriki
Tokyo Metropolitan Institute of Gerontology
Tokyo, Japan

and

Lynn S. Baker
Veterans Administration
Wadsworth Medical Center
Los Angeles, California

PLENUM PRESS • NEW YORK AND LONDON

Library of Congress Cataloging in Publication Data

Naito Symposium on Aging, Tokyo, 1978.
Aging phenomena.

(Advances in experimental medicine and biology; v. 129)
Includes index.
1. Aging – Congresses. I. Oota, Kunio. II. Naitō Kinen Kagaku Shinkō Zaidan.
III. Title. IV. Series.
QP86.N34 1978 599.03'72 80-16223
ISBN-13: 978-1-4684-3736-2 e-ISBN-13: 978-1-4684-3734-8
DOI: 10.1007/ 978-1-4684-3734-8

Proceedings of the Naito Foundation Symposium
on Aging, held in Tokyo, Japan, August 27–29, 1978.

A Division of Plenum Publishing Corporation
227 West 17th Street, New York, N.Y. 10011

FOREWORD

The problem of senescence, as reflected in the history of religion and philosophy, has long been one of the greatest concerns of humankind. In contrast, gerontology as a branch of science is still comparatively young. During the past decade, concomitant with rapid progress in our understanding of the basic life sciences, vast stores of knowledge about biological aging have been accumulated. This knowledge, however, arising from many scientific disciplines and focused on varying levels of biologic organization, seems almost random and covers everything from molecules to human societies. Theories advanced to interpret the facts and to understand the mechanisms involved in senescence have remained in individual, rather than general, territories.

It has long been felt by some gerontologists that it was time for the various specialists to step back and take a generalist view of gerontology, to reconsider and reevaluate the fruits of their analytical pursuits at different levels within a broader context. Some others may think it still premature. It seemed, however, that the majority of those who gathered in Tokyo on the occasion of the XIth International Congress of Gerontology were of the opinion that there was much to be gained in looking for interrelationships among the facts and theories originated in the different levels of investigation in an attempt to observe and appreciate the biological drama of senescence as an entity. In spite of the unusual late summer heat and heavy schedules during the post-congress period, the Naito Symposium was attended by no less than 170 people from a variety of disciplines.

In the symposium, the organizer and participants tried to clarify the status of our present knowledge in the individual areas, to determine exactly what the gaps are in our current understanding, and to help point the way toward new paths for future research and, hopefully, our next breakthroughs. Thanks to the enthusiasm of colleagues from all over the world, the Naito Symposium was felt to be a success: a number of new facts were presented, some fresh strategic points discussed, and certain new ways of reasoning proposed. Looking back, however, the two full days were not enough time to arrive at a full understanding of biological aging. They were sufficient, however, for us to realize the importance of further attempts at unifying our knowledge and to be optimistic that future efforts will, indeed, be fruitful.

On behalf of the organizing committee, I would like to take this opportunity to express my deep-felt thanks to the Naito Foundation, both for sponsoring the project and for their warm hospitality, which was essential to the success of the meeting.

KUNIO OOTA, M.D.
August, 1979
Tokyo

INTRODUCTION: AN OVERVIEW

The theme of the Naito Symposium on Aging is "A Reevaluation of Interrelationships among Aging Phenomena in Different Levels of Organization." Inasmuch as aging is the most complex and multifaceted of all life processes, reevaluation must be performed recurrently and thoughtfully. The Naito Symposium contributes to this process by highlighting several new trends in biogerontological thinking and research.

Three speakers produce evidence against the somatic mutation hypothesis. Permanently tetraploid fibroblast clones produced by cell fusion had the same life span as diploid clones, tending to rule out any direct role of either recessive or dominant mutations in the aging processes of the diploid fibroblast cultures. The absence of any decrease with age of messenger RNA synthesis in most mouse brain regions, except for the specific decrease of mRNA/DNA ratios in the striatum, is consonant with other evidence about the distinctive aging pattern of the dopaminergic nigro-striatal system in mouse and man, and favors hypotheses of genetic program control of aging rather than hypotheses of mutational degradation. The discovery of methionine sulfoxide reductase in mammalian cells, and of its role in reversing peroxidative changes in proteins, tends to strengthen the role of postsynthetic changes in proteins as the basis for the loss of enzyme activity in old age, and to underline enzyme degradation as a major governing factor in the changes of enzyme levels with age. Consistent with these findings, evidence is given that the fidelity of RNA translation does not decrease with age. These lines of evidence imply, not that the somatic mutation hypothesis must be discarded, but rather that it is inadequate in its present form, and needs new kinds of data and a more refined theoretical formulation.

The relation of systemic aging processes to specific ultrastructural and molecular changes in the humoral and neural communication systems is documented in three papers. The almost linear decrease in number of steroid hormone receptors on cell surfaces with age, the decrement of immunological receptors, and the loss of dendritic processes and dendritic spines from cortical neurons suggest that the intercellular communication channels are particularly vulnerable to aging changes, but they also suggest the possibility of exciting new research efforts directed toward assessing the degree of reversibility of these changes.

The equivocal role of the immune system as both a life-sustaining and a senescence-engendering agent is examined from several viewpoints, but space allows me to note only one intriguing observation: the finding that some individuals with deficient immune competence are also deficient in the capacity for certain kinds of DNA repair.

The question of programmed versus random aging also arises in regard to animal cell populations *in vivo*. Certain body cells of developing animals have limited survival due to genetic programming, and genetically programmed cell death is also present in the adult stage. Continued work with exquisitely regulated systems may throw new light on the genetic control of cell proliferation and cell death.

The important problem of the impact of our industrial environment on the aging process is a recurrent theme. In addition to the studies on cellular systems mentioned above, the use of the medaka, or rice fish, *Oryzias latipes*, as a model system for investigating a variety of environmental problems is described, and the nature of the late injury produced in mammals by ionizing radiations is examined. The similarity of the cumulative radiation damage in cultured cells and whole animals is an especially valuable new insight.

This fragmentary account may dimly convey the exciting progress in biogerontological research today, but it cannot adequately convey the vigor and promise of the research being reported by the young Japanese investigators. The next such reevaluation will hear much more from them.

GEORGE A. SACHER
Division of Biological and Medical Research
Argonne National Laboratory
Argonne, IL 60439 USA

CONTENTS

CHANGES IN GENETIC INFORMATION AND AGING

AGING AND INTERCELLULAR COMMUNICATION

AGING IN THE HIGHER HIERARCHY

AGING: SOME PERSPECTIVES

PARTICIPANTS

Organizer:	K. Oota, Japan
Session Chairpersons:	L. Hayflick, United States M. Yamada, Japan H. Tauchi, Japan S. Fujita, Japan P. Ebbesen, Denmark D. Mizuno, Japan M.M.B. Kay, United States M. Iriki, Japan K. Oota, Japan S. Tsurufuji, Japan T. Makinodan, United States C. Finch, United States G. Sacher, United States N. Egami, Japan
Session Speakers:	A. Macieira-Coelho, France Y. Mitsui, Japan A. Shima, Japan K. Brizzee, United States Y. Hayashi (for M. Igarashi), Japan D. Gershon, Israel G. Martin, United States Y. Courtois, France G. Roth, United States T. Tada, Japan P. Ebbesen, Denmark W. Bondareff, United States M. Kay, United States Yu Nagai, Japan A. Ooshima, Japan C. Finch, United States A. Everitt, Australia T. Makinodan, United States T. Noumura, Japan R. Walford, United States N. Egami, Japan R. Cutler, United States

Discussants:

E. Schneider, United States
T. Matsumura, Japan
M. Tomonaga, Japan
T. Yamaguchi, Japan
S. Goto, Japan
D. Mizuno, Japan
S. Aizawa, Japan
S. Kawashima, Japan
Yo Nagai, Japan
I. Yamashima, Japan
T. Ohno, Japan
S. Murota, Japan
T. Matsamura, Japan
K. Hirokawa, Japan
H. Imura, Japan
S. Kawashima, Japan
F. Bourliere, France
T. Sugahara, Japan
T. Yamakawa, Japan
T. Hidaka, Japan
T. Sado, Japan

Opening Remarks:

H. Kumagai, Japan

Closing Remarks:

G. Sacher, United States
K. Oota, Japan

KINETICS OF THE PROLIFERATION OF HUMAN FIBROBLASTS DURING SERIAL SUBCULTIVATION *IN VITRO*

A. Macieira-Coelho

Department of Cell Pathology
Institut de Cancerologie et d'Immunogénétique
(INSERM U-50)
94800 Villejuif, France

INTRODUCTION

The studies of the kinetics of cell proliferation *in vitro* have been plagued by the tendency to establish clear-cut limits to the behavior of cells in regard to the division cycle. Investigators in the field have predominantly thought in terms of compartments instead of gradients, measured instants instead of variations during long periods of time, and expressed the results in terms of means instead of distributions.

Mean generation times aren't always valid because there can be differences up to several days between the shortest and the longest interdivision times; and cells considered arrested in certain periods of the division cycle can actually be cells whose progress is merely slowed down.

Inevitably, this led to overly simplified ideas, such as considering only cycling and non-cycling cells, or believing that the rates of entrance into the cycle are constant. This type of thinking can be particularly fallacious when analyzing the proliferation of human fibroblasts during their life span *in vitro*.

We attempted to elucidate the kinetics of the proliferation of human fibroblasts, taking into account the parameters mentioned above (1-8). In 1966, when we first started to explore this virtually unknown field, our aim was to find out which of the following three hypotheses would fit the data (1): a) Only a small fraction of the cell population in phase III cultures is dividing at unaltered rate, but the majority of the cells are unable to divide. b) The entire

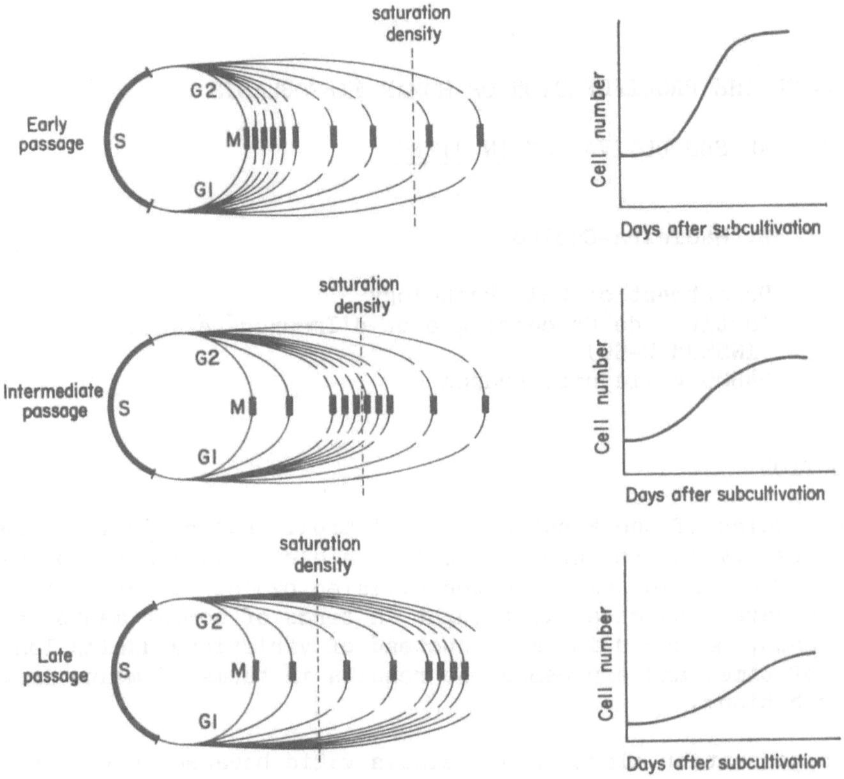

Fig. 1. Illustration of a model of kinetics of the proliferation of human fibroblasts (see text below).

population is uniformly growing at a slow rate, possibly because of selective interferences with one of the stages in the division cycle. c) The cell population has become strongly heterogeneous, and the cells show a spectrum between the two extremes, i.e., complete inhibition and a normal division cycle.

RESULTS AND DISCUSSION

The data collected favored the last hypothesis, and more recently (8) we proposed a model that could explain our data and that of others, while at the same time having the advantage of being free of mathematical formulas. The model is illustrated in Figure 1, where three different periods of the cell population life span are represented. On the left side of the figure, each circle and ellipse represents the generation time of a cell. In early passages, most cells in the population are postulated to have short division cycles. Some cells already exist with long generation times (ellipses) which are extended mainly at the expense of G1 and G2. There is no gross prolongation of the S period and mitosis (4). Since the saturation density is high (vertical dashed line), most cells are able to complete their cycle before this density is reached. At this stage, the growth curve of the population (right hand side of the figure) has a short lag period, a phase of logarithmic growth with a steep slope, and a high saturation density reached within 3-4 days.

Towards the middle of the life span (intermediate passage), there are still cells with short generation times, but most cells have division cycles between the two extremes. Since the saturation density is lower, an increased number of cells will not have time to complete their cycle. Thus, during a prolonged labeling with tritiated thymidine (^{3}H-TdR), an increased number of cells will appear as unlabeled. At this stage, the slope of the logarithmic portion of the growth curve will be less steep and the cells will reach a lower saturation density, although still within 3-4 days.

Towards the end of the life span (late passage), most cells have very long generation times, and since the saturation density is very low, a still greater number of cells do not have time to complete the cycle between subcultivation and confluency. Thus, even more cells will remain unlabeled after growing in the presence of ^{3}H-TdR. The growth curve will be characterized by a long lag phase, a period of short logarithmic growth with a shallow slope, and a low saturation density reached only after 7-10 days.

In Figure 1, the prolongations of G1 and G2 are identical, but it is possible that one is predominant. It should be emphasized that when one speaks about the prolongation of G1 or G2, it applies only to cells that are moving through the cycle. Since the cells that are arrested due, for instance, to the effects of saturation density seem to be all in G1, a distinction should and can be made when measuring the prolongation of the G1 and G2 periods; otherwise, cells that are arrested will be taken as prolonged in G1. This is particularly true for the latter period, which is usually measured indirectly. Methods that allow the analysis of cells in motion along the cycle should be distinguished from those measuring only instants (5,6).

In addition, another important parameter becomes more pronounced at higher population doubling levels: an increased heterogeneity in the initiation of the cell cycle. The cells become more erratic with aging <u>in vitro</u> (2). While in young cultures between subcultivation and resting phase, the number of cells entering the S period increases progressively to a maximum and then decreases to very low levels, in old cultures there is a burst of cells entering S, then the percentage of cells synthesizing DNA goes down and up again before it decreases at confluency (2). This heterogeneity in the initiation of division can lead an investigator to consider as non-dividers cells that still have the potential to enter the cell cycle in a more unpredictable way. This erratic behavior has been confirmed by direct examination of the cells with time lapse cinematography (9), and is suggested from measurements of the rate of entrance into the division cycle (10).

The model we described herein takes into consideration all the data previously published on the kinetics of the proliferation of human fibroblast populations, and may be helpful in understanding cell division during in vitro aging, as well as in other cell systems.

REFERENCES

1. A. Macieira-Coelho, J. Ponten, and L. Philipson, The division cycle and RNA synthesis in diploid human cells at different passage levels in vitro, Exp. Cell Res. 42:673 (1966).
2. A. Macieira-Coelho, J. Ponten, and L. Philipson, Inhibition of the division cycle in confluent cultures of human fibroblasts in vitro, Exp. Cell Res. 43:20 (1966).
3. A. Macieira-Coelho, Influence of cell density on growth inhibition of human fibroblasts in vitro, Proc. Soc. Exp. Biol. Med. 125:548 (1967).
4. A. Macieira-Coelho and J. Ponten, Analogy in growth between late passage human embryonic and early passage human adult fibroblasts, J. Cell Biol. 43:374 (1969).
5. A. Macieira-Coelho and L. Berumen, The cell cycle during growth inhibition of human embryonic fibroblasts in vitro, Proc. Soc. Exp. Biol. Med. 144:43 (1973).
6. A. Macieira-Coelho, Cell cycle analysis in mammalian cells, in: "Tissue Culture: Methods and Applications," P. F. Kruse, Jr. and M. K. Patterson, Jr., eds., Academic Press, New York (1973).
7. A. Macieira-Coelho, Are non-dividing cells present in ageing cell cultures? Nature 248:421 (1974).
8. A. Macieira-Coelho, Kinetics of the proliferation of human fibroblasts during their lifespan in vitro, Mech. Ageing Dev. 6:341 (1977).
9. P. M. Absher, R. G. Absher, and W. D. Barnes, Genealogies of clones of diploid fibroblasts. Cinematographic observations of cell division patterns in relation to population age, Exp. Cell Res. 88:95 (1974).
10. G. L. Grove and V. J. Cristofalo, The transition probability model and the regulation of proliferation of human diploid cell cultures during aging, Cell Tissue Kinet. 9:395 (1976).

NEW APPROACHES TO CHARACTERIZATION OF AGING HUMAN FIBROBLASTS AT INDIVIDUAL CELL LEVEL

Youji Mitsui[1], Koji Matsuoka[1], Shinichi Aizawa[2], and Koichi Noda[3]

[1]Laboratory of Pharmacology, [2]Laboratory of Nutrition, and [3]Laboratory of Ultrastructure Research, Tokyo Metropolitan Institute of Gerontology 35-2 Sakaecho, Itabashiku, Tokyo-173, Japan

SUMMARY

Considering the heterogeneity of cell populations and other critical problems in mass cultured senescent human fibroblasts, we proposed several new approaches for studying true cellular aging, as follows.

1) To establish a correlation among aging indexes at the individual cell level, we demonstrated a relationship among ^{3}H-thymidine incorporation activity, nuclear size, cell volume, and DNA contents at individual cell level.

2) To fractionate homogenous cell populations and examine the relationship between their life spans and aging indexes, we separated human cells into relatively homogenous populations by the sedimentation velocity method, and found that life span of fractionated cells was almost identical among various fractions, irrespective of their great differences in cell volume and ^{3}H-thymidine incorporation indexes. This suggests that some aging indexes, such as cell volumes and ^{3}H-thymidine incorporation activity, are reversible cell properties, and are not specific properties at the individual cell level.

3) To find age-specific cell properties in fractionated senescent cell populations, we performed a quantitative analysis with an image analyzer on electromicroscopic pictures of fractionated small and large cell populations from young and senescent cultures. We discovered that the differences between young and senescent cultures in nuclear size, mitochonria size and number of lysosomes are due

solely to the presence of large cells in senescent cultures, and that an increase in the constricted endoplasmic reticulum is a common phenotype of fractionated senescent cell populations. This suggests that there is some loss of function in endoplasmic reticulum or changes in the membrane system.

4) To examine age-specific changes in membrane system at the individual cell level, we found that the amount of absorption of concanavalin A-bound red blood cells to fibroblast surfaces increases linearly with <u>in vitro</u> passage. Further examination of individual cells indicated that this passage-related change in surface membrane is not dependent on cell cycle phase, surface area, or metabolic age, but certainly is dependent upon division age.

Finally, these findings should be confirmed by using cells from human donors of different ages.

We conclude that our approaches are important for elucidating the true mechanisms of cellular aging.

INTRODUCTION

The finite life span of cultured human diploid fibroblasts has been suggested as a manifestation of aging at the cellular level (1). The inverse relationship between human donor age and the <u>in vitro</u> life span of skin fibroblasts has confirmed the validity of using cultured diploid fibroblasts as a model system for human cellular aging (2,3). The precise characterization of senescent cells is essential for the elucidation of the mechanisms of <u>in vitro</u> cellular aging.

Phase III cells, a term originally used by Hayflick (1), usually represent senescent cell populations, one of the characteristics of which is a decrease in proliferation capacity. Phase III cells have been called late passage cells, terminal phase cells, degenerative phase cells, or senescent cells, depending on the research interest. Although there have been extensive examinations of phase III cells, a total integrated picture of the features of phase III cells remains obscure. Phase III cells are not homogenous cell populations in terms of proliferation capacity (4,5), cell volume (6), nuclear size (7,8), or morphology (9). Therefore, some properties of phase III cells are not necessarily characteristic of senescent cells, and rapidly dividing cell populations among phase III cells apparently look like young cell populations (7,10). This finding calls for new approaches to find more accurate indexes of cellular aging at the level of the individual cells.

In this paper, we will first summarize the recent information on the properties of phase III cells, and point out the crucial problems involved in studying true senescent cells. Finally, we will propose several approaches to these problems, capable of providing some insights into the mechanisms of cellular aging.

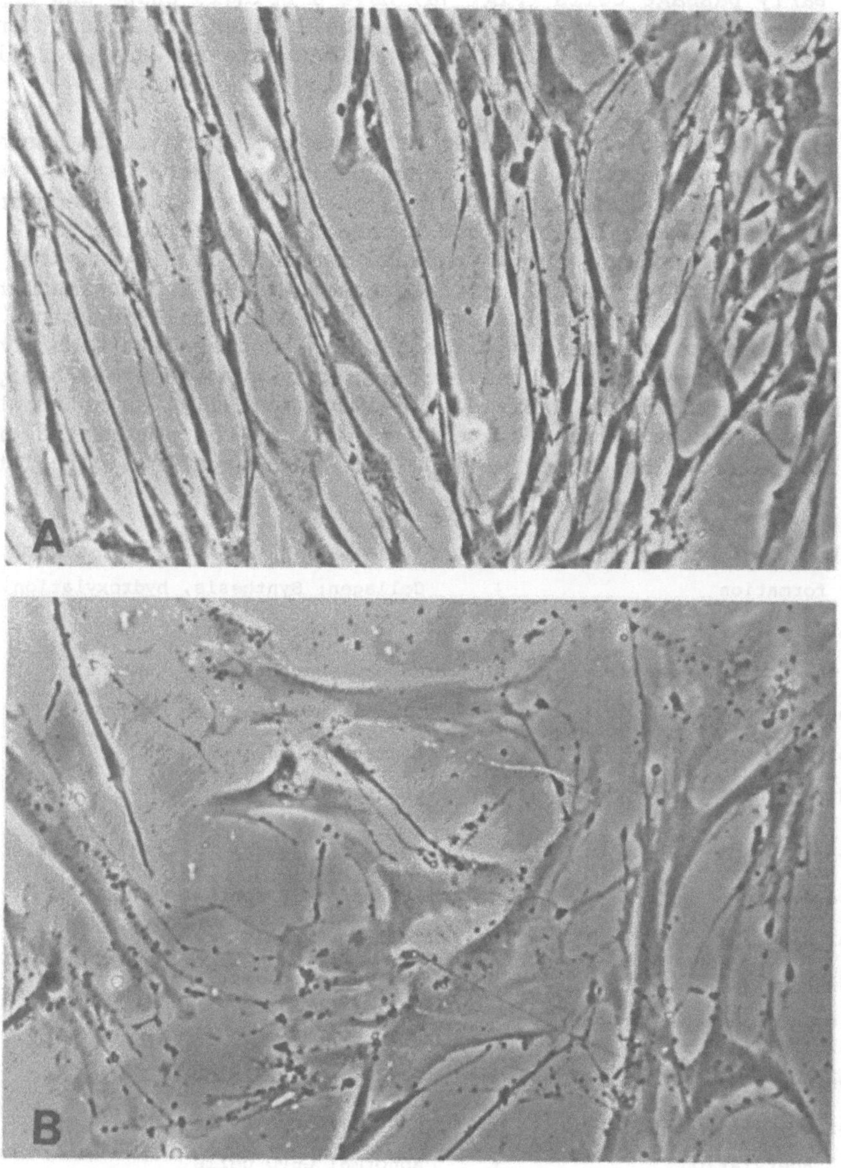

Fig. 1. Morphological features of human fibroblasts under a light microscope.
A: early passage cells (15 pdl)
B: late passage cells (65 pdl)

SUMMARIZED FEATURES OF PHASE III CELLS

A typical example of the morphology of human diploid fibroblasts as revealed by an Olympus light microscope is seen in Figure 1. Most of the early passage cells (Fig. 1a) have a spindle shape and rapidly proliferate, resulting in a criss-cross cell layer. On the other hand, late passage cells (Fig. 1b) sometimes have an enlarged, flattened shape, and cease to proliferate at low cell density.

Although a considerable number of works comparing early passage cells and late passage cells have been published, efforts to integrate these observations with findings on cellular aging phenomena have been scarce. In Table 1, the biochemical and cytological changes in cell properties with passage are listed. In summary, the characteristics of phase III cells seem to be: 1) a decreased growth rate; 2) an increase in cell size; 3) a decreased cell function; and 4) an increase in abnormality. Since these studies have been performed on mass cultured cells, they reflect only average properties, which may vary widely in individual cells. Actually, as noted above (p. 6), an increase in heterogeneity is a fifth characteristic of phase III cells. Therefore, we lack knowledge about the correlation

Table 1. Changes in Cell Properties with *in vitro* Cell Aging

Colony formation	↓	Collagen: Synthesis, hydroxylation and degradation	↓
% labeled cell with ^{3}H-thymidine	↓	Mucopolysaccharide synthesis	↓
Duration of the G_1 phase	↑	Glucose utilization	↑
Growth rate	↓	Lactate dehydrogenase	↓
DNA polymerase	↓	Transaminases	↓
Thymidine kinase	↓		
Cell volume	↑	Surface negative charge	↓
Surface area	↑	LETS protein content	↓
Nuclear size	↑	Cell movement	↓
Microfibril	↑	Neutral proteolytic enzyme	↓
Protein, glycogen, lipid contents	↑	Phagocytosis	↓
RNA synthesis	↓	Polyploidy	↑
Chromatin template activity	↓	Aneuploid cells	↑
Histone acetylation	↓	Abnormal G6PD cells	↑
RNA content	↑	Lysosomal enzyme	↑
		Chromatin associated degradation enzymes	↑

correlation among these changes in cell properties at the individual cell level.

THE CORRELATION AMONG AGING INDEXES AT THE INDIVIDUAL CELL LEVEL

We have reported the close relationship between modal cell volume and population doubling time at various passage numbers (6). The fractionation by sedimentation velocity of small and large cells from the same culture has provided indirect evidence for the close correlation among cell volume, nuclear size, and proliferation capacity (7). As shown in Figure 2, cell nuclei are heterogenous in size, and a direct relationship between nuclear size and proliferation capacity can be examined in individual cells using autoradiography. Figure 3 shows the nuclear size distribution of labeled cells and unlabeled cells at middle and late passage cultures incubated with ^{3}H-thymidine for various time intervals, ranging from 17 hours to two weeks.

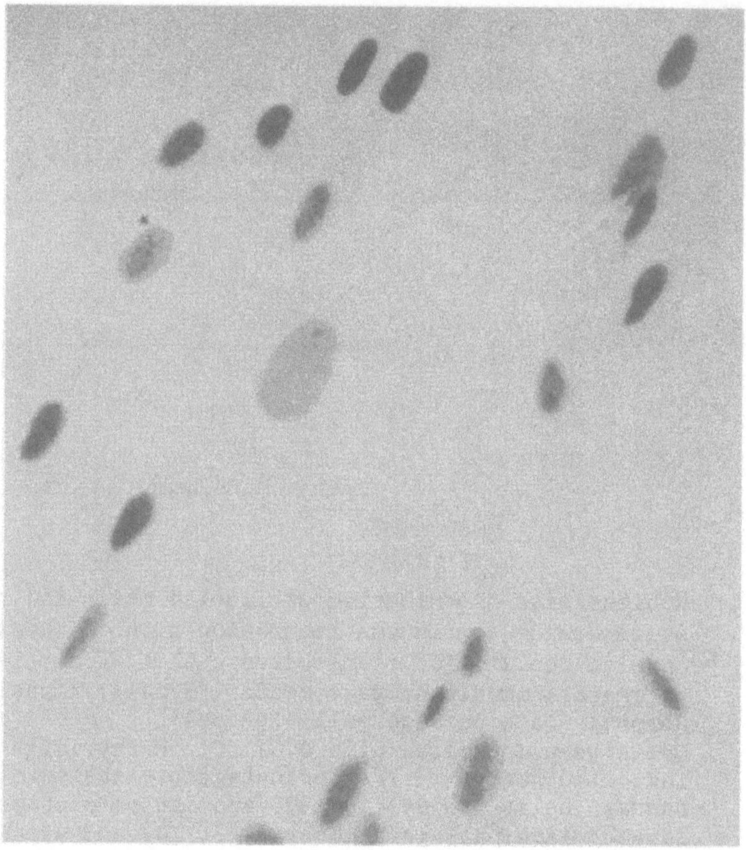

Fig. 2. Nuclei of middle passage cells stained with giemsa. Note the heterogeneity in size.

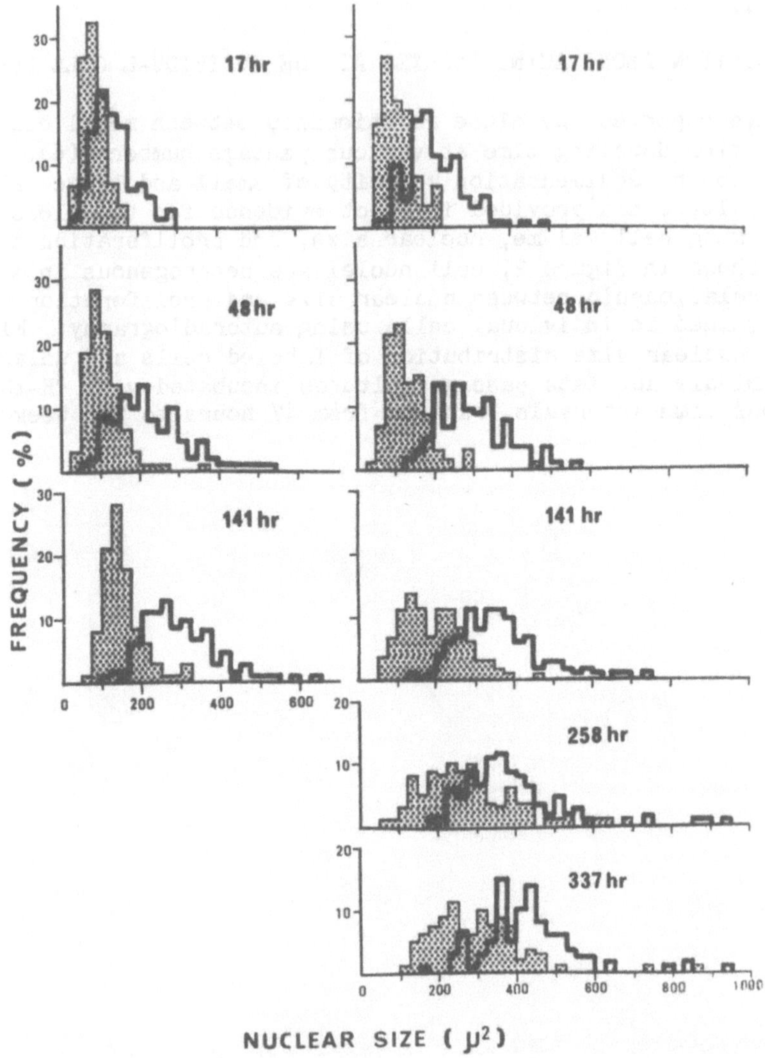

Fig. 3. Nuclear size distribution of labeled cells and unlabeled cells during continuous incubation with ^{3}H-thymidine. Labeled nuclei: [shaded box] ; unlabeled nuclei: [open box] ; left column of graphs: middle passage cells (35 pdl); right column of graphs: late passage cells (53 pdl).
Cells were incubated with 0.01 μCi ^{3}H-thymidine for the indicated periods. The percentage of labeled middle passage cells was 84, 96, 99, and the percentage of labeled late passage cells was 47, 70, and 91 at 17, 48, and 141 hrs, respectively.

It is apparent that at any given incubation time, the unlabeled cell nuclei are larger than labeled cell nuclei. Moreover, with increasing incubation time, there is a definite shift in the nuclear size distribution to larger sizes for both the labeled and unlabeled cell populations. These findings, when one considers that unlabeled, slowly dividing cells become labeled with increasing incubation time, lead to the conclusion that the more slowly dividing cells have larger nuclear sizes. Non-dividing cells were identified as the cells with maximum nuclear size which remained unlabeled even after the total number of unlabeled cells per dish ceased to decrease during incubation with ^{3}H-TdR. Non-dividing cells at terminal phase, which remained unlabeled even after 10 days of incubation, had a mean nuclear size of 430 μm^2, while the rapidly dividing cells at both middle and terminal phase, which were labeled within 17 hours, had a mean nuclear size of 100 μm^2.

Figure 4 shows the relationship between DNA content and the size of individual, terminal phase cell nuclei. Since this terminal phase culture was examined after it reached confluency at low cell density, only a few S phase cells with an intermediate amount of DNA between 2C and 4C were observed. As can be seen in Figure 4, non-dividing cells with nuclei of a maximum size of more than 400 μm^2 had 4C or 8C DNA. On the other hand, small cells with a nuclear size smaller than 200 μm^2 had 2C DNA. We consider these small cells to be rapidly cycling cells, as is indicated by their nuclear size distribution when labeled within 17 hours.

Thus, we conclude that phase III cells can be divided into three types of cell population in terms of proliferation capacity. These

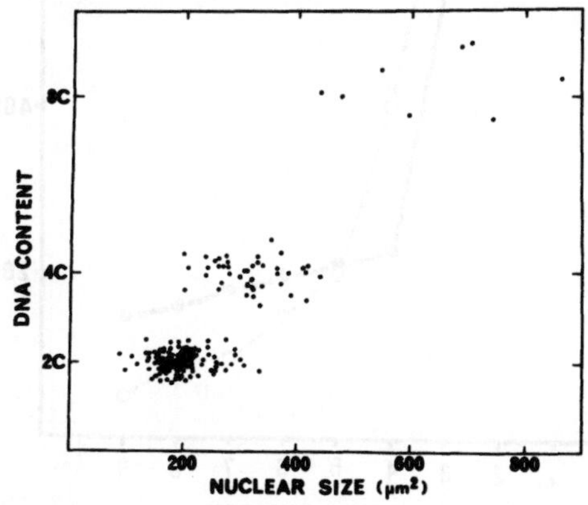

Fig. 4. DNA content and nuclear size of individual cells at terminal phase culture. The relative DNA content was determined with a scanning microphotometer after Feulgen staining.

types are terminal senescent cells (non-dividing), resting senescent cells (slowly dividing), and cycling senescent cells (rapidly dividing). However, cycling cells among phase III cells in our study were apparently identical to cycling cells in early passage cultures in terms of cell volume, nuclear size, and ^{3}H-TdR incorporating activity. Therefore, a question arises as to how cycling senescent cells are different from resting senescent cells, or from the cycling cells in early passage culture. Thus, our second approach was to examine aging indexes in relatively homogenous cell populations.

AGING INDEXES AND LIFE SPAN OF FRACTIONATED CELL POPULATIONS

We have previously reported that the cell separation method obtains relatively homogenous cell populations in terms of cell volume using sedimentation velocity (6,7,8). Figure 5 shows that the largest cell population (fraction 1) obtained using this technique had the highest percentage of unlabeled cells, while the smallest

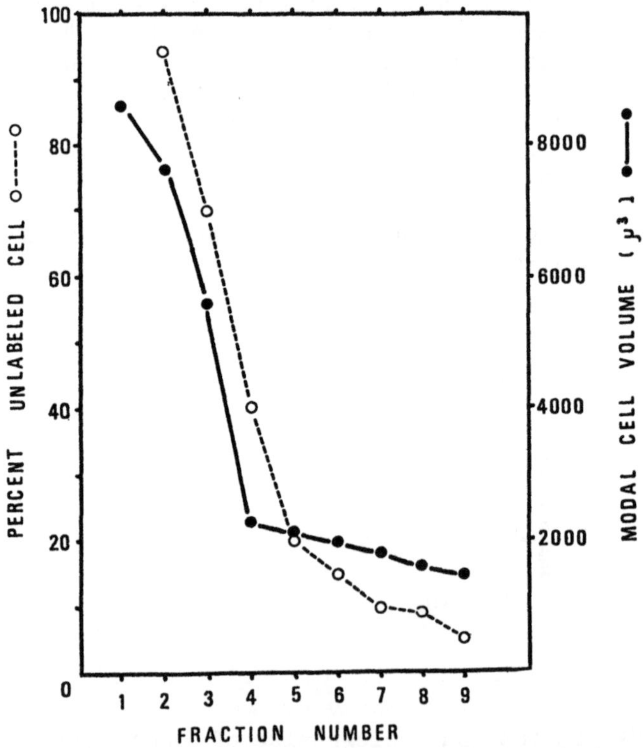

Fig. 5. Cell volume and the percent of unlabeled cells in fractionated late passage cell populations. ^{3}H-thymidine was added to the culture for 24 hrs, and cells were fractionated by the sedimentation velocity method.

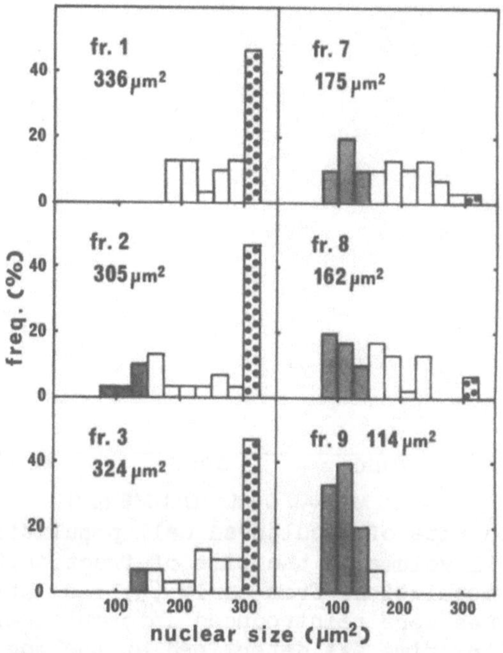

Fig. 6. Nuclear size distribution of fractionated middle passage cell populations.
Nuclear size was examined 24 hrs after the fractionated cell populations were reintroduced into cultures.
Nuclei larger than 300 μm^2: [dotted] ; nuclei smaller than 150 μm^2: [hatched] . Note that there was no overlapping of nuclear size distribution between fractions 1 and 9.

cell populations (fraction 9) had the lowest percentage of unlabeled cells.

Due to the close correlation between cell volume and ^{3}H-thymidine incorporation activity, we could obtain several cell populations with various cell proliferation capacities. These fractionated cell populations differing in size and proliferation capacity were reintroduced into cultures, and their proliferation capacity and life span thereafter were examined. Shortly after their reintroduction into cultures, the nuclear size distribution of each fraction was examined. As can be seen in Figure 6, fraction 1 had the largest nuclear size distribution (mean: 336 μm^2), while fraction 9 had the smallest nuclear size distribution (mean: 114 μm^2). It should be noted that there was no overlapping in terms of nuclear size between fractions 1 and 9. However, after 3 days in tissue culture, fractions that differed markedly at the time of fractionation returned to a relatively uniform cell volume and proliferation capacity for both early and late passage cultures (Fig. 7). Thus, the small rapidly

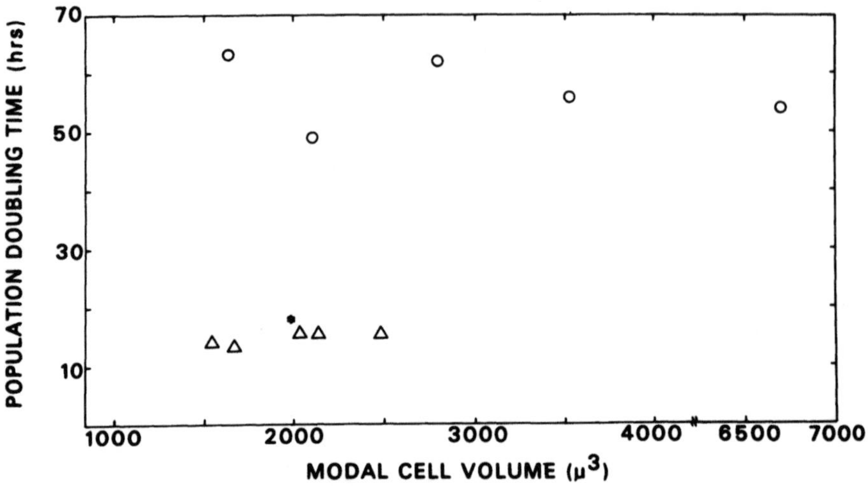

Fig. 7. Growth rate of recultured cell populations as a function of cell volume at the time of fractionation. Fractionated cell populations from early (Δ) and late (O) passage cultures were reintroduced into cultures, and population doubling time was determined at the log phase of growth. Unseparated early passage control cells (*Δ) were also examined as above.

dividing cell population in the late passage culture was found not to be identical with the small rapidly dividing cell population in the early passage culture. Furthermore, in order to examine the life span of fractionated cell populations, a middle passage cell culture was fractionated first at the 29th population doubling level (pdl), then both fraction 1 and 9 and the unseparated cells were recultured for a further seven pdls. Fractions 1 and 9 were again fractionated at the 36th pdl, yielding fractions 1, 2, and 3 from the recultured fraction 1, and fractions 9 and 10 from the recultured fraction 9. As can be seen in Figure 8, no significant difference between the _in vitro_ life span of each of the fractionated cell populations and the parallel control culture was observed.

These results indicate that: 1) rapidly dividing cell populations in late passage cultures have a much shorter life span than rapidly dividing cells in early passage cultures, in spite of their similarity on some aging indexes; and that 2) rapidly dividing cell populations have almost the same life span as slowly dividing cell populations in the same culture. These findings may suggest that the proliferation capacity and the cell volume of individual cells in a given culture are temporary properties. Thus, size and proliferative capacity might be modifiable characteristics capable of changing with

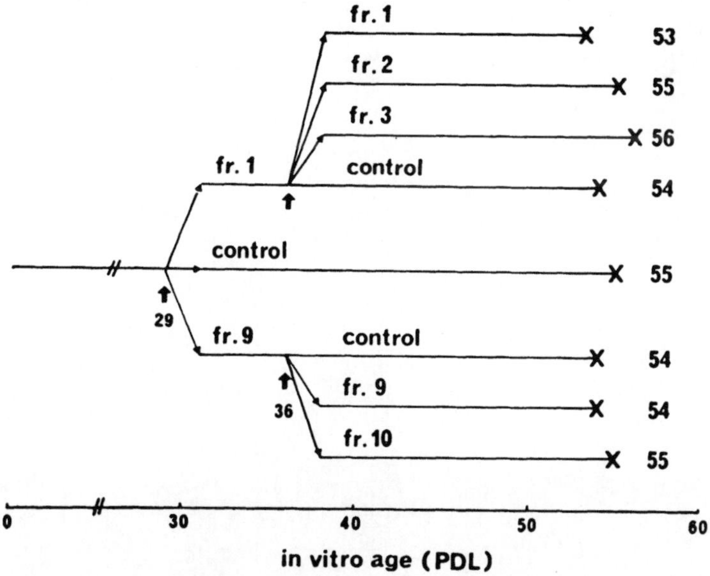

Fig. 8. Life span of fractionated cell populations. After the separation of fractions 1 and 9 at the 29th pdl, they were recultured for a further 7 pdls and fractionated again at the 36th pdl.

cell division. These results support the program theory of aging rather than the mutation or error theory.

We were next concerned to know how small and large cells in late passage cultures are different from those in early passage cultures in terms of cell properties other than ^{3}H-thymidine incorporation capacity, cell volume and nuclear size. Therefore, our third approach was to try to draw a common phenotype of aging from the fractionated cell populations.

QUANTITATIVE ANALYSIS WITH AN IMAGE ANALYZER AND ELECTROMICROSCOPIC PICTURES OF FRACTIONATED YOUNG AND OLD CELLS

Immediately after fractionating cells using the sedimentation velocity method, small (fraction 8) and large (fraction 1) cell populations from old cultures and a small cell population from young cultures were fixed with osmic acid and processed for electromicroscopic observation.

The size of the nuclei of each fraction can be seen in Figure 9. The largest cells had the largest nuclear size, and small cells from old cultures had nuclei of the same size as those of small cells from young cultures. Irregularity in nuclear size, which has been

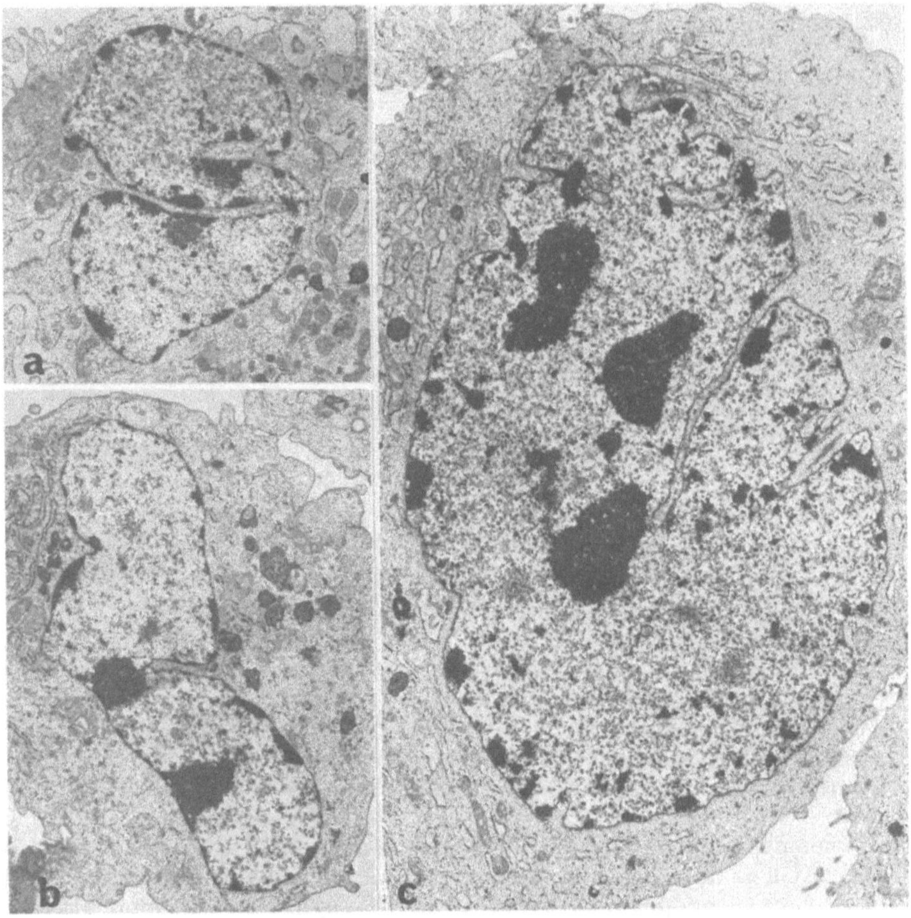

Fig. 9. Electron microscopic pictures (x 6,000) of nuclei from fractionated cells.
a. from fraction 8 of early passage cells;
b. from fraction 8 of late passage cells;
c. from fraction 2 of late passage cells.

suggested as a characteristic of old cultures, was determined by the formula,

$$\frac{1}{2\sqrt{\pi}} \cdot \frac{L}{\sqrt{S}}$$

L, the length of the nuclear periphery, and S, the area of the nucleus, were measured with an image analyzer and electron microscopic pictures.

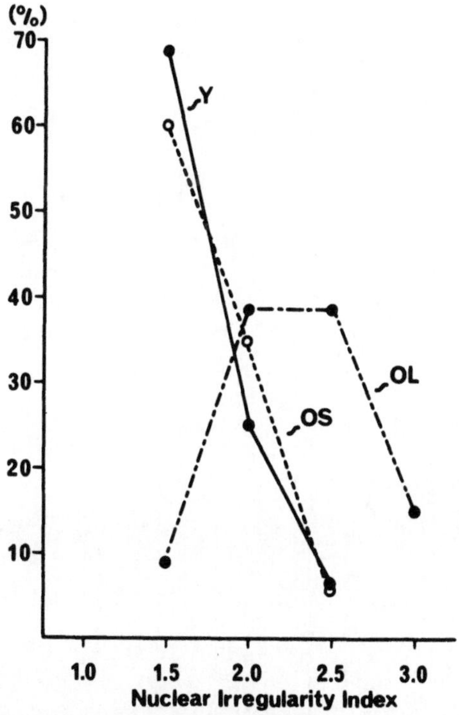

Fig. 10. Irregularity of nuclear shape.
Ordinate: percentage of cells with a given irregularity index from the total number of cells examined (35 cells).
Abscissa: the nuclear irregularity index represented by the formula

$$\frac{1}{2\sqrt{\pi}} \cdot \frac{L}{\sqrt{S}} .$$

Y: fraction 8 of early passage cells; OS: fraction 8 of late passage cells; OL: fraction 2 of late passage cells.

Figure 10 shows that passage-related differences in nuclear irregularity are due solely to the presence of large nuclei with increased irregularity. Thus, nuclear irregularity was found not to be a common phenotype of senescent cells. Figure 11 gives the features of the mitochondria (M) and endoplasmic reticulum (ER) in young small and old large cells. Swelling M were observed in 14% of each group of small and large cells. The total area of M per cell was much larger in old large cells than in young small cells. However, the percentage of M area to area of cytoplasm showed no difference among the different fractions (Fig. 12). A similar analysis was performed on the number and size of the fractions' lysosomes, which indicated that the changes in M and lysosomes are a function of cytoplasm size and are not age-specific.

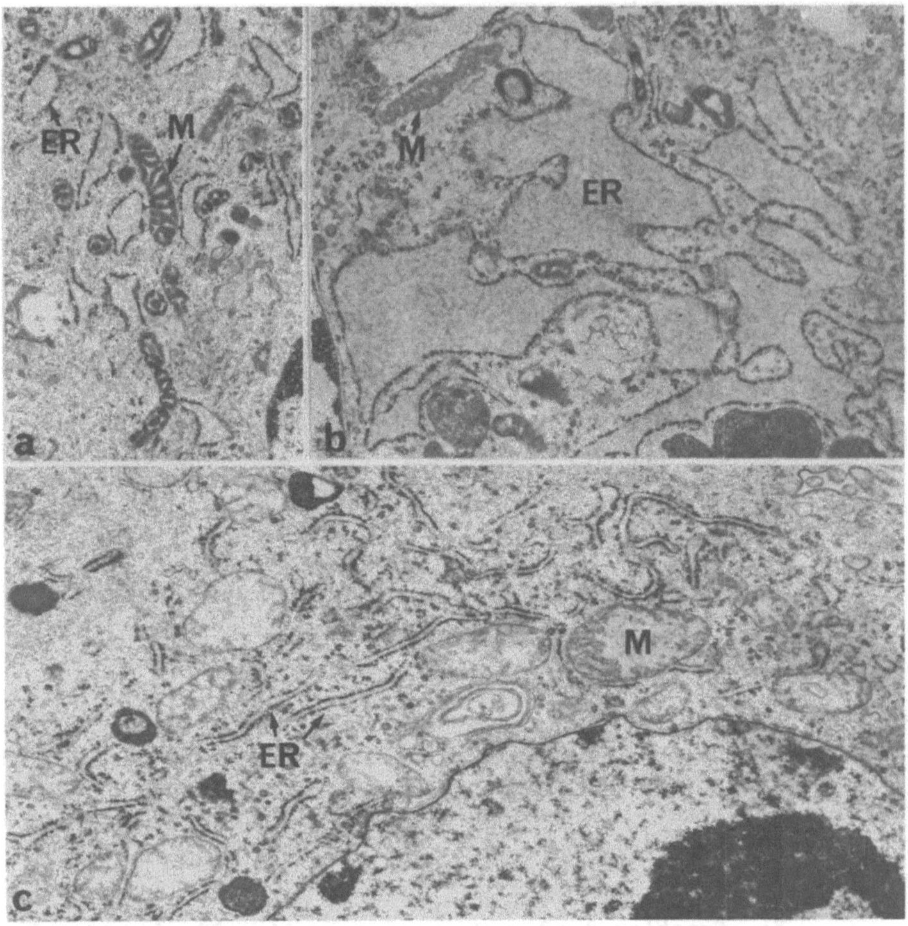

Fig. 11. Electron microscopic pictures (x 15,000) of cytoplasm from fractionated cells.
M: mitochondria; ER: endoplasmic reticulum; a and b: fraction 8 of early passage cells; c: fraction 2 of late passage cells. Note the constricted ER and enlarged M in the late passage cells.

On the other hand, constricted ER were observed in both old small and large cell fractions as compared with dilated ER in young small cells (Fig. 11). In fact, an examination of the length of the short axis of the largest ER in each cell (Fig. 13) suggested that ER constriction in old cultures is an age-related change. This was further confirmed by examining monolayer cultured young and old cells. These facts suggest some loss of function on the part of ER or changes in the membrane system. Therefore, our fourth approach was to examine changes in the surface membrane of individual cells.

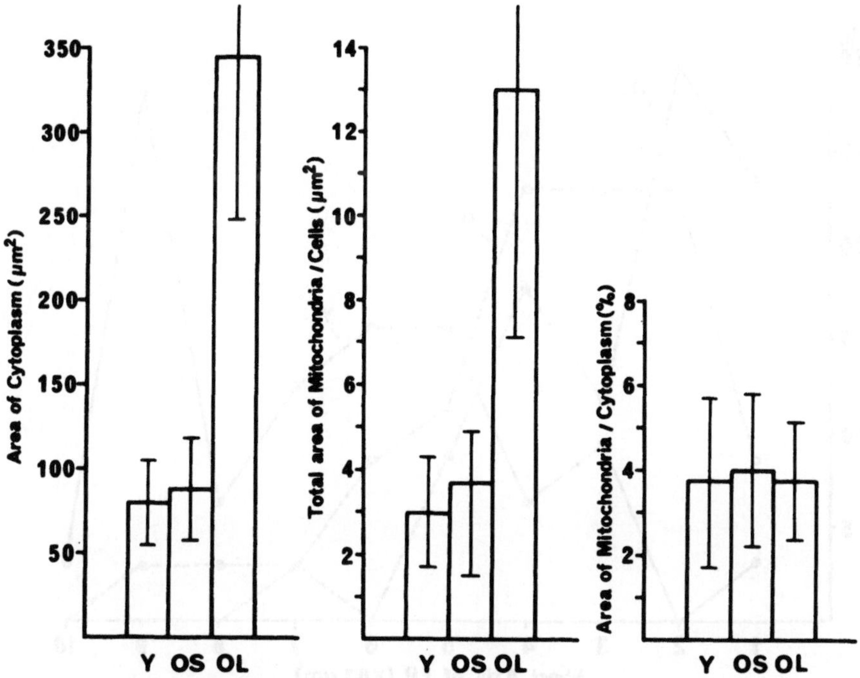

Fig. 12. The amount of area for cytoplasm and mitochondria in fractionated cells. The single line bar extending above each column represents standard deviation of the mean value of each index. Y, OS, and OL are as in Fig. 10.

AGE-RELATED CHANGES IN CELL SURFACE MEMBRANES

The adsorption of Concanavalin A treated red blood cells to the surface of fibroblasts can be examined at the individual cell level (11). As can be seen in Figure 14, early passage cells adsorbed only a few Concanavalin A-coated red blood cells, while, interestingly enough, both small and large cells in senescent culture had a high hemadsorption activity.

Pulse labeled cells with ^{3}H-thymidine at the S phase had a hemadsorption almost identical to that of unlabeled cells at the G_1 or G_2 cell cycle phase. Inhibitors of DNA and protein synthesis, as well as a low serum concentration, had only slight effects on the hemadsorption activity in contrast with their marked effects on nuclear size.

Three strains of human embryo lung fibroblasts (WI-38, IMR-90, and TIG-1) showed a linear increase in hemadsorption per mg protein of fibroblast as a function of population doubling level

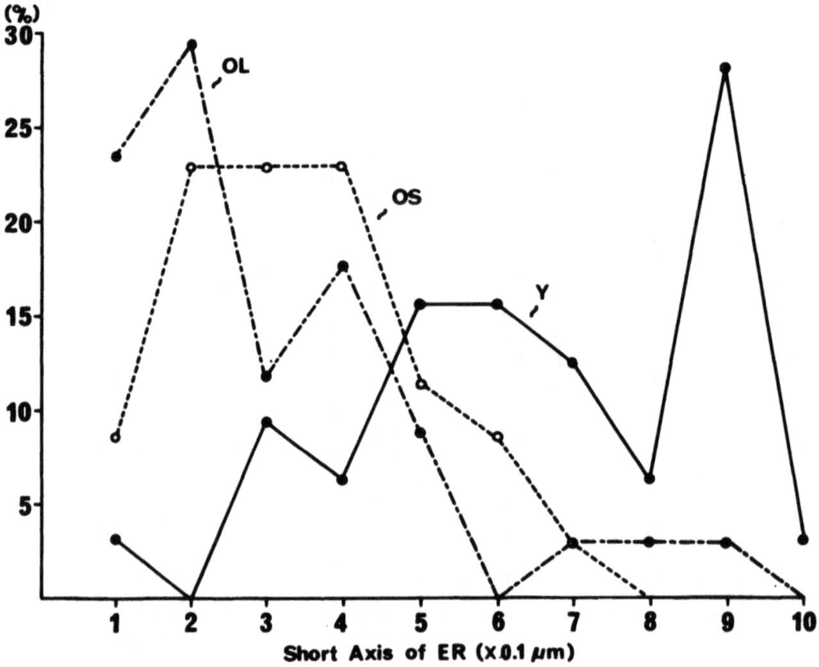

Fig. 13. Length of the short axis of ER of fractionated cells. Ordinate: percentage of cells with a given ER short axis from the total number of cells examined. Abscissa: the length of the short axis of the largest ER in each cell. There were few dilated ER per cell, if any, in some late passage cells.

(see Fig. 15). Since the amount of ^{3}H-Concanavalin A binding to fibroblast surfaces does not change throughout the life span of human fibroblasts, the changes in the adsorption of Concanavalin A-coated red blood cells to fibroblast surface was concluded to reflect a continuous change in the Concanavalin A receptor modulating system with aging (12).

A linear progressive type of change, rather than a catastrophe type of change, is very important for gaining insight into the cellular mechanisms of aging. In this sense, the clarification of the molecular basis of surface changes is under extensive investigation and is expected to reveal features important for our understanding of cellular aging. However, we think that another examination we are now carrying out, on the relation of the increased nuclear protein in senescent cells to a decline in replication capacity (13,14), will also provide an important key for disclosing the mechanisms of cellular aging.

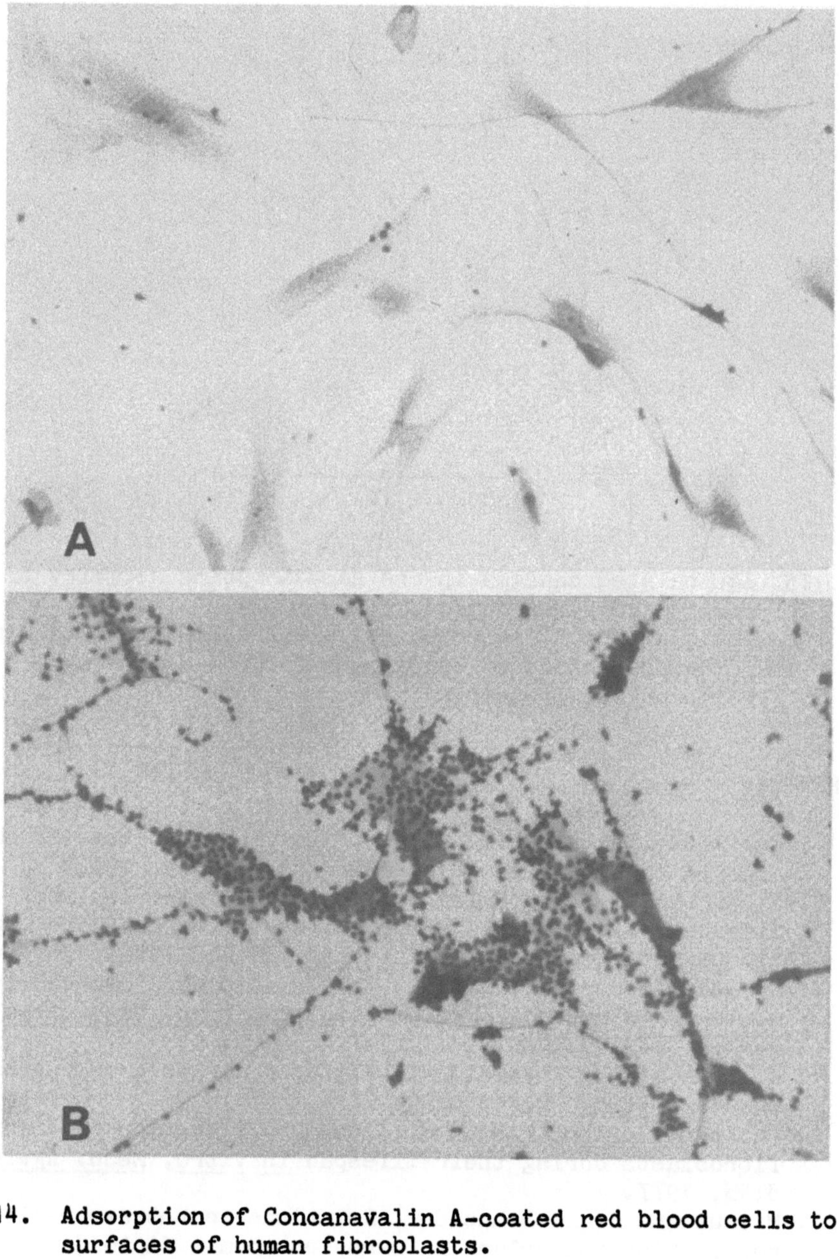

Fig. 14. Adsorption of Concanavalin A-coated red blood cells to surfaces of human fibroblasts.

A: early passage cells; B: late passage cells. Each round dot, or speck, on the cells shows a red blood cell.

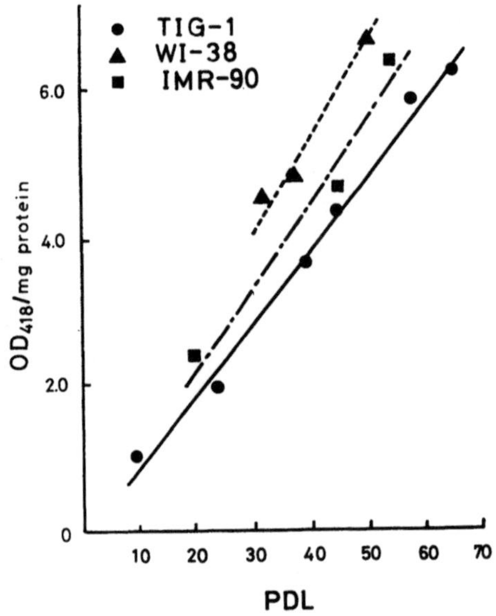

Fig. 15. Age-related changes in the hemadsorption activity of three strains of human diploid fibroblasts.
The amount of adsorbed red blood cells was determined by the absorbance of hemoglobin (O.D. 418) per mg of fibroblast protein.

REFERENCES

1. L. Hayflick, The limited number of in vitro lifetime of human diploid cell strains, Exp. Cell Res. 37:614, 1965.
2. G. M. Martin, C. A. Sprague, and C. J. Epstein, Replicative lifespan of cultivated human cells: Effect of donor age, tissue, and genotype, Lab. Invest. 23:86, 1970.
3. E. L. Schneider and Y. Mitsui, The relationship between in vitro cellular aging and in vivo human age, Proc. Natl. Acad. Sci. USA 73:3584, 1976.
4. V. J. Cristofalo, Thymidine labelling index as a criterion of aging in vitro, Gerontology 22:9, 1976.
5. A. Macieira-Coelho, Kinetics of the proliferation of human fibroblasts during their lifespan in vitro, Mech. Ageing Dev. 5:45, 1977.
6. Y. Mitsui and E. L. Schneider, Relationship between cell replication and volume in senescent human diploid fibroblasts, Mech. Ageing Dev. 5:45, 1976.
7. Y. Mitsui and E. L. Schneider, Increased nuclear sizes in senescent human diploid fibroblast cultures, Exp. Cell Res. 100:147, 1976.

8. Y. Mitsui and E. L. Schneider, Characterization of fractionated human diploid fibroblast cell population, Exp. Cell Res. 103:23, 1976.
9 J. J. Wolosewick and R. K. Porter, Observations on the morphological heterogeneity of WI-38, Am. J. Anat. 149:197, 1977.
10. L. N. Kapp and R. R. Klevecz, The cell cycle of low passage and high passage human diploid fibroblasts, Exp. Cell Res. 101:154, 1976.
11. Y. Mitsui, S. Aizawa, and K. Matsuoka, The relation of cell nuclei and surface membranes to the capacity of cell proliferation in human diploid fibroblasts, in:"Proceedings of XIth International Congress of Gerontology," Excepta Medica, The Netherlands, p. 149, 1979..
12. S. Aizawa, Y. Mitsui, and F. Kurimoto, Cell surface changes accompanying aging in human diploid fibroblasts. II. Two types of age-related changes revealed by Concanavalin A-mediated red blood cell adsorption, Exp. Cell Res., in press.
13. H. Sakagomi, Y. Mitsui, S. Murota, and Y. Yamada, Two dimensional electrophoretic analysis of nuclear acidic proteins in senescent human fibroblasts, Cell Struc. Funct. 4:215, 1979.
14. Y. Mitsui, H. Sakagami, S. Murota, and Y. Yamada, Age-related decline in Hi histone fraction in human diploid fibroblast cultures, Exp. Cell Res., in press.

CHANGE OF RESPONSIVENESS TO GROWTH STIMULATION OF NORMAL CELLS DURING AGING

Tadao Ohno

National Institute of Radiological Sciences
Anagawa, Chiba-shi
260 Japan

INTRODUCTION

The sole determinant of life span of normal diploid cells *in vitro* has been considered to be the intrinsic doubling number of the cells (1,2,3). Recent investigations, however, suggest that extracellular factors can affect the proliferative potential of the cells. For example, hydrocortisone (4) and epidermal growth factor (5) elongate the life span of fibroblasts and keratinocytes, respectively. *In vivo* experiments also suggest that the milieu in old animals reduces the growth potential of hematopoietic stem cells (6). However, quantitative relationships between cellular growth potential and factors which are supposed, or have been known, to influence cellular growth potential are obscure. This report describes the relationship between the amount of growth stimulating factors and cellular growth potential in the course of aging *in vitro*, and discusses a possible growth property of divergent cells in a cell population.

METHODS AND RESULTS

Response of Human Lung Fibroblasts to Dialyzed Serum

Figure 1 shows the growth rate of human lung fibroblasts (IMR-90) determined for various dialyzed serum concentrations at different population doubling levels (PDL) (7). By extrapolating the linear part to the level of 1 PDL-increase for 4 days and by plotting the extrapolated dialyzed serum concentrations versus the PDL, curve A in Figure 2 was obtained. The ordinate of Figure 2 is the log scale of the dialyzed serum concentration, and the curve slopes upward. Therefore, the cells require more and more dialyzed serum to maintain

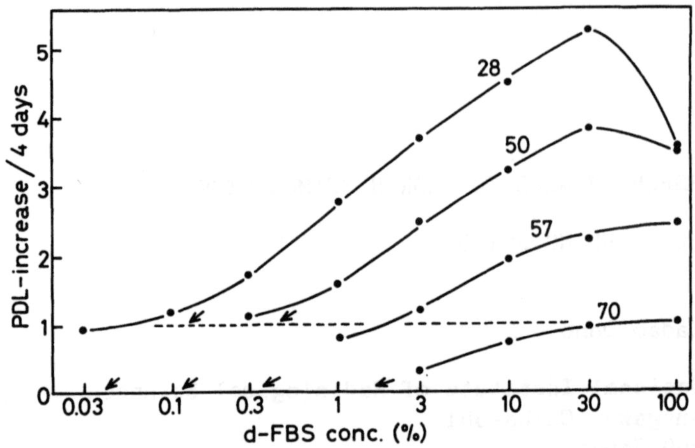

Fig. 1. Effect of dialyzed fetal bovine serum (d-FBS) concentration on the growth rate of IMR-90 cells at different population doubling levels (PDL).

Figures attached on each curve are PDLs of the cells tested. Arrows indicate extrapolation of the linear part of each curve to 1-PDL increase or no-PDL increase per 4 days (Ohno, 1979).

a constant growth rate as the PDL increases. This means that the cells must lose responsiveness to serum growth factors in an accelerated manner during aging in vitro.

This property of the cells may provide a mechanism for the previously observed phenomenon that large-volume cells, which have been supposed to be the non-dividing cells in the population, could divide as well as the small-volume cells, which have been confirmed as actively dividing cells (see Mitsui, this volume). If one part of a population of cells divides more rapidly than others by consuming serum growth factors, the former must lose their responsiveness to serum growth factors before the latter does. The latter groups, which have not divided, now get relatively more opportunities to respond to the serum growth factors. Since the large-volume cells are considered to be the cells that remain in the intermitotic state for a longer period and are, therefore, the cells that divide less frequently than small-volume cells, the large-volume cells can divide as well as, or rather better than, the small-volume cells when the large-volume cells are separated and cultured in fresh medium containing sufficient amounts of growth factors.

By further extrapolating the linear part of the curves in Figure 1 to a no PDL-increase level, maximum dialyzed serum concentrations incapable of promoting cell division were obtained (Fig. 2, Curve B). Curve B has a slope similar to that of curve A, and suggests

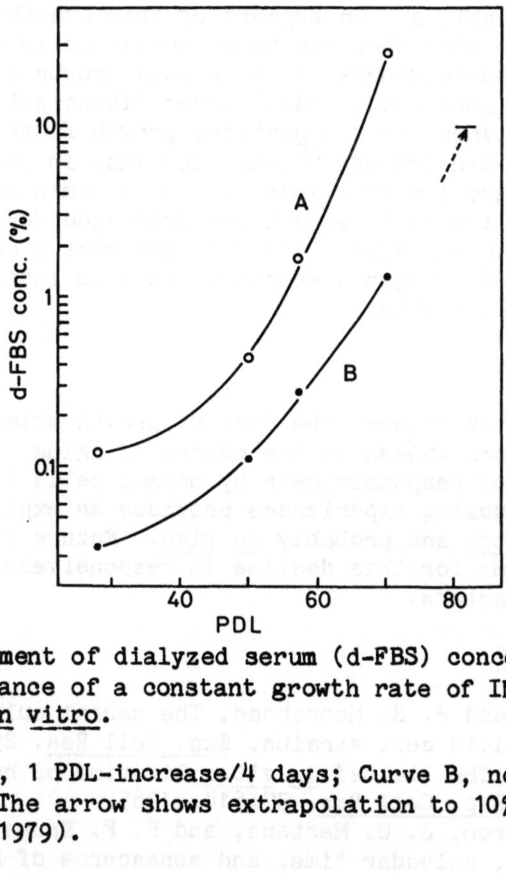

Fig. 2. Requirement of dialyzed serum (d-FBS) concentration for maintenance of a constant growth rate of IMR-90 cells during aging in vitro.

Curve A, 1 PDL-increase/4 days; Curve B, no PDL-increase/4 days. The arrow shows extrapolation to 10% d-FBS level (Ohno, 1979).

that the cells will stop their growth at higher concentrations of dialyzed serum as the cells age. Therefore, it is possible to predict the cellular life span in vitro when the cells are cultured at a limited concentration of the dialyzed serum, e.g., addition of 0.3% or 10% dialyzed serum will result in 58 or 80-85 PDL. The observed life spans of the cells cultured at 0.3% and 10% dialyzed serum were 54 and 76 PDL, respectively, which corresponds well with the predicted life span. These facts suggest that the loss of cellular responsiveness to serum growth factors and the level of these growth factors in the milieu of the cells are the strict determinants of the cellular life span in vitro.

Response of Normal Cells to Growth Factors

Cell populations in older animals must contain the cells with more doubling experience than those in younger animals. If the progressive cellular loss of responsiveness to growth promotors in vivo takes place concomitantly with division of the cells, as in vitro (Fig. 2), it offers a mechanism for aging, at least in proliferative cell populations. In support of this hypothesis, Swierenga et al. (8) demonstrated that rat thigh muscle cells progressively lost mitogenic responsiveness to rat plasma growth factors as the age of the cell donor increased. Adult human fibroblasts showed lower mitogenic responsivness to the platelet growth factor than fetal fibroblasts (9). Binding of ^{125}I-labeled insulin and insulin-stimulated glucose metabolism of primary cultured human skin fibroblasts were reduced when the cells were taken from aged donors (10). Furthermore, Makinodan and Adler (11) reported that T cells showed striking decline of mitogenic responsiveness to lectins in mice aged from 3 months to 24 months.

CONCLUDING REMARKS

The relationship between the size of growth stimulation and cellular growth responsiveness in the course of aging in vitro has been presented. Loss of responsiveness by normal cells concomitant with an increase in doubling experiences provides an explanation for cellular aging in vitro and probably in vivo. Future studies should focus on mechanisms for this decline in responsiveness by normal cells to growth factors.

REFERENCES

1. L. Hayflick and P. S. Moorehead, The serial cultivation of human diploid cell strains, Exp. Cell Res. 25:585, 1961.
2. L. Hayflick, The limited in vitro lifetime of human diploid cell strains, Exp. Cell Res. 37:614, 1965.
3. R. T. Dell'Orco, J. G. Mertens, and P. F. Kruse, Jr., Doubling potential, calendar time, and senescence of human diploid cells in culture, Exp. Cell Res. 77:356, 1973.
4. V. J. Cristofalo, Metabolic aspects of aging in diploid human cells, in "Aging in Cell and Tissue Culture," E. Holeckova and V. J. Cristofalo, eds., Plenum Press, New York (1970).
5. J. G. Rheinwald and H. Green, Epidermal growth factor and the multiplication of cultured human epidermal keratinocytes, Nature 265:421, 1977.
6. J. W. Albright and T. Makinodan, Decline in the growth potential of spleen-colonizing bone marrow stem cells of long-lived aging mice, J. Exp. Med. 144:1204, 1976.
7. T. Ohno, Strict relationship between dialyzed serum concentration and cellular life span in vitro, Mech. Ageing Dev. 11:179, 1979.
8. S. H. H. Swierenga, J. F. Whitfield, and A. L. Boynton, Age-related and carcinogen-induced alterations of the extracellular growth factor requirements for cell proliferation in vitro, J. Cell Physiol. 94:171, 1978.

9. J. R. B. Slayback, L. W. Y. Cheung, and R. P. Geyer, Comparative effect of human platelet growth factor on the growth and morphology of human fetal and adult diploid fibroblasts, Exp. Cell Res. 110:462, 1977.
10. H. Orimo and H. Ito, Glucose intolerance in the aged, Jap. J. Geriat. 13:157, 1976.
11. T. Makinodan and W. Adler, The effects of aging on the differentiation and proliferation potentials of cells of the immune system, Fed. Proc. 34:153, 1975.

MULTINUCLEATION AND POLYPLOIDIZATION OF AGING HUMAN CELLS IN CULTURE

Toshiharu Matsumura

Department of Cancer Cell Research
Institute of Medical Science
University of Tokyo
Shirokanedai, Minato-ku
Tokyo 108, Japan

INTRODUCTION

Multinucleated cells and polyploid cells appear widely in liver, salivary glands, and other mammalian organs. In liver, the multinucleation and polyploidization of hepatocytes are the functions of development, nutrition, regeneration and aging (1,2,3,4). A schematic genealogy of cells has been proposed for the development of multinucleation and polyploidization in rodent liver (2).

Multinucleation and polyploidization appear also in cultured cells. The subject of this paper will be limited to cultured cells from normal human donors that have limited life span (5), unless otherwise mentioned. This is because cells with infinite proliferation potential are different in many respects from cells with finite proliferation potential, and therefore cannot accurately reflect the process of cellular aging. Multinucleated cells have been observed in a human lung culture in its late passages (6). Polyploid cells were noticed both in early and late passages of human lung cell cultures (7,8,9) and in human kidney cell cultures (10).

In a previous study in which human lung cells were cultivated for weeks after the cessation of their rapid proliferation, multinucleated cells were observed to comprise around 50% of total cell population (11). In another study, in which epithelial-like cells from fetal human liver were proliferated in culture, multinucleated cells were noticed early in the primary and secondary cultures (12). The purpose of this short paper is to summarize the results obtained recently in the two systems of human lung cell culture and human

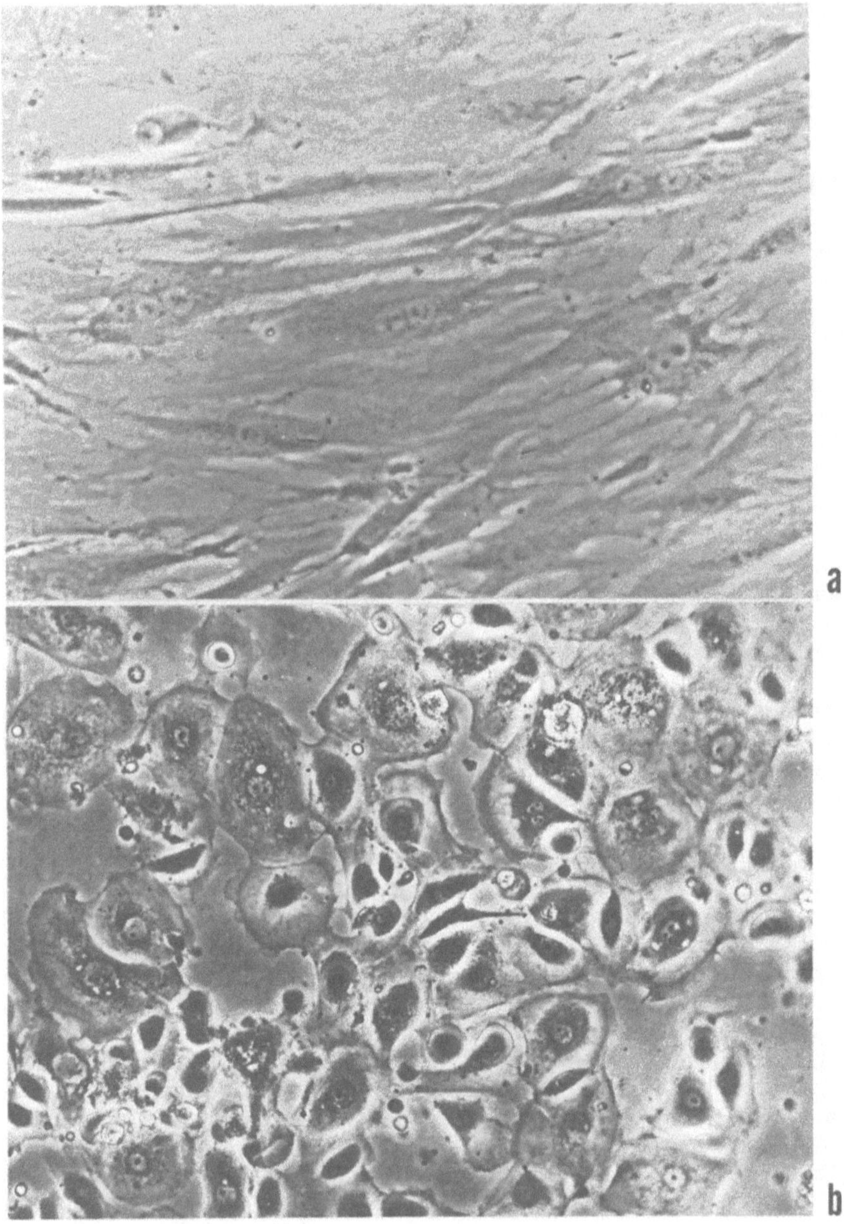

Fig. 1. Phase-Contrast Micrographs of Cultured Human Lung WI-26 Cells (Fig. 1a, x280) and Cultured Human Liver Cells (Fig. 1b, x480). WI-26 cells were cultivated, after their rapid proliferation, for 26 additional weeks without appreciable further proliferation. The liver cells obtained from a human fetus were cultivated for 13 days in a primary culture. This population of the liver cells was proliferating. Binucleated cells are noticeable in both Figures 1a and 1b.

liver cell culture (details to be published elsewhere by Matsumura and Nitta, and by Matsumura and Miyashita), to present a working hypothesis by the author on the multinucleation and polyploidization of cultured cells, and to try to make an assessment of the hypothesis with special reference to cellular aging in culture.

MATERIALS AND METHODS

Lung Cell sytem and Liver Cell System

Human lung cells (WI-38 and WI-26) were cultivated for weeks following the conclusion of their rapid proliferation phase, as described previously (11). These cells will subsequently be referred to as senescent cells. Epithelial-like cells from fetal human liver were cultivated in a chemically defined medium supplemented with 10% fetal bovine serum, and in the presence of irradiated feeder cells (12). Liver cells were passaged by trypsinization. These liver cells produced colonies similar to those produced by keratinocytes (13), and the proportion of clonogenic cells in a given cell population was small. Both the senescent human lung cells and the liver cells in early passages were examined for the proportion of multinucleated cells, for their nuclear DNA content by Feulgen staining and microspectrophotometry, and for their entrance into S phase by continuous labelling with tritiated thymidine and autoradiography. Detailed methods will be described elsewhere by Matsumura and Nitta, and by Matsurmura and Miyashita.

MODE OF MULTINUCLEATION AND POLYPLOIDIZATION

Figure 1a shows the morphology of a typical senescent human lung cell population. Multinucleated cells comprised around 30 to 50% of the cell population. These were predominantly binucleated cells. The nuclei in both mononucleated and binucleated cells contained DNA levels of around one, two, or four times that of the usual amount. The two nuclei in a single binucleated cell generally contained equivalent amounts of DNA. With respect to the DNA content and the number of nuclei, the senescent cells could be divided into six major groups, as shown in Figure 2. Although detailed data are not presented in this paper, the senescent cells showed the following properties: the number of labelled mononucleated cells and labelled binucleated cells increased during continuous exposure to tritiated thymidine; the rate of entrance into S phase, however, was considerably slower than that of proliferating (phase II) cells; no clonogenic cells were found in the senescent population when the cells in a given senescent population were kept for weeks or months and showed a slight increase or decrease in cell number.

In a proliferating (phase III) cell population, a small proportion of multinucleated cells was detected. The proportion of these cells increased with increasing population doubling levels. When

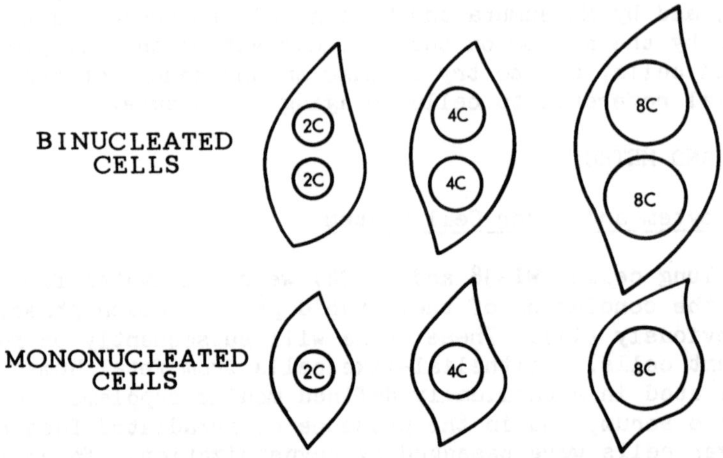

Fig. 2. Schematic presentation of major classes of senescent human lung cells. In a cell drawn in a spindle-like shape, there are one or two nuclei, drawn as circles. The number in a circle shows the amount of DNA in a nucleus. It should be noted that, in an actual cell population, a nucleus with a DNA content between, or more than, the amounts indicated in this figure can also be present. In addition, there are some cells with more than two nuclei, or with nuclei demonstrating irregular morphology, although they are in the minority.

proliferating (phase II) cells were grown in colonies for two weeks in the presence of 10% serum, and then incubated in the presence of 0.5% serum, no appreciable cell proliferation occurred after the first two weeks, but multinucleated cells comprising 10 to 20% of the cell population appeared after 6 to 8 weeks. The proportion of multinucleated cells was higher in small colonies than in large colonies.

Figure 1b shows the morphology of human liver cells in primary culture. They are similar in morphology to those classified as immature liver cells (14). Multinucleated cells comprised about 10% of the total cell population. These were also predominantly binucleated cells. The two nuclei in a single binucleated cell contained equivalent amounts of DNA. A nucleus in either a mononucleated or a binucleated cell contained DNA levels that varied from the usual quantity to twice the usual quantity. Labelled mononucleated cells and binucleated cells accumulated during continuous exposure to tritiated thymidine. When liver cells were trypsinized and plated, a small proportion of the cells formed colonies of varying sizes within two weeks of incubation. The proportion of multinucleated cells was higher in small colonies than it was in large colonies.

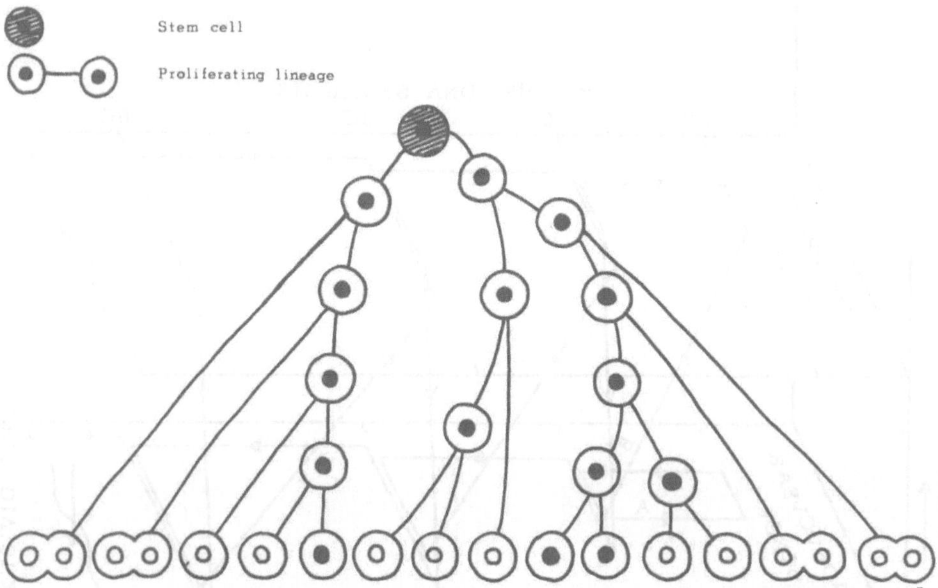

Fig. 3. A hypothetical scheme for the proliferation and multinucleation of cultured human liver cells. The cells at the bottom are the descendants of a single cell, shown at the top. Clonogenic cells are represented by cells with filled nuclei. Nonclonogenic cells are represented by cells with open nuclei.

DISCUSSION

Cell Cycle and "Cell Spiral" Model. Experimental studies using pulse labelling and cinemicrography will tell much about the mode of multinucleation and polyploidization in culture. While these studies are in progress, this author would like to interpret the results summarized above by presenting a hypothetical model. In Figure 3, a model of proliferation and multinucleation of human liver cells in culture is described schematically. In this model, it is hypothesized that: a clonogenic cell is diploid; a nonclonogenic cell is a descendent of a clonogenic cells; and that the latter cell contains either a single nucleus or two nuclei. This model can qualitatively explain all of the above results for both human liver and lung cells. The quantitative terms in both systems, such as the proportion of clonogenic cells in a culture or the time required for a direct descendant of a clonogenic cell in a cell population to become a binucleated cell, may differ, however.

For senescent human lung cells, some of which are polyploid, a further model of multinucleation and polyploidization is shown in

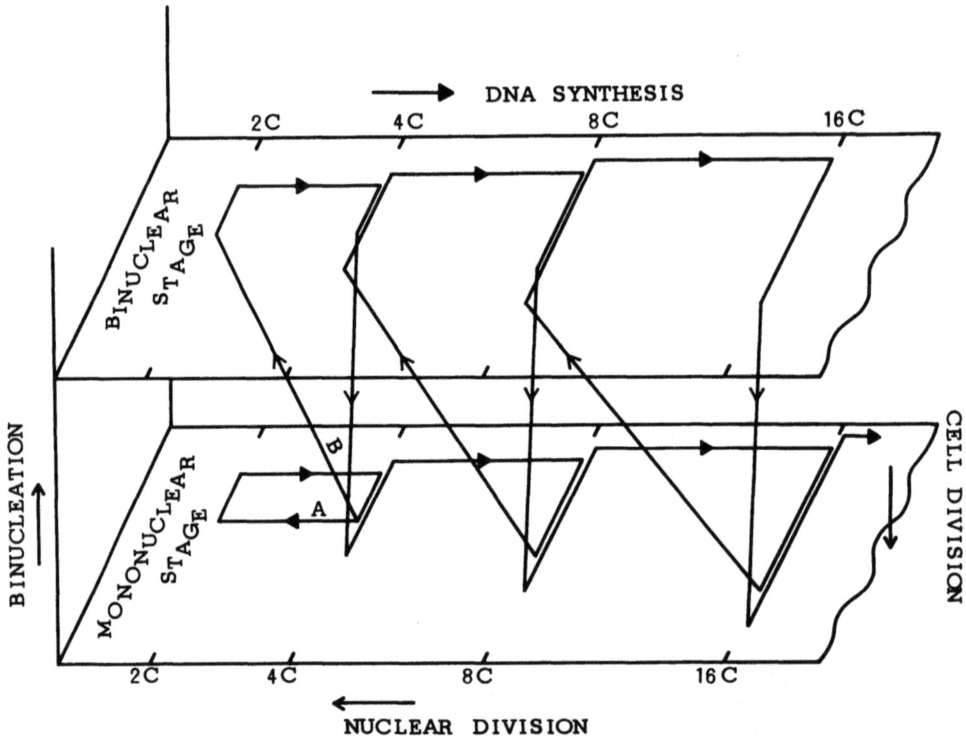

Fig. 4. Cell cycle and "cell spiral" model of _in vitro_ cellular aging. A cell cycle in which a clonable cell remains is shown by "A" at the bottom left. When a cell leaves this cycle (by an unknown mechanism), it follows the path indicated by "B," referred to as "cell spiral" in the text.

Figure 4. In Figure 4, it is hypothesized that: a clonogenic cell is diploid and proliferates by turning a cell cycle; that there is an unknown mechanism by which a cell leaves the cycle, follows another path, which is referred to as a "cell spiral," and never returns to the cell cycle; and that the cell in the "spiral" shuttles back and forth between a mononuclear and a binuclear stage, synthesizes DNA in between, and moves up to a polyploid state. It should be noted that there may be several ways other than that described in Figure 4 to explain how a cell might shuttle between the mononuclear and the binuclear stages, synthesizing DNA in between. Leaving the cell cycle may not mean instant commitment, since commitment could possibly happen while a cell is still cycling. For senescent human lung cells, spiralling cells may be destroyed or removed from a culture by such outside influences as trypsinization. Removal of spiralling cells from a senescent population may cause the loss of a culture. No evidence was found that human liver cells undergo polyploidization in culture. Possibilities were that the period of observation was too short to detect polyploid cells, that polyploidizing cells were removed from a culture by outside influences such as trypsinization, or that there were mechanisms preventing a cell from spiralling further.

Previously reported observations of cultured rat liver cells support the present model. Richman et al. (15) found that a primary culture of rat hepatocytes containing many binucleated cells did not proliferate, but was able to synthesize DNA upon a hormonal stimulation. It is possible that those hepatocytes were not in cell cycle, but in "cell spiral." Proliferating clones of liver epithelial-like cells have been obtained in culture. They have some of the differentiated functions of hepatocytes (16). Careful studies permitted the maintenance of diploid clones of mononuclear cells (17,18). Although they should not directly be compared with human liver cells because the former have infinite proliferation potential, one could speculate that those diploid clones are transformed in such a way that they remain in a permanently cycling state and never "spiral."

SUMMARY

In conclusion, evidence has been presented to show that multinucleation and polyploidization are common, if not ubiquitous, phenomena observable both in proliferating human cell populations in culture, and in cell populations which have already passed through their proliferative phase in culture. A hypothetical model is presented, the essence of which postulates the existence of a regularly controlled cell life, including DNA synthesis, out of cell cycle.

AKNOWLEDGEMENT

The author gratefully acknowledges Dr. L. Hayflick and Dr. H. Katsuta for their kind introduction aging study in culture.

REFERENCES

1. H. Tauchi and T. Sato, Some micromeasuring studies of hepatic cells in senility, J. Gerontol. 17:254 (1962).
2. C. Nadal and F. Zajdela, Polyploidie somatique dans le foie de rat. I. Le role des cellules binucleees dans la genese des cellules polyploides, Exp. Cell Res. 42:99 (1966).
3. D. N. Wheatley, Binucleation in mammalian liver: Studies on the control of cytokinesis in vivo, Exp. Cell Res. 74:455 (1972).
4. W. Ya. Brodsky and I. V. Uryvaeva, Cell polyploidy: Its relation to tissue growth and function, Int. Rev. Cytol. 50:275 (1977).
5. L. Hayflick and P. S. Moorhead, The serial cultivation of human diploid cell strains, Exp. Cell Res. 25:585 (1961).

6. A. Maciera-Coelho, J. Ponten, and L. Philipson, Inhibition of the division cycle in confluent cultures of human fibroblasts in vitro, Exp. Cell Res. 43:20 (1966).
7. E. Saksela and P. S. Moorhead, Aneuploidy in the degenerative phase of serial cultivation of human cell strains, Proc. Natl. Acad. Sci. 50:390 (1963).
8. M. C. Yoshida and S. Makino, A chromosome study of non-treated and an irradiated human in vitro cell line, Japan J. Human Gen. 5:39 (1963).
9. Z. K. Kadanka, J. D. Sparkes, and H. G. Macmorine, A study of the cytogenetics of the human cell strain WI-38, In Vitro 8:353 (1973).
10. R. C. Miller, W. W. Nichols, J. Pottash, and M. M. Aronson, In vitro aging: Cytogenetic comparison of diploid human fibroblasts and epitheliod cell lines, Exp. Cell Res. 110:63 (1977).
11. T. Matsumura, Z. Zerrudo, and L. Hayflick, Senescent human diploid cells in culture: Survival, DNA synthesis and morphology, J. Gerontol., (1977) (in press).
12. T. Matsumura and S. Miyashita, Characteristics of human liver epithelial-like cells proliferating in culture, Proc. Japan Cancer Assoc., 37th Annual Meeting 120 (1978).
13. J. G. Rheinwald and H. Green, Epidermal growth factor and the multiplication of cultured human epidermal keratinocytes, Nature 265:421 (1977).
14. H. Imai, Human embryonic liver cell in culture. A preliminary report, Okayama Igakkai Zasshi 89:237 (1977).
15. R. A. Richman, T. H. Claus, S. Pilkis, and D. L. Friedman, Hormonal stimulation of DNA synthesis in primary cultures of adult rat hepatocytes, Proc. Natl. Acad. Sci. USA 73:3579 (1976).
16. A. Ichihara, Relation of the characteristics of liver cells during culture, differentiation, and carcinogenesis, in: "Control Mechanisms in Cancer," W. E. Criss, T. Ono, and J. R. Sabine, eds., Raven Press, New York (1976).
17. J. Bausher and W. I. Schaeffer, A diploid rat liver cell culture. I. Characterization and sensitivity to alfatoxin B_1, In Vitro 9:286 (1974).
18. H. Masuji, H. Nakabayashi, and J. Sato, Long-term cultivation of two diploid epithelial cell lines derived from normal rat liver cells, Acta Med. Okayama 28:281 (1974).

MECHANISM OF AGE-DEPENDENT DECREASE IN SULFATION OF CHONDROITIN SULFATE

Sei-itsu Murota*, Atsushi Honda*,**, Midori Abe*, and Yo Mori**

*Department of Pharmacology, Tokyo Metropolitan Institute of Gerontology, Itabashi-ku, Tokyo 173 and
**Department of Biochemistry, Tokyo College of Pharmacy, Hachioji-shi, Tokyo 192-03, Japan

INTRODUCTION

A number of investigators have been concerned with the relationship between extracellular substances and aging (1,2). It is generally recognized that the amount of hexosamine-containing substances in tissue decreases with age, while the insoluble collagen content in the tissue increases with age (3). Recently, it has been reported that the decrease in elasticity of cartilage with age is related to the content and structure of the proteoglycan in the matrix (4).

The main purpose of the present study was to determine what causes these age-dependent alterations in both the amounts of hexosamine-containing substances in tissues and the changes in the structure of chondroitin sulfate chains of proteoglycan macromolecules. This paper discusses the age-dependent decrease in sulfation of chondroitin sulfate in rat costal cartilage. A part of this work has been published elsewhere (5).

METHOD AND RESULTS

Changes in Glycosaminoglycan Content with Aging

The amount of glycosaminoglycan (GAG) in dry costal cartilage tissue from Sprague-Dawley male rats of various ages (young, 3 months; middle, 12-18 months; and old, 23-24 months) decreased with aging, while the GAG content in mg DNA (unit cartilage cell) remained the same with aging. These results can be explained by the finding that the total number of cartilage cells decreased with aging.

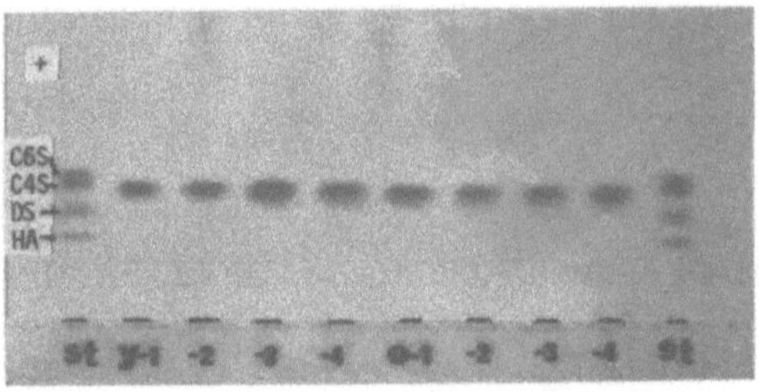

Fig. 1. Electrophoresis of glycosaminoglycan from young (3 months; y-1 to y-4) and old (23 months; 0-1 to 0-4) rat costal cartilage.
Electrophoresis was carried out in 0.3 M calcium acetate (pH 7.25) at a constant current of about 1 mA/cm for 3 hr (6). The strips were stained with 0.5% Alcian Blue in 3% acetic acid. Hyaluronic acid (HA), chondroitin 4-sulfate (C4S), chondroitin 6-sulfate (C6S), and dermatan sulfate (DS) were used as reference standards. Similar electrophoretic patterns were obtainted in the middle-aged (15 months) rat glycosaminoglycan samples.

Chondroitin Sulfate in Rat Costal Cartilage

Electrophoretic analysis demonstrated that chondroitin 4-sulfate was the major glycosaminoglycan of rat costal cartilage irrespective of age (3, 15, and 23 months), as shown in Figure 1. This result was in agreement with that reported in the literature (7), but was quite different from the results reported in the literature for human (8,9) and rabbit (10) costal cartilage, i.e., there is an age-dependent decrease in the ratio of chondroitin 4-sulfate to chondroitin 6-sulfate. This means that rat costal cartilage is suitable for examining the influence of aging on the biosynthesis of chondroitin sulfate.

Age-Dependent Alteration in the Biosynthetic Activities of Cartilage

In an attempt to determine the cause of an age-dependent alteration in the tissue contents of GAG, we examined the influence of aging on the biosynthetic activity of cartilage in the production of hexosamine-containing substances. Rat costal cartilage of different ages was incubated with radioactive precursors, ^{3}H-glucosamine or ^{35}S-sulfuric acid, and newly synthesized hexosamine-containing substances, i.e., glycosaminoglycan (GAG) and glycopeptide (GP), were prepared and analyzed. The radioactivity uptake of GAG per mg dry cartilage tissue indicated that there was an apparent decrease in the incorporation of ^{35}S-sulfate into GAG with age (a statisticallv significant difference existed between 100-day- and 350-day-old rats: $p < 0.01$, but no significant difference existed between

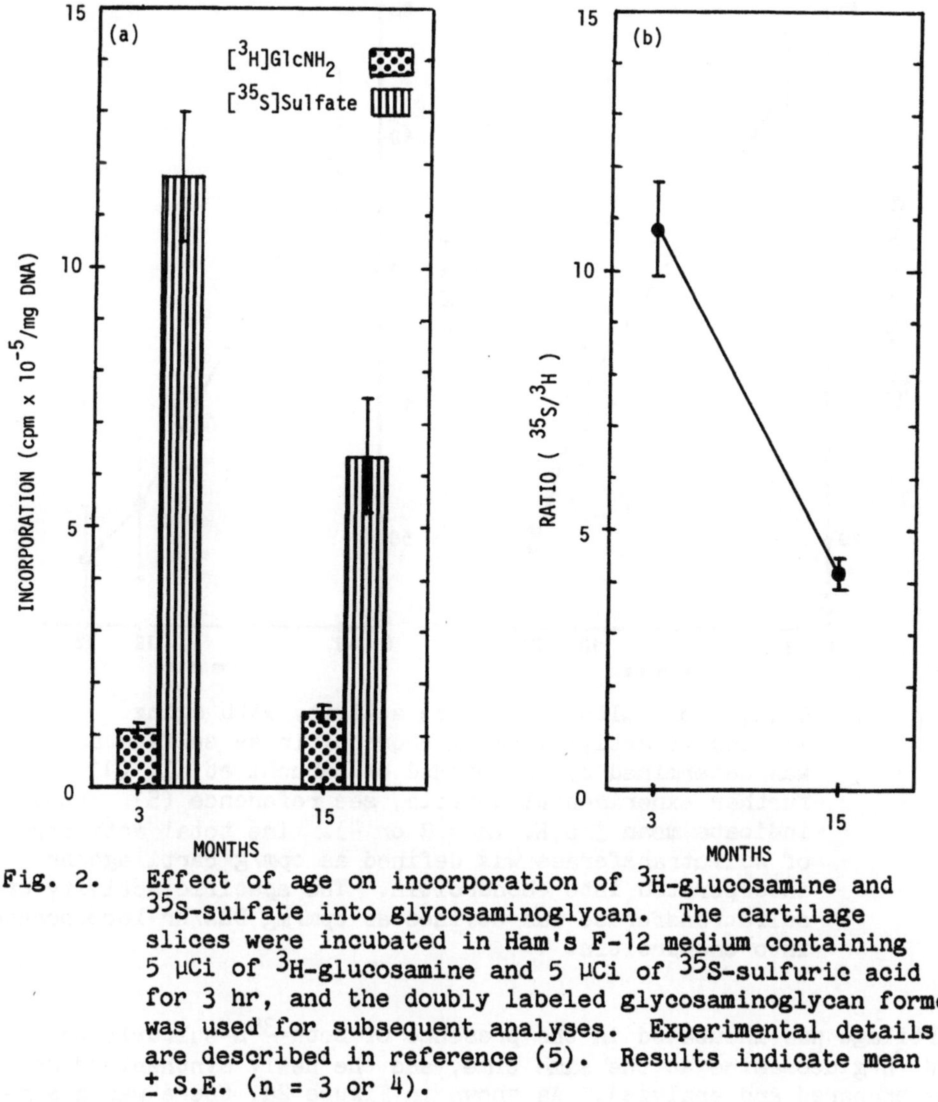

Fig. 2. Effect of age on incorporation of ^{3}H-glucosamine and ^{35}S-sulfate into glycosaminoglycan. The cartilage slices were incubated in Ham's F-12 medium containing 5 μCi of ^{3}H-glucosamine and 5 μCi of ^{35}S-sulfuric acid for 3 hr, and the doubly labeled glycosaminoglycan formed was used for subsequent analyses. Experimental details are described in reference (5). Results indicate mean ± S.E. (n = 3 or 4).

350-day- and 710-day-old rats), while the incorporation of ^{3}H-glucosamine into GAG did not show a change with age. On the other hand, the incorporation of ^{3}H-glucosamine into GP occurred only to a minor extent, and this level remained unchanged with age. The incorporated ^{35}S-radioactivity level in GP was negligible.

To confirm the above mentioned findings, that the ^{35}S-sulfate incorporation was much more affected by aging than the ^{3}H-glucosamine incorporation, a double isotope method was used. Rat costal

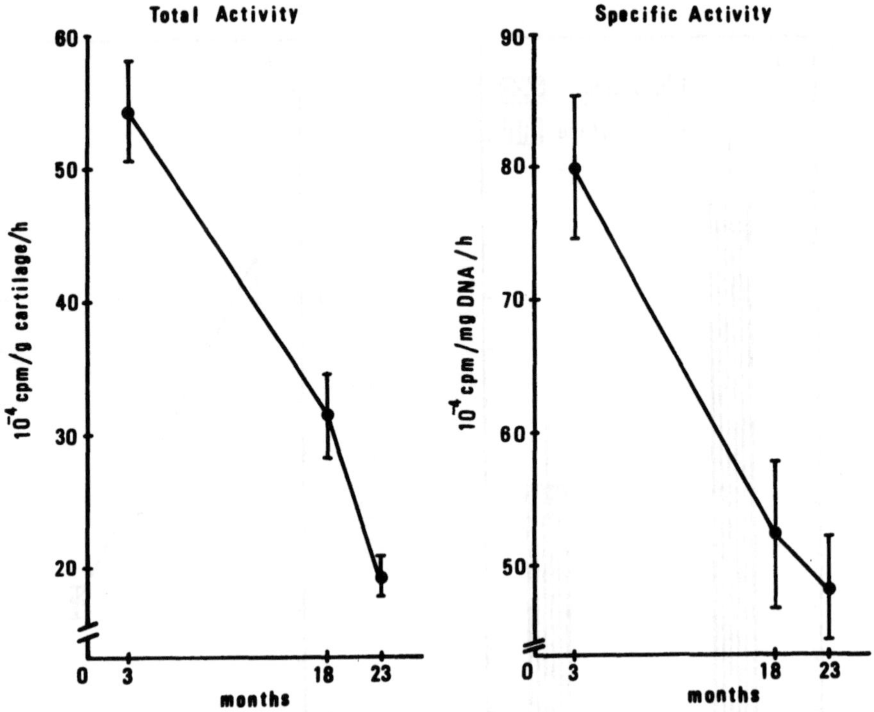

Fig. 3. Changes of sulfotransferase activity with aging. The enzyme activity using chondroitin as sulfate acceptor was determined by the method of Habuchi et al. (11). For further experimental details, see reference (5). Results indicate mean ± S.E. (n = 3 or 4). The total activity of sulfotransferase was defined as cpm/g cartilage/hr incorporated into chondroitin. The specific activity of sulfotransferase was defined as cpm/mg DNA/hr incorporated into chondroitin.

cartilage was incubated in the presence of both ^{35}S-sulfuric acid and ^{3}H-glucosamine at the same time, and the newly synthesized GAG was prepared and analyzed. As shown in Figure 2a, there was a significant decrease in the specific radioactivity of ^{35}S-sulfate per mg DNA (unit cartilage cell), whereas the specific radioactivity of ^{3}H-glucosamine per mg DNA (unit cartilage cell) did not change significantly in the young (3 months) and the middle-aged (15 months) rats. The ratio of radioactivity of ^{35}S-sulfate to ^{3}H-glucosamine, then, decreased significantly between 3 months and 15 months of age, as shown in Figure 2b.

The above result suggested that the biosynthesis of the repeating disaccharide units in the chondroitin sulfate molecule was affected little with aging, but the sulfation of the chondroitin sulfate chain decreased with the process of aging.

Changes in Sulfotransferase Activity with Aging

Sulfation of chondroitin sulfate by 3'-phosphoadenosine 5'-phosphosulfate (PAPS) was first described by D'Abramo and Lipmann (12). Later, direct transfer of a sulfate group from ^{35}S-PAPS to both chondroitin sulfate and chondroitin by sulfotransferase was demonstrated *in vitro* (13-16). DeLuca et al. (17) showed that sulfation occurred on the polysaccharide, along with, or immediately following, polymerization. In our laboratory, an attempt was made to examine the changes in sulfotransferase activity with aging. This enzyme is known to be responsible for the sulfation process in chondroitin sulfate biosynthesis. At present, however, the true sulfate acceptor of sulfotransferase in the biosynthesis of proteochondroitin sulfate has not been fully elucidated. Therefore, the enzyme activity was determined using chondroitin as sulfate acceptor (11). As was expected, both the total sulfotransferase activity and the specific activity per mg DNA (unit cartilage cell) decreased significantly with age, as shown in Figure 3. Similar results were also obtained when female rats were used. It is possible that this change can be attributed to a decrease in the enzyme activity of individual chondrocytes with aging. Furthermore, the decrease in sulfotransferase activity of cartilage cells with age was parallel to a reduction in the incorporation of ^{35}S-sulfate in chondrocytes with age. Recently, Hart (18) reported that the specific activity of glycosaminoglycan-sulfotransferase with each exogenous acceptor (e.g., keratan sulfate) changed only slightly during chick corneal development. It is interesting to note, however, that a difference exists in the activity of sulfotransferase between the processes of development and aging. Moreover, the analysis of disaccharide units formed after chondroitinase ABC digestion of ^{35}S-chondroitin or ^{35}S-endogenous acceptor, produced in the enzymic reaction mixtures (the enzyme source from 3-month-old rats), showed that the percentage of incorporation of ^{35}S sulfate into ΔDi-4S (ΔGlcUA-GalNAc-4S) was about 90% (Honda et al., unpublished data). Similar results were obtained when the enzyme source from old (23-month-old) rat costal cartilage was used. These results indicated that the sulfotransferase in rat costal cartilage specifically catalyzed the transfer of sulfate from ^{35}S-PAPS to position 4 of acetlygalactosamine residue of chodroitin or endogenous acceptor. It may then be said that chondroitin, used as a sulfate acceptor, behaved similarly to *in vivo* rat costal cartilage, in that the sulfotransferase specified the position for introduction of a sulfate group.

Changes in Degree of Sulfation and Molecular Size of Chondroitin Sulfate with Aging

Analysis of disaccharide units, formed after chondroitinase ABC digestion (19) of ^{3}H-labeled GAG isolated from young (3 months) and old (23 months) cartilage, showed that the percentages of incorporation of ^{3}H-glucosamine into ΔDi-OS (ΔGlcUA-GalNAc) increased significantly (from 7.7% to 13.6%) with age. This result suggested that the appearance of nonsulfated positions in the structure of the chondroitin sulfate chain increased with age.

On the basis of gel chromatography on Bio-Gel A-1.5m, no significant difference in the approximate molecular size of chondroitin sulfate was observed between the young (3 months) and old (23 months) samples. This finding suggested that aging did not affect the average chain length of chondroitin sulfate, and was consistent with the findings of Inerot et al. (4) and Šimůnek and Muir (20). It is, therefore, not unreasonable to assume that the bionsynthesis of the repeating disaccharide units in the chondroitin sulfate chain is affected little by the aging process.

DISCUSSION

Cartilage proteoglycan is composed of a protein core to which a large number of highly negatively charged chondroitin sulfates and a relatively small number of keratan sulfates are covalently attached, in the model proposed by Heinegård and Hascall (21). Recently, Inerot et al. (4) indicated that the structural change of proteoglycan macromolecules of articular cartilage with age was probably due to a diminishing of the chondroitin sulfate-rich region, whereas the hyaluronic acid-binding region and the keratan sulfate-rich region remain comparatively constant. This change in the proteoglycan macromolecular structure is believed to result in a decrease in the elasticity of the older cartilage.

In our study, sulfation of the chondroitin sulfate chain was found to decrease with age. Moreover, the number of non-sulfated positions in the structure of the chondroitin sulfate chain of rat costal cartilate proteoglycan increased with aging. The decrease in sulfation may result from either defective sulfation enzymes or an enhanced sulfatase activity, or a combination of both. At the present time, however, there is little direct evidence for the involvement of sulfatases in aging (22,23). The fact that the sulfotransferase activity decreased with aging, as shown in our study, must be directly related to the decrease in the biosynthetic sulfation of chondroitin sulfate.

It is of biological significance to relate the decreased sulfation of chondroitin sulfate in aged rats to the change in the elastic properties of cartilage with age, since negatively charged sulfate groups of the chondroitin sulfate chains in the proteoglycan molecule may play an important role for the interaction between proteoglycan and collagen. It is also important to consider that the sulfate group of proteochondroitin 4-sulfate binds with Ca^{2+} to function as a store of Ca^{2+}, and prevents the cartilage from calcifying (24,25).

Further, the degree of sulfation of chondroitin sulfate chains in proteoglycan molecule must be one of the major factors in the organization of the multimolecular-structures in the cartilage matrix.

REFERENCES

1. H. G. Vogel, ed., "Connective Tissue and Ageing," Excerpta Medica, Amsterdam (1973).
2. D. A. Hall, ed., "The Aging of Connective Tissue," Academic Press, London (1976).
3. H. Boström, in: "Aging of Connective and Skeletal Tissue," A. Engel and T. Larson, eds., Nordiska Bokhandelsforlag, Stockholm (1969).
4. S. Inerot, D. Heinegård, L. Audell, and S.-E. Olsson, Articular-cartilage proteoglycans in aging and osteoarthritis, Biochem. J. 169:143 (1978).
5. A. Honda, M. Abe, S.-I. Murota, and Y. Mori, The effect of aging on the synthesis of hexomsamine-containing substances from rat costal cartilage: A decrease in sulfation of chondroitin sulfate with aging, J. Biochem. 85:519 (1979).
6. N. Seno, K. Anno, K. Kondo, S. Nagase, and S. Saito, Improved method for electrophoretic separation and rapid quantitation of isomeric chondroitin sulfates on cellulose acetate strips, Anal. Biochem. 37:197 (1970).
7. Y. H. Liau, N. I. Galicki, and M. I. Horowitz, Heterogeneity of rat rib chondroitin sulfate and susceptibility to rat gastric chondrosulfatase, Biochim. Biophys. Acta 539:315 (1978).
8. M. B. Mathews and S. Glagov, Acid mucopolysaccharide patterns in aging human cartilage, J. Clin. Invest. 45:1103 (1966).
9. H. Iwata, The determination and fine structures of chondroitin sulfate isomers of human cartilage and pathological tissues, J. Jap. Orthop. Assoc. 43:455 (1969).
10. H. J. Mankin and A. Z. Thrasher, The effect of age on glycosaminoglycan synthesis in rabbit articular and costal cartilages, J. Rheumatol. 4:343 (1977).
11. O. Habuchi, T. Yamagata, and S. Suzuki, Biosynthesis of the acetylgalactosamine 4,6-disulfate unit of squid chondroitin sulfate by transsulfation from 3'-phosphoadenosine 5'-phosphosulfate, J. Biol. Chem. 246:7357 (1971).
12. F. D'Ambramo and F. Lipmann, The formation of adenosine-3'-phosphate-5'-phosphosulfate in extracts of chick embryo cartilage and its conversion into chondroitin sulfate, Biochim. Biophys. Acta 25:211 (1957).
13. S. Suzuki and J. L. Strominger, Enzymatic sulfation of mucopolysaccharides in hen oviduct. I. Transfer of sulfate from 3'-phosphoadenosine 5'-phosphosulfate to mucopolysaccharides, J. Biol. Chem. 235:257 (1960).

14. S. Suzuki and J. L. Strominger, Enzymatic sulfation of mucopolysaccharides in hen oviduct. II. Mechanism of the reaction studied with oligosaccharides and monosaccharides as acceptors, J. Biol. Chem. 235:267 (1960).
15. S. Suzuki and J. L. Strominger, Enzymatic sulfation of mucopolysaccharides in hen oviduct. III. Mechanism of sulfation of chondroitin and chondroitin sulfate A, J. Biol. Chem. 235:274 (1960).
16. H. C. Robinson, The sulfation of chondroitin sulfate in embryonic chicken cartilage, Biochem. J. 113:543 (1969).
17. S. DeLuca, M. E. Richmond, and J. E Silbert, Biosynthesis of chondroitin sulfate: Sulfation of the polysaccharide chain, Biochemistry 12:3911 (1973).
18. G. W. Hart, Glycosaminoglycan sulfotransferases of the developing chick cornea, J. Biol Chem. 253:347 (1978).
19. H. Saito, T. Yamagata, and S. Suzuki, Enzymatic methods for the determination of small quantitites of isomeric chondroitin sulfates, J. Biol. Chem. 243:1536 (1968).
20. Z. Šimůnek and H. Muir, Changes in the protein-polysaccharides of pig articular cartilage during prenatal life, development and old age, Biochem. J. 126:515 (1972).
21. D. Heinegård and V. C. Hascall, Aggregation of cartilage proteoglvcans. III. Characteristics of the proteins isolated from trypsin digests of aggregrates, J. Biol. Chem. 249:4250 (1974).
22. R. Silberberg and P. Lesker, Enzyme activity in aging articular cartilage, Experientia 27:133 (1971).
23. Å. Wasteson, U. Lindahl, and A. Hallén, Mode of degradation of the chondroitin sulfate proteoglycan in rat costal cartilage, Biochem. J. 130:729 (1972).
24. J. D. Salvo and M. Schubert, Specific interaction of some cartilage protein-polysaccharides with freshly precipitating calcium phosphate, J. Biol. Chem. 242:705 (1967).
25. R. D. Campo, C. D. Tourtellotte, and R. J. Bielen, The protein-polysaccharides of articular, epiphyseal plate and costal cartilages, Biochim. Biophys. Acta 177:501 (1969).

HYDRODYNAMIC PROPERTIES OF COLLAGEN FIBRIL AND AGING

Toshiharu Matsumura

Department of Cancer Cell Research
Institute of Medical Science
University of Tokyo
Shirokanedai, Minato-ku, Tokyo 108
Japan

INTRODUCTION

One biochemical approach to aging research has been to isolate bodily structural components, study their physiochemical properties, and establish the molecular basis for bodily changes during the aging process. This approach has been particularly fruitful in the field of connective tissue research, ever since soluble collagen was first isolated from tendon, and synthetic fibrils were reconstituted from the soluble collagen in vitro (1). When, in addition to soluble collagens and soluble ground substances, connective tissue components with high order structures, observable as collagen fibril, collagen fiber, and collagen fiber bundle (2) are isolated and characterized, such age-related changes as shrinkage temperature and tensile strength of skin (3) may be able to be expressed in terms of the physiochemical properties of their structural components.

Collagen fibril is one of those structural units in connective tissue where collagen molecules assemble in a regular fashion. They have an familar cross striation pattern when observed by an electronmicroscope. The fact that the average diameter, and the variability of diameter, of collagen fibril increases during mammalian aging was described by Banfield (4) and Schwarz (5). In the last ten years, the presence of an intrafibrillar structural unit, tentatively called either collagen filament or collagen microfibril, has been predicted with evidence resulting from electronmicroscopy (6), sequence analyses (7), and X-ray diffraction (8). The structure of the predicted microfibril consists of a five-fold helix of collagen molecules related by a 1D (length of the unit striation pattern) stagger.

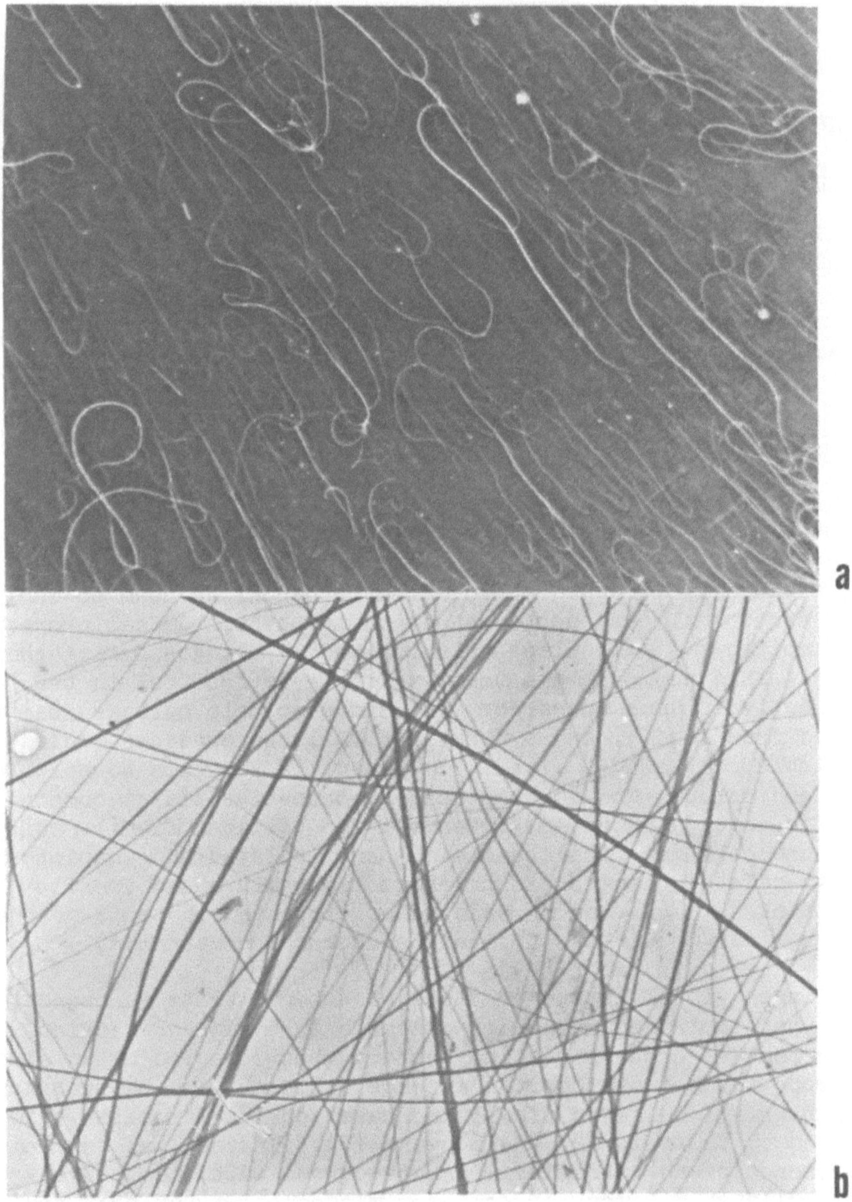

Fig. 1a. Phase contrast micrograph of sea cucumber (Stichopus japonicus) collagen fibrils. A drop of the fibril suspension was smeared and dried on a glass slide (x 310).

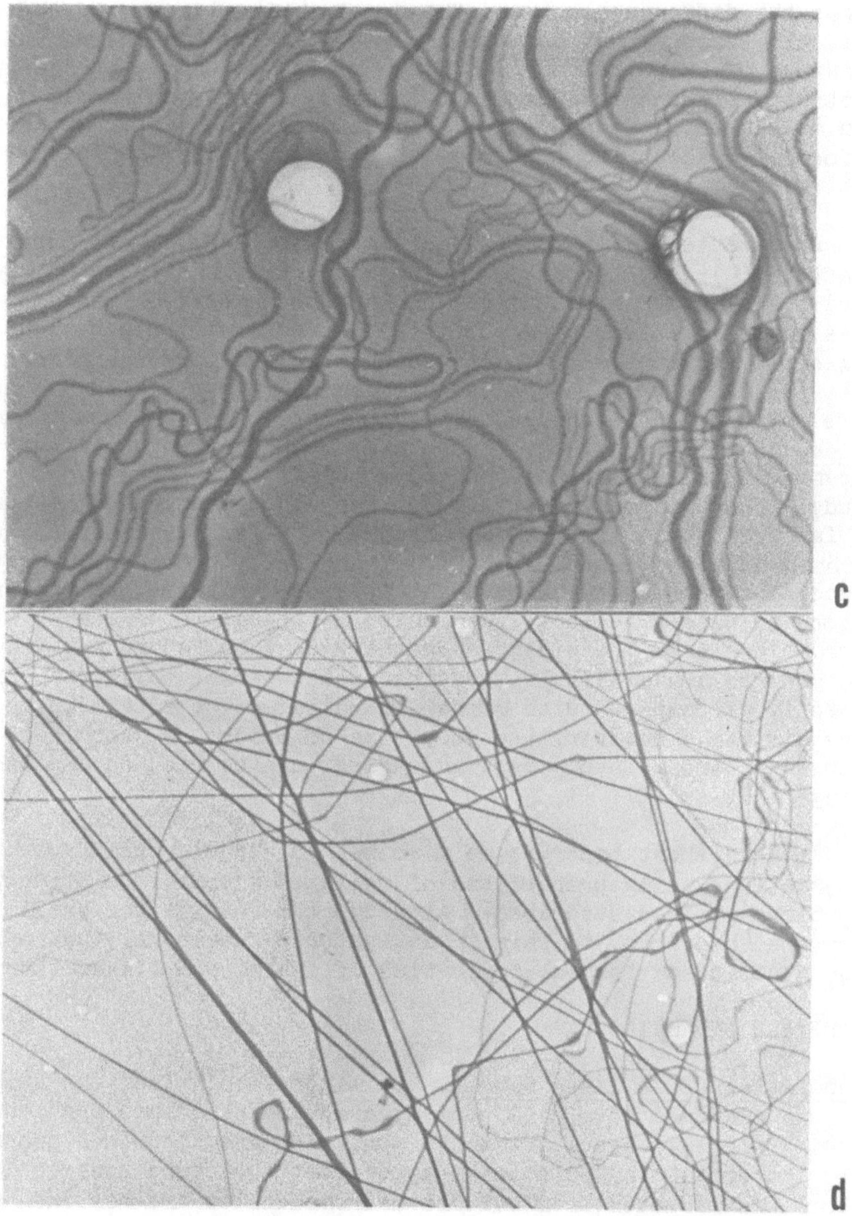

Fig. 1b-d. Electron micrographs of native (b), denatured (c), and partially denatured (d) collagen fibrils. An aliquot of fibril suspension was kept in the cold without incubation (b), incubated at 55°C for 10 min (c), or at 47°C for 60 min (d), and processed for electron-microscopy following pseudo-replica technique and uranyl acetate staining (x 8000).

Since the difference between the denaturation temperature of collagen molecule (around body temperature for mammals) and the shrinkage temperature of skin (around 60°C for mammals, depending on age) predicts the presence of weak and cooperative interactions among collagen molecules, a hydrodynamic study of collagen fibril would provide information about its predicted structure and the thermodynamic properties of connective tissues.

Preparations of mammalian collagen fibril have been obtained by Banfield (9) and Steven (10). Those preparations, however, were not used for hydrodynamic studies, perhaps because the preparation process may have interrupted the intact structure. Preparations of collagen fibrils have also been obtained from various echinodermal animals (11,12,13). Figure 1a shows collagen fibrils with a spindle-like shape and heterogeneous sizes obtained from the sea cucumber, Stichopus japonicus (14). There are advantages in using the sea cucumber fibrils and other echinodermal fibrils for a hydrodynamic study: there is only a single collagen type, and no collagenase has so far been found in echinoderms; the fibrils are quite insoluble both in acid and neutral solutions; and the fibril can be kept in suspension for days without precipitation, which allows the investigators to handle a fibril suspension as though it were a solution of macromolecules. The disadvantages are that no laboratory-grown echinoderms are available, and that echinodermal collagens cannot directly be compared with mammalian collagens, even though they are very similar. However, the body size of Stichopus japonicus, which increases during development and aging, can be used as a parameter of aging (15).

In this short paper, some viscometric and electromicroscopic observations using prepartions of collagen fibril from Stichopus japonicus will be described. Although the results are preliminary, they are the first, to this investigator's knowledge, that show the hydrodynamic and thermal properties of isolated collagen fibril.

MATERIALS AND METHODS

Preparation of Collagen Fibril. Collagen fibril from the sea cucumber was prepared in a cold room by a method described previously (13). Briefly, tissue fragments were disaggregated in a neutral salt solution containing EDTA and β-mercaptoethanol, and then collagen fibril was isolated from soluble macromolecules and residual particles by centrifugation. The isolated fibril was resuspended in neutral salt solution, dialyzed against water with the pH adjusted to 8.0 with a trace amount of Tris-HCL buffer. For viscometry, the suspension of isolated fibrils was passed through a sintered-glass filter to remove remaining aggregates of fibrils.

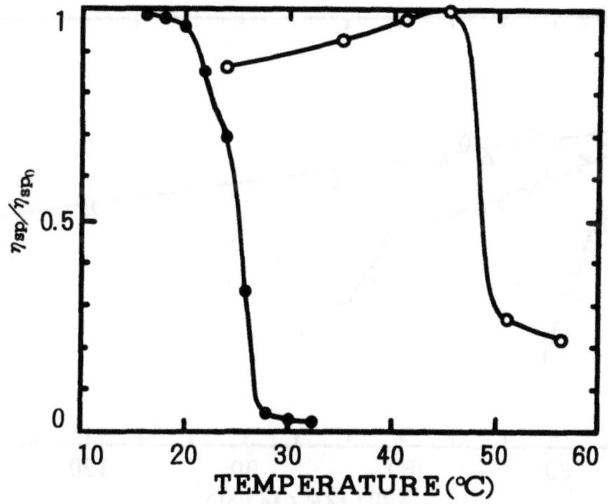

Fig. 2. Viscosity changes of collagen fibril suspensions and of a solution of solubilized collagen. The fraction of specific viscosity at a temperature (η sp) to the maximal value of the specific viscosity observed during the experimental range of temperature (η sp_0) is shown as a function of increasing temperature (ca. 0.12°C/min). A fibril suspension was treated with Pronase (50 μg/ml) at 4°C overnight, and then the solubilized collagen was isolated from Pronase solution by acid precipitation and resolubilization (detailed methods to be described elsewhere). Capillary viscometers with a flow of about 100^{-1} sec were used.

RESULTS

Thermal Denaturation of Collagen Fibril. Individual collagen fibrils in the preparation obtained above show a striation pattern under an electronmicroscope (Fig. 1b). After an incubation of the fibril suspension at 55°C for 10 minutes the cross striation pattern was completely lost and the fibrils were swollen (Fig. 1c). No significant amount of collagen protein was lost from the denatured fibril into the water following this short incubation. After a 60-minute incubation at 47°C, the collagen fibrils lost their cross striation pattern in some areas, whereas it was retained in most areas of the fibrils (Fig. 1d).

The viscosity of collagen fibril suspension decreased between 46°C and 50°C when the suspension was incubated with increasing temperature (Fig. 2). This temperature range is about 20°C higher than that for the viscosity change of solubilized collagen (see legend for Fig. 2). Profiles of the isothermal decline of viscosity varied to a certain extent, depending on the preparations used. Some examples

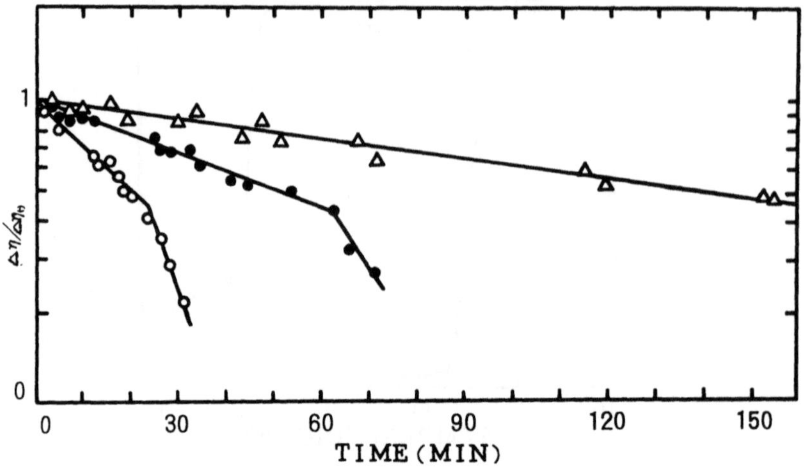

Fig. 3. Isothermal decline of viscosity of collagen fibril suspensions. From the specific viscosities of the initiation of incubation ($\eta sp\ t = o$), at an incubation time ($\eta\ sp\ t$), and after complete denaturation ($\eta sp\ d$) which was attained by keeping the suspension at 50°C for 10 min, the fraction of viscosity change to the total viscosity decrement ($\Delta\eta/\Delta\eta o = \frac{\eta sp\ t - \eta sp\ d}{\eta sp\ t = o - \eta sp\ d}$) is presented as a function of incubation time. The value ($\Delta\eta/\Delta\eta o$) was measured for a preparation of fibril suspension at 47°C (o——o) and at 46°C (●——●), and for another preparation at 48°C (Δ——Δ).

are shown in Figure 3. The profile consisted of one or two consecutive phases, hereafter referred to as phase A and phase B. In both phases, the difference between specific viscosity at time t and that after full denaturation declined exponentially. The kinetic constant for phase B was larger than that for phase A.

DISCUSSION

<u>The Structural Bases of Thermal Denaturation</u>. The electron microscopic and viscometric results as described above present conclusive evidence that the thermal shrinkage of connective tissue is an event happening within the collagen fibril, consisting of a cooperative denaturation of the ordered structure within the fibril. An isothermal profile of viscosity changes (Fig. 3) suggests that the denaturation consists of one or two first-order reactions, depending on the preparations used. Electronmicroscopic results show that, at least for some preparations, the denaturation does not happen throughout the entire fibril at once (Fig. 1c). A simple hypothesis that can explain all of the above results is that there is a

subfibrillar structural unit which denatures in a first-order reaction with the kinetic constant of phase B, and that the accumulation in a fibril of a certain number of denatured subfibrillar units leads to the denaturation of the entire fibril. For other fibril preparations that showed only one phase of isothermal viscosity change, the subfibrillar units may be tightly packed by an interaction among the subfibrillar units within a fibril, so that the fibril denatures as a first-order reaction with the kinetic constant of phase A. If this is the case, then the size of a collagen fibril, which is known to be a function of age, will influence the kinetic constant and period of phase A, but not of phase B. The two-phase viscosity change for some preparations might also be indicative of a loss of structural intactness during fibril preparation. Substantiation of the above hypothesis awaits further experimental work, as does the determination of thermodynamic parameters of fibril denaturation.

ACKNOWLEDGEMENT

The assistance of Professor Haruhiko Noda is gratefully acknowledged.

REFERENCES

1. J. Nageotte, Coagulation fibrillaire in vitro du collagène dissous dans un acide dilué, Compt. Rend. Acad. Sci. 184:115 (1927).
2. A. J. Cruise, The structure and deformation of collagen fibers. II. The morphology of collagen fibers, J. Soc. Leather Chemists 40:321 (1965).
3. D. M. Rusmussen, K. G. Wakim, and R. K. Winkelmann, Effect of aging on human dermis: Studies of thermal shrinkage and tension, in: "Advances in Biology of Skin, Vol. VI, Aging," W. Montagna, ed., Pergamon Press, Oxford (1964).
4. W. G. Banfield, Width and length of collagen fibrils during the development of human skin, in granulation tissue and in the skin of adult animals, J. Gerontol. 10:13 (1955).
5. W. Schwarz, Morphology and differentiation of the connective tissue fibres, in: "Connective Tissue," R. E. Tunbridge, M. Keech, J. F. Delafresnaye, and G. C. Woods, eds., Blackwell Scientific Publications, Oxford (1957).
6. J. W. Smith, Molecular pattern in native collagen, Nature 219:157 (1968).
7. B. L. Trus and K. A. Piez, Molecular packing of collagen: Three-dimensional analysis of electrostatic interactions, J. Mol. Biol. 108:705 (1976).
8. A. Miller, Molecular packing in collagen fibrils, in: "Biochemistry of Collagen," G. N. Ramachandran and A. H. Reddi, eds., Plenum Press, New York (1976).

9. W. G. Banfield, Occurrence of tapered collagen fibrils from human sources with observations on mesenchymal neoplasms, Proc. Soc. Exp. Biol. Med. 81:658 (1952).
10. F. S. Stevens, he Nishihara technique for the solubilization of collagen: Application to the preparation of soluble collagens from normal and rheumatoid connective tissue, Ann. Rheum. Dis. 23:300 (1964).
11. T. Matsumura, M. Shinmei, and Y. Nagai, Disaggregation of connective tissue: Preparation of fibrous components from sea cucumber body wall and calf skin, J. Biochem. 73:155 (1973).
12. T. Matsumura, M. Hasegawa, and M. Shigei, Collagen biochemistry and phylogeny of echinoderms, Comp. Biochem. Physiol. 62B:101 (1978).
13. T. Matsumura, Shape, size and amino acid composition of collagen fibril of the starfish Asterias amurensis, Comp. Biochem. Physiol. 44B:1197 (1973).
14. T. Matsumura, Collagen fibrils of the sea cucumber, Stichopus japonicus: Purification and morophological study, Connective Tissue Res. 2:117 (1974).
15. K. Mitsukuri, "otes on the habits and life-history of Stichopus japonicus Selenka, Annot. Zool. Japan 5:1 (1903).

ALTERNATE CELLULAR MODELS FOR AGING STUDIES

Edward L. Schneider*

Section on Cellular Aging and Genetics
Laboratory of Cellular and Molecular Biology
Gerontology Research Center
National Institute on Aging
National Institutes of Health
Baltimore, Maryland 21224, USA

Studies such as those described by Drs. Macieira-Coelho and Mitsui lead to increased insight into the mechanisms of the limited proliferative capacity of human diploid fibroblasts. While I suggest that these elegant studies of the *in vitro* passage of human cells be continued, I urge the development of alternate models for the study of cellular aging. In our laboratory, we have examined human diploid cells as a function of *in vitro* passage and the age of the donor of these cells. The first studies in this latter area were conducted by Drs. Hayflick, Goldstein, Martin, and their co-workers (1-3). These investigators demonstrated the diminished proliferative potential of cell cultures with the increasing age of the donor. At the Gerontology Research Center in Baltimore, we have been fortunate to be able to conduct our studies on skin fibroblast cultures derived from young and old volunteer members of the Baltimore Longitudinal Study. We have examined the total replicative ability of these skin fibroblast cultures, as well as many of the parameters analyzed by Drs. Mitsui and Macieira-Coelho as a function of *in vitro* passage (4).

Our results confirm the findings of Dr. Martin that cell cultures from young donors have greater numbers of total population replications and delayed onsets of senescence than parallel cultures obtained from old donors (Table 1). The percent replicating cells was determined by incubating cell cultures for 24 hours with

*Dr. Schneider's current address: Davis Institute on Aging, 700 Delaware Street, Denver, Colorado 80204, USA.

Table 1. Summary of Studies Conducted on Skin Fibroblast Cultures Derived from Young and Old Human Subjects[a]

Replication Parameter	Young Subjects (20-35 yrs)		Old Subjects (65 + yrs)	
Onset of Senescent Phase (PD)[b]	35.2 ± 2.1	(23)[c]	22.5 ± 1.7	(21)
In Vitro lifespan (PD)	44.6 ± 2.5	(23)	33.6 ± 2.1	(21)
Cell population replication rate (hrs.)	20.8 ± 0.8	(18)	24.3 ± 0.9	(18)
Percent replicating cells[d]	87.7 ± 1.6	(7)	79.6 ± 2.5	(7)
Cell number at confluency ($x\ 10^4$ cells/cm^2)	7.31 ± 0.42	(18)	5.06 ± 0.52	(18)
Percent cells able to form colony ≥ 16 cells[e]	69.0 ± 3.3	(9)	48.0 ± 4.4	(8)
Sister chromatid exchanges/cell[f]	67.9 ± 1.6	(7)	56.1 ± 1.4	(6)

[a]The results of these studies have been originally published in ref. 4, 5, and 7.

[b]PD = Population doublings

[c]Numbers within brackets indicate number of cell cultures examined, values are mean ± standard error of the mean.

[d]Determined by incubating cells for 24 hours with tritiated thymidine and then measuring the frequency of labeled nuclei by autoradiography.

[e]Two weeks after plating at low cell densities

[f]Cell cultures were incubated for 48 hours with 7.5 ng/ml mitomycin C. Fifteen cells from each culture were analyzed for SCE.

tritiated thymidine, and then determining the percent labeled nuclei by autoradiography. Cell population doubling time and the cell number at confluency were measured from cell culture growth curves. For each measure of cell replication, cell cultures from old donors had diminished capabilities when compared to parallel cultures from young donors (Table 1).

Studies of individual cells have been conducted in collaboration with Dr. James Smith and Olivia Pereira-Smith (5). Analysis of the colony size distributions of young and old donor skin fibroblast cultures indicates that cells from young donors form larger colonies more frequently than do cell cultures from old donors (Table 1).

We have recently completed studies of sister chromatid exchanges (SCE). These studies indicate that mitomycin-C induced SCE are diminished as a function of *in vitro* passage (6) and the age of the cell culture donor (7) (Table 1). A number of other collaborative studies have been completed on cell cultures from young and old donors, including studies of macromolecular synthesis using a viral probe (8) and examination of insulin and EGF receptors (9).

In summary, a number of the alterations that are found as a function of *in vitro* passage can also be seen as a function of donor age. At the Gerontology Research Center, we have 800 relatively healthy volunteers who visit our Center every year and a half for a comprehensive series of physiological and psychological testing. Thus, we can examine the relationship between *in vitro* and *in vivo* measurements.

Finally, I would like to urge the combination of *in vitro* and *in vivo* studies. We have taken this approach in our studies of SCE which have been conducted *in vitro* in human cells and well as *in vivo* in rodent cell populations (10).

REFERENCES

1. L. Hayflick, The limited *in vitro* lifetime of human diploid cell strains, *Exp. Cell Res.* 37:614 (1965).
2. S. Goldstein, J. W. Littlefield, and J. S. Soeldner, Diabetes mellitus and aging: Diminished plating efficiency of cultured human fibroblasts, *Proc. Nat. Acad. Sci. USA* 64:155 (1969).
3. G. M. Martin, C. A. Sprague, and C. J. Epstein, Replicative lifespan of cultivated human cells: Effect of donor age, tissue, and genotype, *Lab. Invest.* 23:86 (1970).
4. E. L. Schneider and Y. Mitsui, The relationship between *in vitro* cellular aging and *in vivo* human age, *Proc. Nat. Acad. Sci. USA* 73:3584 (1976).
5. J. R. Smith, O. M. Pereira-Smith, and E. L. Schneider, Colony size distributions as a measure of *in vivo* and *in vitro* aging, *Proc. Nat. Acad. Sci. USA* 75:1353 (1978).
6. E. L. Schneider and R. E. Monticone, Aging and sister chromatid exchange II. The effect of *in vitro* passage level of human fetal lung fibroblasts on baseline and mutagen-induced sister chromatid exchange frequencies, *Exp. Cell Res.* 115:269 (1978).
7. E. L. Schneider and B. Gilman, Sister chromatid exchanges and aging III. The effect of donor age on mutagen induced sister chromatid exchange, *Hum. Genet.*, in press (1979).
8. D. B. Danner, E. L. Schneider, and J. Pitha, Macromolecular synthesis in human diploid fibroblasts: A viral probe examining the effect of *in vivo* aging, *Exp. Cell Res.* 114:63 (1978).

9. M. D. Hollenberg and E. L. Schneider, Receptors for insulin and epidermal growth factor-urogastrone in adult human fibroblasts do not change with donor age, Mech. Ageing Dev., in press (1979).
10. D. Kram, E. L. Schneider, R. R. Tice, and P. Gianas, Aging and sister chromatid exchange. I. The effect of aging on mitomycin-C induced sister chromatid exchange frequencies in mouse and rat bone marrow cells in vivo, Exp. Cell Res. 114:471 (1978).

AGING OF HEPATOCYTES

Akihiro Shima

Department of Experimental Radiology
Shiga University of Medical Science
Ōtsu, Shiga 520-21
Japan

INTRODUCTION

The purpose of this paper is not to survey current knowledge on aging of hepatic cells in general, but to summarize some of our own results that are concerned with the age changes in DNA content-based polyploidization of hepatocytes of three kinds of laboratory animals: mouse (1), fish (2), and house shrew (3).

The major technique used throughout the experiment was a strictly controlled Feulgen-DNA cytofluorometry combined simultaneously with tritiated thymidine autoradiography (4,5,6). As a parameter of age changes in hepatocytes, we measured the changes in DNA contents of hepatocytes which had been suggested by the extensive micromorphometric studies on human livers by Tauchi and Sato (7,8,9).

AGING OF MOUSE HEPATOCYTES

The C57BL/6 male mice used in our experiments had a mean life span of 24 months and a maximum life span of 31 months under our laboratory conditions (1). Figure 1 summarizes the change in relative frequency of each nuclear ploidy class as a function of animal age. The nuclei in S phase are not included in this figure. All measurements were done without regard to binuclearity, which is well known to occur in the liver of rodents and humans during aging. The decrease in percentage of 2C (diploid) nuclei occurred as early as 1 month of age, and the reduction continued steadily up to 28 months. This decrease in the percentage of 2C nuclei is accompanied by a marked increase in the percentage of 4C nuclei after about 1 month of age. However, the percentage of 4C nuclei stayed at almost the same

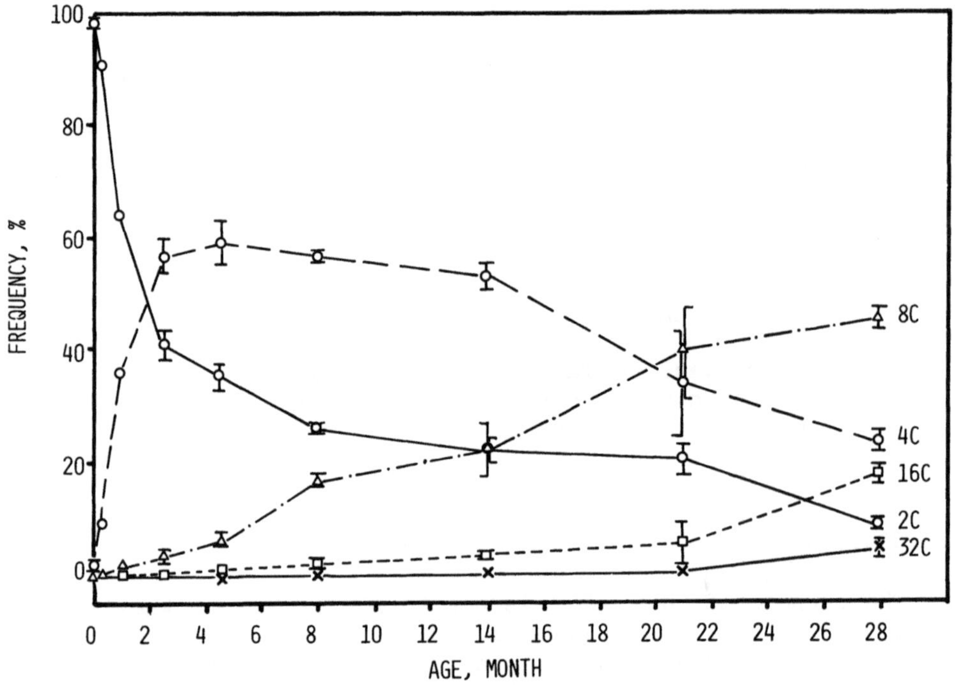

Fig. 1. Changes in relative frequency of mouse hepatocytes of various ploidy classes. Reproduced from Shima and Sugahara (1).

level from 2.5 months to 14 months of age, and thereafter it climbed toward 24 percent at 28 months of age. The percentage increase in 8C and 16C nuclei, and probably even in 32C nuclei, might be persistent throughout the life of the mice.

The clear age dependency in hepatocyte polyploidization can be shown in another, simpler, way by introducing the term, "Polyploidization Index," (P.I.), as shown in Figure 2. The Polyploidization Index is defined by dividing the summation of percentage of polyploid nuclei by percentage of diploid nuclei, because diploid (2C) nuclei might be possibly regarded as the basic unit in somatic cells. A straight line could be fitted between logarithms of age in months and P.I., by least square method, with a correlation coefficient $r = +0.892$. These results do not tell anything about the mechanism(s) of the age-dependent polyploidization in mouse hepatocytes. However, the present results could be of use as basic data for further research into the mechanism(s).

As the next step following the phenomenalistic description of age-dependent polyploidization of mouse hepatocytes, it would be

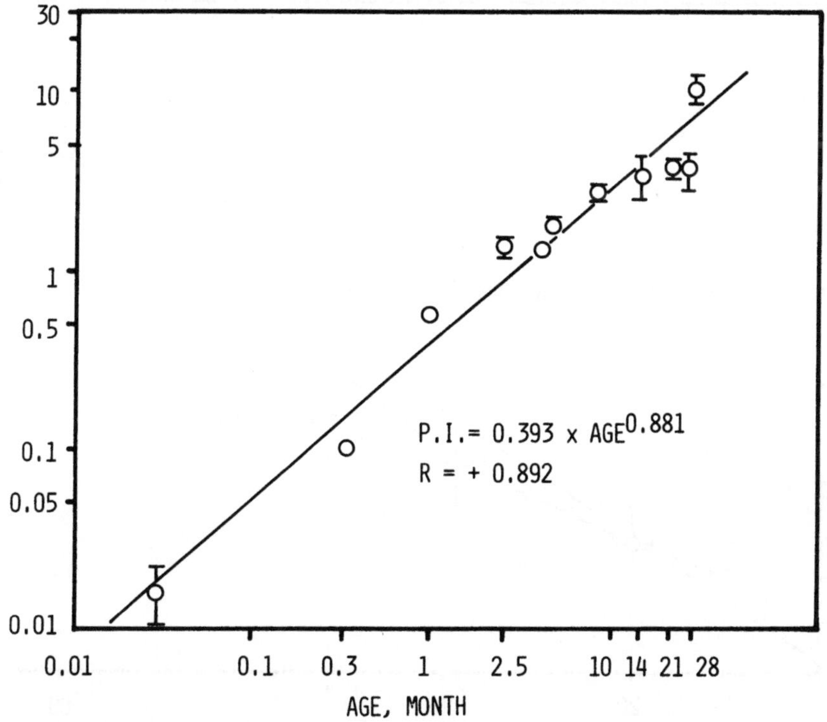

Fig. 2. Relationship between age in months and degree of polyploidization of mouse hepatocytes. Polyploidization Index (P.I.) = % polyploids/% diploids; r, correlation coefficient. Reproduced from Shima and Sugahara (1).

quite natural for one to attempt to learn what the differences are among hepatocytes of various ploidy classes. To begin with, we compared the template-primer activities of DNA among hepatocytes of various ploidy classes (10), by utilizing the enzymatic method originally developed by Modak et al. (11-14). In the method they originated, the paraffin sections of animal tissues were used to react with exogenously added DNA polymerase. However, we used methanol-fixed smears of the liver in order to avoid possible artifacts derived from routine histological procedures, and also to make it possible to combine grain counting method with Feulgen-DNA cytofluorometry simultaneously. The details of the present procedures have already been described (15). Briefly, methanol-fixed smears of the liver were allowed to react with exogenously added DNA polymerase I of E. coli in the presence of ^{3}H-TTP, three other dNTP's and other co-factors. E. coli DNA polymerase can be utilized to nick DNA with 3'-OH end as well as the gapped DNA (16). The specimens were then stained with Feulgen nuclear reaction and dipped into a nuclear emulsion to prepare autoradiographs. The DNA content measurement and

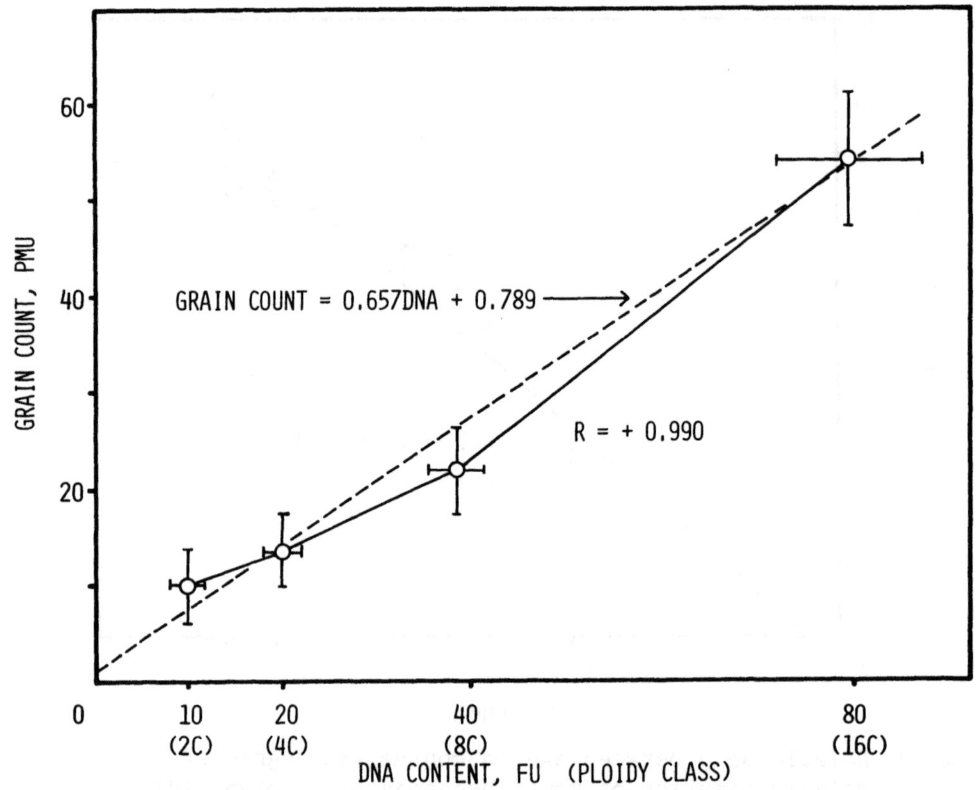

Fig. 3. Template-primer activity of 12-month-old mouse hepatocytes of various ploidy classes detected by E. coli DNA polymerase I. FU, fluorescence unit; PMU, photo-multiplier unit. Reproduced from Shima, Egami and Sugahara (10).

grain counting were done simultaneously on each hepatocyte nucleus. Since no grain could be found on nuclei wihout denaturing treatments of the specimens, all preparations were treated with 0.01 N HCl at 25°C for 30 min prior to incubation with the reaction mixture.

The results shown in Figure 3 were obtained from livers of 12-month-old C57BL/6 male mice (10). The grain count was in an almost linear relationship with the amount of DNA, i.e., nuclear ploidy classes. However, if the grain count was divided by the DNA content, something like "specific" template-primer activities could be obtained, as shown in Figure 4 (10). It appears evident that no principal difference in such "specific" activities could be found among four ploidy classes of the hepatocytes. In summary, the number of sites in the nucleus which were sensitive to 0.01 N HCl and which could also react with exogenously added DNA polymerase I of E. coli might be doubled when the ploidy class of hepatocyte ascends from one

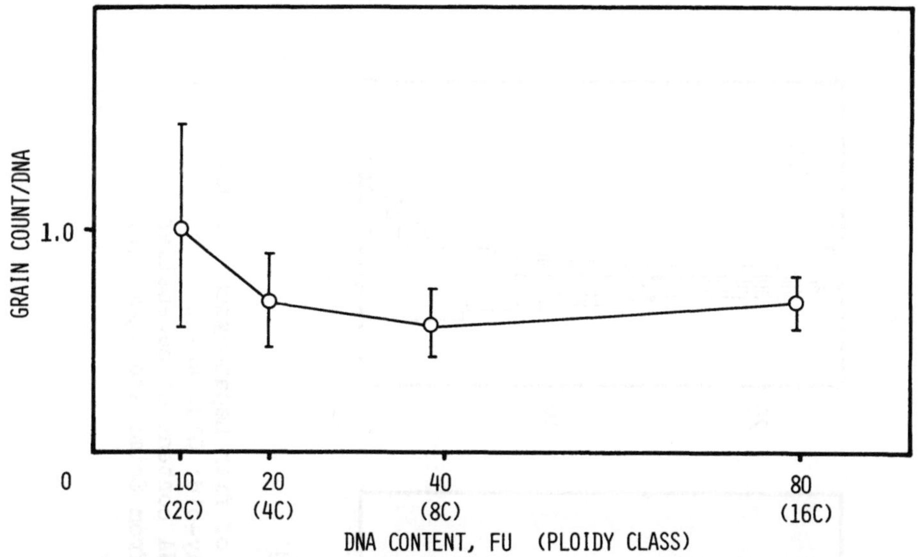

Fig. 4. Specific template-primer activity of 12-month-old mouse hepatocytes of various ploidy classes detected by E. coli DNA polymerase I. Reproduced from Shima, Egami and Sugahara (10).

class to the next higher class, i.e., through polyploidization. In addition, the type of DNA damage that can be detected by E. coli DNA polymerase I might not be primarily responsible for age-dependent polyploidization of mouse hepatocytes.

AGING OF FISH HEPATOCYTES

The age-related changes in the DNA contents of hepatocytes were also examined using male Japanese killifish Medaka, Oryzias latipes, which is one of the best known poikilothermal laboratory animals. The life table of the fish has already been established with mean and maximum life spans of 1000 days and 1838 days, respectively (17,18). The results summarized in Figure 5 indicate that: (a) there is no principal difference among the frequency distributions of nuclear DNA contents of young (about 100-day-old), medium (about 450-day-old), and old (about 1200-day-old) fish, and (b) the distributions of DNA contents are continuous from 2C (= 10 FU) to 4C range, irrespective of age (2). The first point indicates that no systematic polyploidization occurs in hepatocytes of the fish during aging, and the second point suggests that almost the same fraction of hepatocytes might be in S phase of 2C cell cycle in young, medium, and old fish, at least judging from our previous data on mouse hepatocytes (1). In order to examine the second point, the fish were injected with tritiated thymidine and autoradiographs were prepared with the

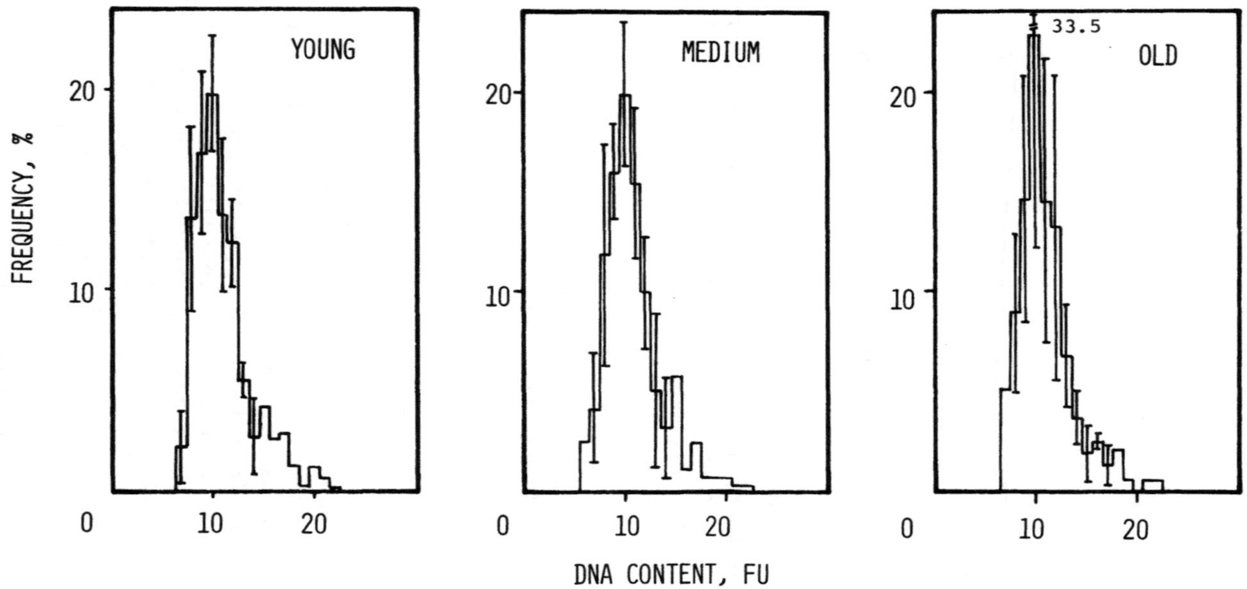

Fig. 5. Frequency distribution of DNA contents of fish hepatocytes. Young, about 100-day-old; Medium, about 450-day-old; Old, about 1000-day-old. 10 FU is equal to the DNA content of cerebellar internal granule neurons. Reproduced from Shima and Egami (2).

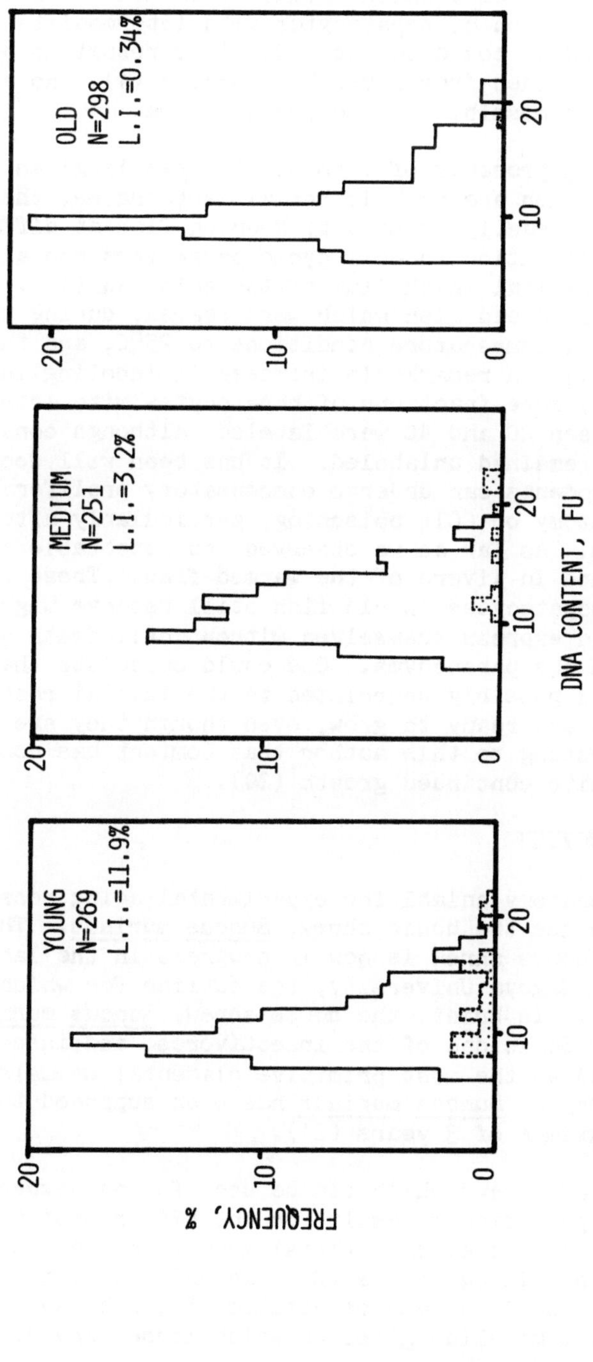

Fig. 6. DNA labeling of fish hepatocytes after a two-hour *in vivo* pulse with tritiated thymidine. Dotted histogram indicates labeled nuclei. N, number of nuclei measured; L.I., labeling index. Reproduced from Shima, Egami and Sugahara (10).

results shown in Figure 6 (10). The labeling index decreased, from 12 percent in young fish to 0.3 percent in old ones, with advancing age of the fish. Another point which should be marked in Figure 6 is that only the minor fraction of hepatocytes with intermediate DNA contents between 2C and 4C could be labeled. This result is quite different from that obtained from mouse hepatocytes (1). No answer for this discrepancy is possible at the present time.

Another interesting property of fish hepatocytes is given in Figure 7 (10). Since fish are poikilothermal vertebrates, the cell cycle parameters can be easily changed by keeping fish at different temperatures. Such alteration in cell cycle parameters has already been reported for intestinal epithelium of the goldfish (19). Therefore, we transferred old fish which were reared, during winter days, under natural low temperature conditions to 25°C, and the fish were warmed for 10 days. A remarkable increase in labeling index was evident, and also many more fractions of hepatocytes with intermediate DNA contents between 2C and 4C were labeled, although considerable fractions still remained unlabeled. It has been well documented that hepatocytes of rodents can undergo compensatory proliferation after partial hepatectomy or CCl_4 poisoning, particularly after large-scale cell loss. As far as we observed, no detectable signs of pycnosis could be found in livers of the warmed fish. These results might indicate that hepatocytes in old fish still reserve high growth potentials which could express themselves without cell death and probably cell loss in the parenchyma. One could speculate that the present findings could possibly be related to the initial response of the warmed fish which are ready to grow, even though they are old. Finally, it is interesting to this author that Comfort has concluded that fish do age despite continued growth (20).

AGING OF SHREW HEPATOCYTES

As the third laboratory animal for experimental aging research, we have just begun to use the house shrew, *Suncus murinus*. The domestication of the house shrew is now in progress in the laboratory of Professor Kondo of Nagoya University, the outline for which can be found in reference 21. In brief, the house shrew, *Suncus murinus*, belongs to the Family Soricidae of the insectivores; and insectivores are generally accepted as the most primitive placental mammals. The average life expectancy of *Suncus murinus* has been supposed to be 2 years or so with a maximum of 3 years (21).

Since the number of shrews which can be used for our experiment is still small, only preliminary results on the DNA content distribution of hepatocytes and cerebellar internal granule neurons of 1- and 2-year-old males are now in our hands (3). In order to simplify the comparison with mice, the liver and cerebellum of the house shrew were stamped onto the same slide glass on which mouse cerebellum was

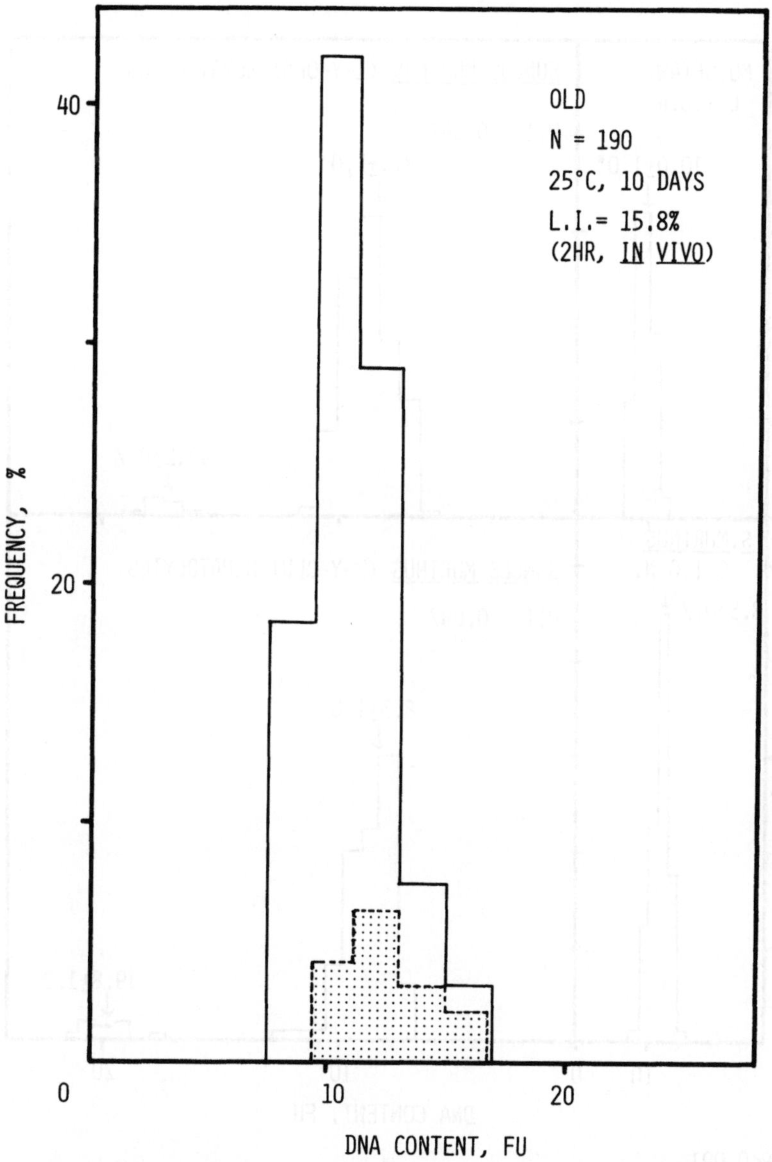

Fig. 7. Increased labeling of hepatocytes of old fish transferred from low temperature to 25°C. Dotted histogram, labeled nuclei. Reproduced from Shima, Egami and Sugahara (10).

stamped, which provided a standard. As shown in Figure 8, the mean DNA content of cerebellar internal granule neurons of the house shrew was 8.5 FU, while that of the mouse was 10.0 FU. This consistent

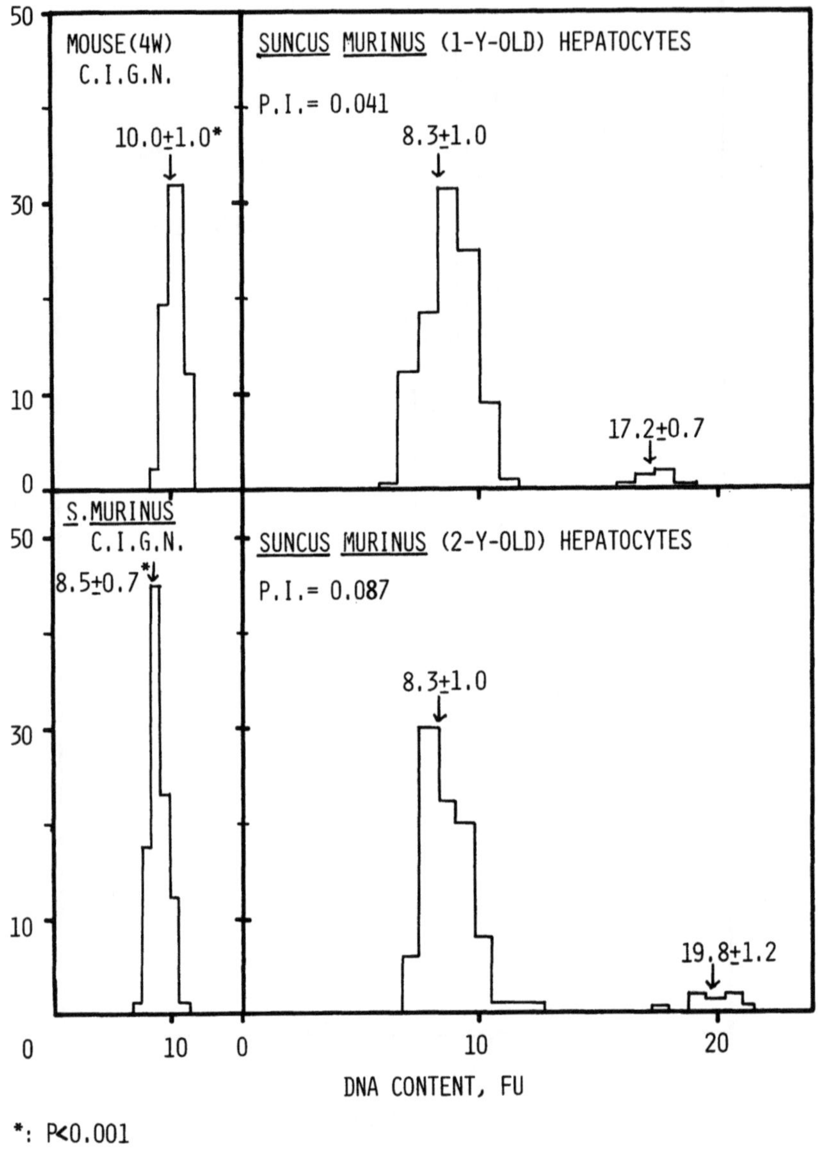

Fig. 8. Frequency distribution of DNA contents of neurons and hepatocytes of mouse and house shrew (Suncus murinus). C.I.G.N., cerebral internal granule neurons; FU, fluorescence unit. P.I., polyploidization index (= % polyploids/% diploids). Reproduced from Shima, Shinohara and Kondo (3).

difference ($p < 0.001$) indicates that the genome size of the house shrew is significantly smaller than that of the mouse.

Two other points should be made. The frequency distribution histograms of DNA contents of shrew hepatocytes, characterized by major 2C peak and minor 4C peak, are almost identical between two age groups; and the hepatocyte nuclei with intermediate DNA contents are equally almost absent. Whether the nuclei with DNA contents around 17 FU are G_2 nuclei of diploid cells or G_1 nuclei of tetraploids is not yet clear. Further studies utilizing larger numbers of the shrews of various ages and combining autoradiography are now in progress. There preliminary results indicate that, in the house shrew, almost all the hepatocytes seemed to be diploid, at least in 1- and 2-year-old animals; which is to say that few polyploids occur.

CONCLUSION

Judging from the DNA content measurements, mouse hepatocytes are most prone to undergo polyploidization with advancement of the animal age, while fish hepatocytes are the least likely to do so, and shrew hepatocytes are probably somewhere between the two. Our attempt to find uniformity in the aging of hepatic cell resulted in the finding of rather a marked diversity. However, further efforts to search for mechanism(s) responsible for the diversity might allow us to approach the uniformity.

REFERENCES

1. A. Shima and T. Sugahara, Age-dependent ploidy class changes in mouse hepatocyte nuclei as revealed by Feulgen-DNA cytofluorometry, Exp. Gerontol. 11:193 (1976).
2. A. Shima and N. Egami, Absence of systematic polyploidization of hepatocyte nuclei during the ageing process of the male Medaka, *Oryzias latipes*, Exp. Gerontol. 13:51 (1978).
3. A. Shima, S. Shinohara, and K. Kondo, Unpublished data.
4. S. Fujita, T. Ashihara, M. Fukuda, T. Hattori, and S. Yoshida, Combination of Feulgen cytofluorometry with ^{3}H-thymidine autoradiography, Acta Histochem. Cytochem. 6:205 (1973).
5. S. Fujita and M. Fukuda, Irradiation of specimens by excitation light before and after staining with Pararosaniline Feulgen: A new method to reduce non-specific fluorescence in cytofluorometry, Histochemistry 40:59 (1974).
6. S. Fujita, T. Ashihara, and M. Fukuda, Simultaneous measurement of DNA content and grain count on an autoradiograph of Feulgen stained cells, Histochemistry 40:155 (1974).
7. H. Tauchi, On the fundamental morphology of the senile changes, Nagoya J. Med. Sci. 24:97 (1960).
8. T. Sato, T. Miwa, and H. Tauchi, Age changes in the human liver of the different races, Gerontolgia 16:368 (1970).

9. H. Tauchi and T. Sato, Effect of environmental conditions upon age changes in human liver, Mech. Ageing Dev. 4:71 (1975).
10. A. Shima, N. Egami, and T. Sugahara, Comparative study on the polyploidization of hepatocytes of mouse and fish during ageing, in:"Liver and Aging-1978," K. Kitani, ed., Elsevier/ North-Holland Biomedical Press, Amsterdam (1978).
11. S. P. Modak, R. C. von Borstel, and F. J. Bollum, Terminal lens cell differentiation II. Template activity of DNA during nuclear degeneration, Exp. Cell Res. 56:105 (1969).
12. S. P. Modak and F. J. Bollum, Terminal lens cell differentiation III. Initiator activity of DNA during nuclear degeneration, Exp. Cell Res. 62:421 (1970).
13. S. P. Modak and F. J. Bollum, Detection and measurement of single-strand breaks in nuclear DNA in fixed lens sections, Exp. Cell Res. 75:307 (1972).
14. G. B. Price, S. P. Modak, and T. Makinodan, Age-associated changes in the DNA of mouse tissue, Science 171:917 (1971).
15. M. Matsui, A. Shima, and N. Egami, Autoradiographic detection of the template-primer activities of DNA by exogenous DNA polymerases in fixed mouse tissues, J. Fac. Sci., Univ. Tokyo, Sec. IV, 13:399 (1976).
16. R. B. Kelly, N. R. Cozzarelli, M. P. Deutscher, I. R. Lehman, and A. Kornberg, Enzymatic synthesis of deoxyribonucleic acid XXXII. Replication of duplex deoxyribonucleic acid by polymerase at a single strand break, J. Biol. Chem. 245:39 (1970).
17. N. Egami and H. Etoh, Life span data for the small fish, Oryzias latipes, Exp. Geront. 4:127 (1969).
18. N. Egami, Further notes on the life span of the teleost, Oryzias latipes, Exp. Geront. 6:379 (1971).
19. Y. Hyodo-Taguchi and N. Egami, Development of gastrointestinal radiation injury and recovery at different temperatures in fish, in:"Comparative Cellular and Species Radiosensitivity," V. P. Bond and T. Sugahara, eds., Igaku-Shoin, Tokyo (1969).
20. A. Comfort, The effect of age on growth-resumption in fish (Lebiste) checked by food restriction, Gerontologia 4:177 (1960).
21. K. Kondo, S. Oda, H. Takahashi, and R. Izeki, The house shrew: A new laboratory animal for comparative study of aging, in:"Abstracts for Plenary Sessions and Symposia of the XIth International Congress of Gerontology," Tokyo (1978).

THE AGING PROCESS IN THE NEURON*

Kenneth R. Brizzee[1] and Craig Knox[2]

[1]Department of Neurobiology
Delta Regional Primate Research Center
Tulane University Medical Center
Covington, Louisiana 70433

[2]Department of Anatomy
Tulane University Medical Center
New Orleans, Louisiana 70122

INTRODUCTION

The neuron as the ultimate anatomical and physiological unit of the nervous system, and the archetype of postreplicative cells of the body, has perhaps received a greater amount of attention as a model for the study of aging processes than any other cell type. Additional interest in the neuron as a subject for aging studies stems from the view that that these elements, in strategic locations in the nervous system, may function as pacemakers, or the central control elements, of the "time clocks" of aging which may determine the onset and rate of senescence (1).

Several topics pertaining to aging in the neuron, including neurotransmitters, hormonal receptors, age changes in dendritic organization, and neuroendocrine factors, will be covered by other authors in this volume. The present chapter therefore will be confined to a consideration of age changes in neuron cell populations, synapses and synaptic end bulbs, and structural and cytologic changes in these postreplicative cells with age.

CHANGES IN NEURONAL POPULATIONS AND THE NEURON-TO-GLIA RATIO WITH AGE

General Considerations

Of the many age-related structural changes in the brain which

*Supported by NIH RR00164

have attracted the attention of experimental gerontologists, probably none has excited greater interest than the possibility of neuronal "fall-out" (2) with age. Although opinions still differ with regard to the magnitude, rate, and even the occurrence of neuronal loss, there appears to be a consensus among most experimental gerontologists that neuron loss with age does indeed occur in certain regions of the mammalian central nervous system.

Changes in Total Cell Populations in Whole Brain

One investigation of neuron populations in the whole brain of the mouse using the "sonification" technique revealed no significant decline in the numbers of neurons from young adulthood to 24 months of age. However, by 29 months the neuron population decreased significantly to approximately one-third of the original number, while the glial population appeared to increase (3). It was concluded that the shape of the neuron survival curve resembled the shape of the mouse survival curve, and both tended to correspond to the exponential Gompertz plot.

In another recent investigation of possible changes in neuronal number in the whole body employing the "DNA method" in mice, no change in total number of neurons with age was observed (4).

Cerebral Cortex

In a series of human brains, without demonstrable pathology, ranging in age from newborn to 95 years of age, Brody (5) reported a decrease in neurons with age in several regions of the cerebral cortex.

In another study involving an analysis of neuron populations in the brains of two "elderly" men, without any major disease known to be associated with cell loss, a decrease of 44% in neuron number was reported (6). In yet another investigation comparing neuron populations in cerebral cortex in young and old human subjects, a decrease of 22% in the number of neurons in Brodman's area 6, 28% in area 10, 23% in area 21, and 29% in the subiculum was observed (7).

Quantitative histological studies in the cerebral cortex of young adult and aged rhesus monkeys have also revealed a similar but less severe decrease in the packing density in cerebral cortex, especially in area 3 (8). The greatest loss was observed in the granule cell population in lamina IV. Wisniewski et al. (9) also described a loss of neurons in the cerebral cortex in aged rhesus monkeys. In our study (8), it was also shown that the number of glial cells per mm^3 of tissue and the glia/neuron ratio increased significantly with age.

In the cerebral cortex of the albino rat, a quantitative histological study using an automated technique (Leitz Texture Analyzing

System) revealed a significant decrease in neurons in the visual cortex (area 17) (10). It was not possible in that investigation, with the automated equipment, to differentiate vascular cell nuclei from glial nuclei. Hence the "small cell" population included both glial and vascular cell counts. These did not appear to change with age. Earlier studies carried out by manual methods of cell enumeration in our laboratory showed that no neuron loss occurred in the somatosensory area of cerebral cortex of aged as compared with young adult Long-Evans rats (11). In that investigation, a significant increase in the glial population with a concomitant reduction in the neuron-to-glia ratio with age was observed. Such glial increases with age have been observed in cerebral cortex of various species by several workers, including Wahal and Riggs (12), Timiras and Vernadakis (13), Vaughan and Peters (14), Uemura and Hartmen (15,16), and Sturrock (17). It is noteworthy that Sturrock, in an earlier study (18), found a decrease in total numbers of glia in the anterior commissure with age. He tentatively suggested that part of the reason for the differences in glial counts in different structures might be gradual migration of neuroglia from white to gray matter with increasing age (17). We concur with this postulate.

The possibility of subspecies differences in the rate and intensity of the aging process, as evidenced by the difference in neuron loss between Long-Evans (11) and albino (10) rats, clearly indicates a need for additional aging studies giving special attention to subspecies comparisions in relation to the median and maximum life span of each, as well as to environmental conditions during the rearing of the animals.

Cerebellum

In the cerebellum of man, apes, dogs and cats, a decrease in the number of Purkinje neurons per unit volume of tissue has recently been observed in aged as compared to young adult animals (19,20). More recently, Tarnowska-Dziduszko (21) reported atrophy of all 3 layers of the cerebellar cortex, patchy cell losses in the granular layer, and marked loss of Purkinje neurons in aged human tissues. The most recent investigations by Hall et al. (22), which employed automated techniques, also reported a loss of Purkinje neurons in the cerebellum with age.

Basal Ganglia and Thalamus

An 18% decrease in number of neurons in the human anterior thalamic nucleus with age was reported (23). Neuroglial cell populations, reported as mean number of cells per field of view, did not appear to change significantly from age 24 to 64 years in man in various thalamic nuclei (23). Quantitative data on age differences in glial populations in the thalamus at older age levels have not yet been reported.

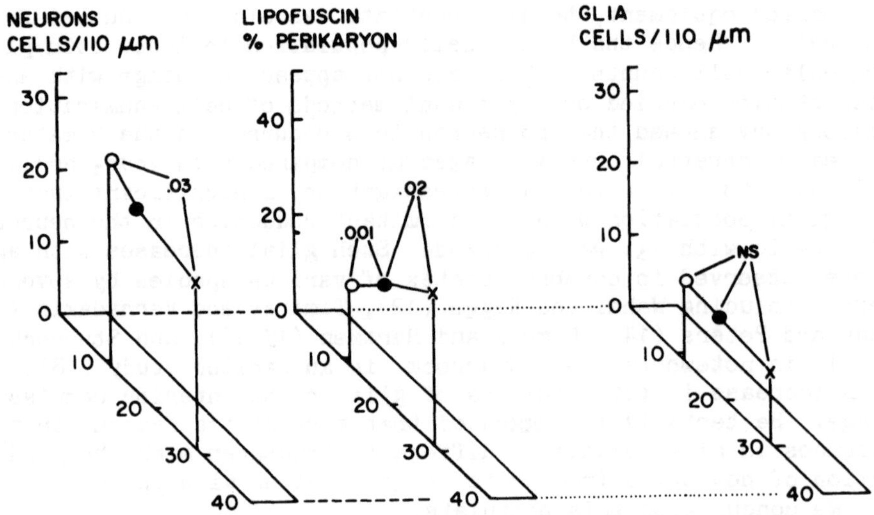

Fig. 1. Age differences in neurons, lipofuscin and glia in hippocampus CA-1 zone. (Brizzee and Ordy, Mech. Ageing Dev., in press, 1978). Reprinted with the permission of the publisher.

In the striatum, Gellerstedt (24) described a loss of small neurons. A recent report (25) supports this finding and, in addition, describes a loss of large neurons in the 65-year-old human putamen with concurrent loss of putamen volume.

Hippocampus

Quantitative histological studies on the CA-1 zone of the hippocampus of Fisher 344 rats of 11, 17, and 29 months of age revealed a significant decrease in number of neurons per unit area of the pyramidal layer between the 11th and 29th months (26) (Fig. 1). Quantitative estimates of the lipofuscin in the neurons increased significantly in the same tissues. Although there is no apparent increase in the glial packing density in the aged rat (26) or human (27), hippocampus, astroglial hypertrophy and increased oligodendroglial satellitosis are prominent features of the hippocampus of the aged rat (28,29).

Brain Stem

No loss in total number of neurons was observed in the ventral cochlear nucleus in man, but the total volume decreased significantly in old age (30). The human abducens nucleus was also observed to exhibit no neuron loss in advanced age (31). A significant decrease in neuronal populations of the substantia nigra (32) and locus coeruleus (33), however, may indicate dysfunction of central monoaminergic systems in aged persons.

Conflicting results on changes in total numbers of neurons in the main nucleus of the human inferior olive have been reported in recent years. Monagle and Brody (34) observed no decrease in number of neurons, while Sandoz (35) reported a significant loss of neurons in this nucleus with age.

Spinal Cord

An investigation of the changes in the total number of large cells in the spinal cord of mice revealed no significant differences at 6, 25, and 50 weeks (37). However, at 110 weeks the number of cells was decreased by 15 to 20%. A loss of up to 38% of ventral horn neurons was described in the aged rat (38).

Nucleus

A decrease in the size of nuclei of cerebellar granule cells in aged chinchillas was reported by Cammermeyer (39), and a similar observation was made with respect to mean nuclear volume in the

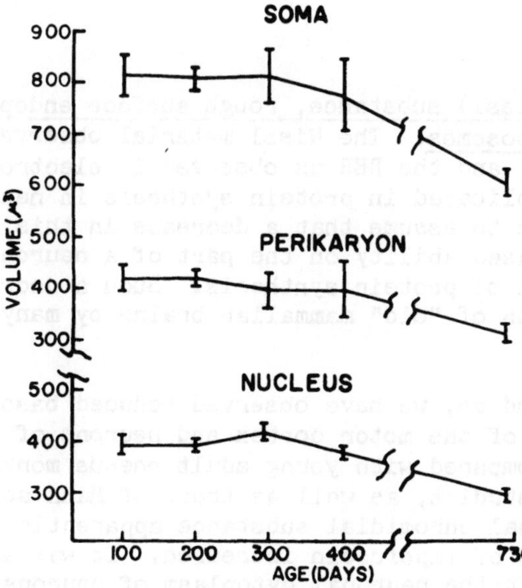

Fig. 2. Decrease in mean soma, perikaryal and nuclear volume in neurons of somatosensory cerebral cortex with age in albino rats. (Brizzee et al., 1962, Pergamon Press). Reprinted with permission of the publisher.

somatosensory area of the rat cerebral cortex by Brizzee et al. (40) (Fig. 2). Lin et al. (41) reported that nuclear volume in female rats decreased with age in several hypothalamic nuclei or areas.

It has been reported by some authors that the neuron nucleus in aged mammals is characterized by a darkening of the culeoplasm, increased basophilia and accumulation of Feulgen-stainable chromatin (42,43). Other authors (23) have described increased pallor of neuron nuclei and a diminution in the amount of Feulgen-stained chromatin in cerebellar granule cell neurons of aged, as compared with young, rabbits and chinchillas (39).

The differentiation between the nucleus and cytoplasm was sharp in neurons of young animals but much less so in some neurons in aged subjects (Fig. 3). The same tendency was noted in human tissues, but the variation was greater than in animals. A loss of regularity of cell outline and absence of a sharp demarcation between nucleus and cytoplasm was observed in senile rhesus monkeys (44) and humans (45).

Fine structural studies have also revealed nuclear inclusions (Fig. 4) which appear to increase in number with age in lateral vestibular nucleus neurons of rats (46). Other studies have indicated that increased numbers of nuclear invaginations (28,46) and decreased numbers of perichromatin granules in pyramidal neurons of the central cortex and in cerebellar granule cells (47) may also be age-related changes in neuronal nuclei.

Perikaryon

Chromidial (Nissl) substance, rough surface endoplasmic reticulum (RER) and free ribosomes. The Nissl material observed at light microscope levels, and the RER as observed in electron micrographs, have long been implicated in protein synthesis in neurons. It appears reasonable to assume that a decrease in this material must result in a decreased ability on the part of a neuron to carry out the vital function of protein synthesis. Such a decrease has been observed in neurons of "old" mammalian brains by many investigators (39,48,49,50).

In our own studies, we have observed reduced basophilia in pyramidal neurons of the motor cortex and neurons of spinal ganglia (44) in aged as compared with young adult rhesus monkeys (Fig. 3A,B; Fig. 5A,B). Our studies, as well as those of Mann and Yates (48), showed that neuronal chromidial substance apparently decreased with age, as the amount of lipofuscin increased. It was also observed, in another study, that the neuronal cytoplasm of neurons of the lateral vestibular nucleus in aged (18 months) rats contained fewer patches of granular endoplasmic reticulum than in young adults (Figs. 6,7) and that the small patches do not consist of parallel cisternase in the older rats (46).

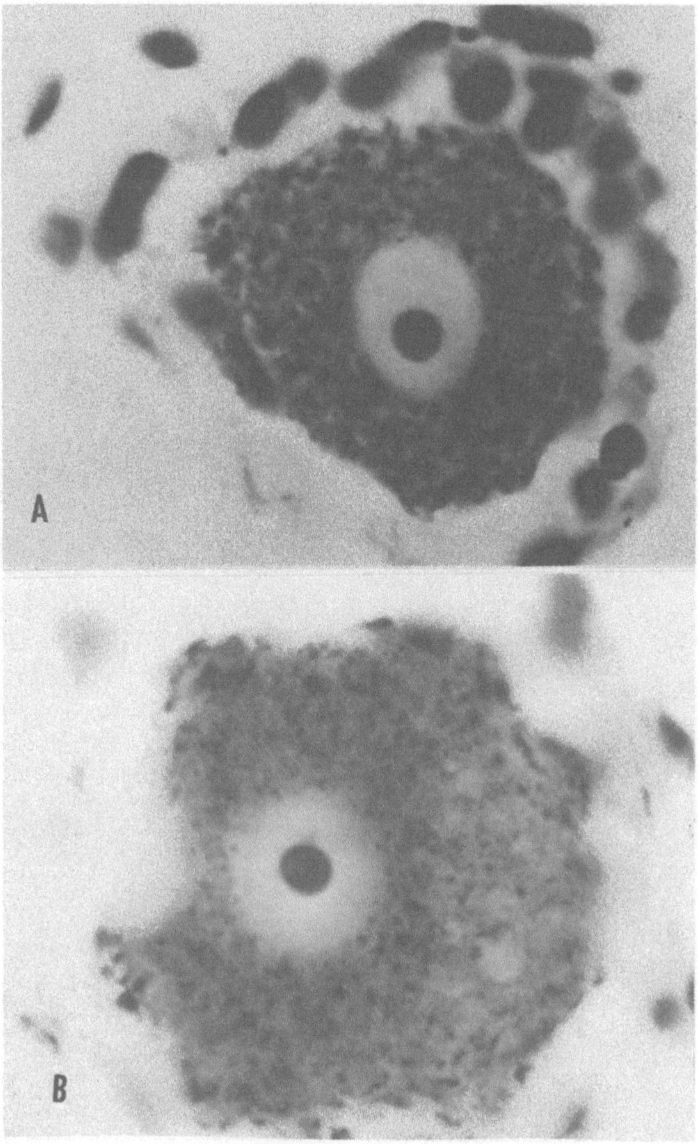

Fig. 3A. Neuron dorsal root ganglion of young adult rhesus monkey showing relatively large densely packed Nissl bodies and marked basophilia. Toluidine blue.
Fig. 3B. Neuron of dorsal root ganglion of aged rhesus monkey showing sparse, relatively fine Nissl bodies and apparent early stage in the formation of vacuoles (arrow). The relatively sharp distinction between the nucleus and cytoplasm observed in the young adult is not seen in the aged animal. Toluidine blue. (Brizzee et al., 1975, Plenum Press). Reproduced with the permission of the publisher.

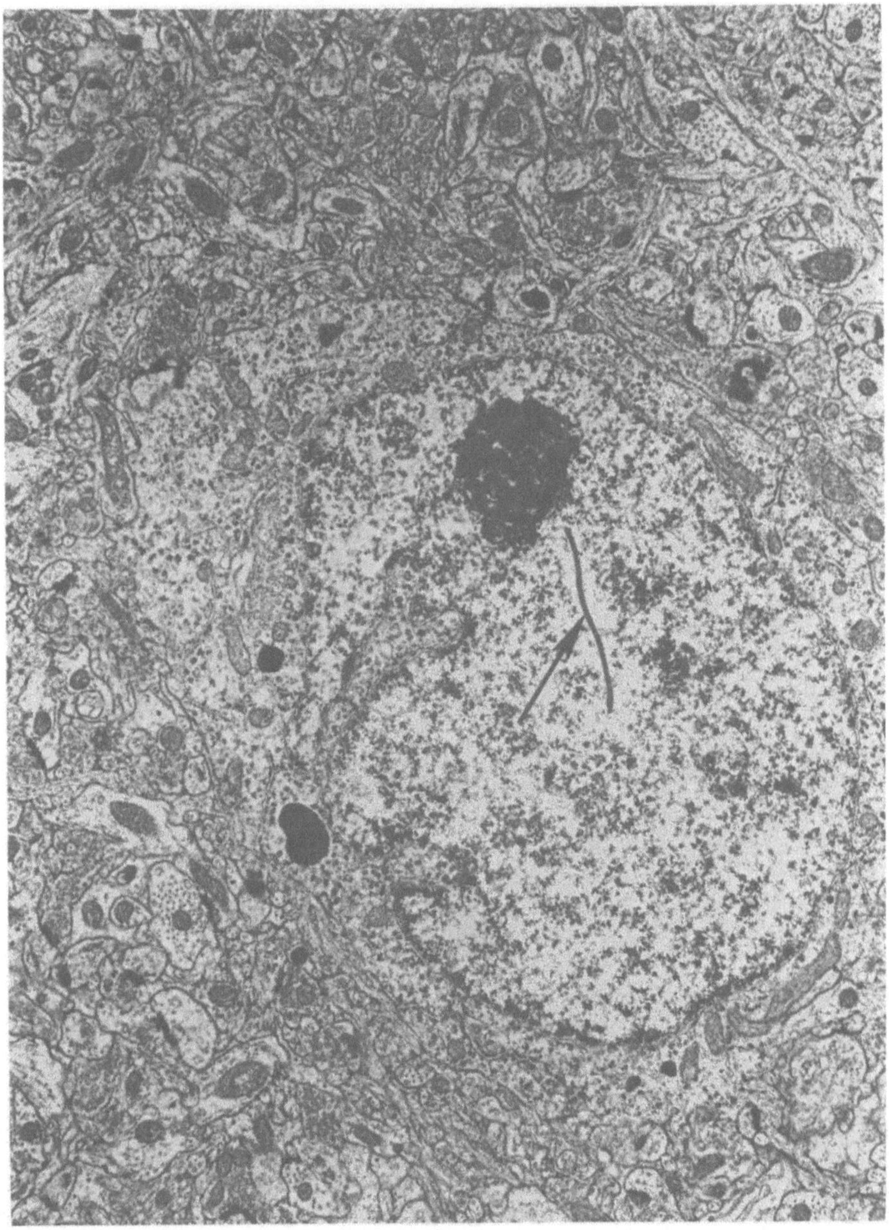

Fig. 4. Nuclei of cerebral cortical neurons in 7-year-old squirrel monkey showing nuclear rodlet inclusion (arrow). X 13,650. Reproduced with the permission of Dr. J. E. Johnson, Jr., National Institute on Aging.

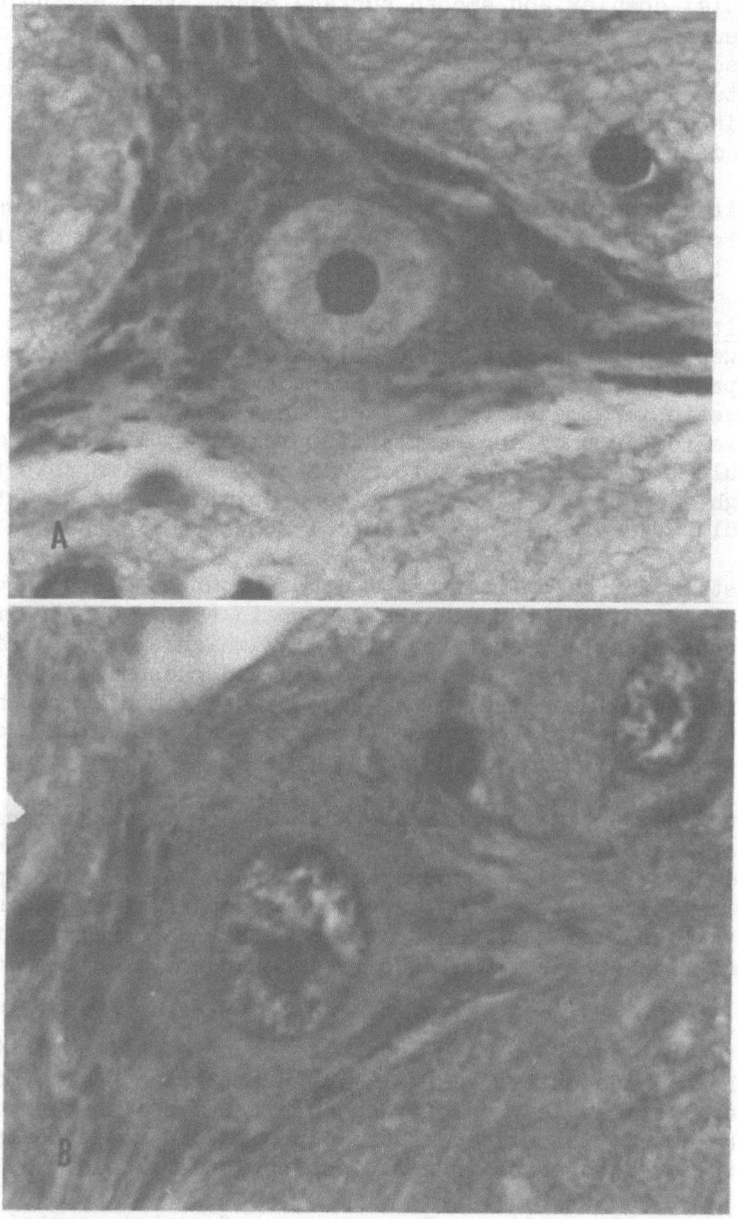

Fig. 5A. Neuron in lamina V of motor cortex of young adult rhesus monkey, showing marked basophilia of Nissl bodies. Toluidine blue.

5B. Neuron of lamina V of motor cortex of aged rhesus monkey showing reduced basophilia and sparcity of the Nissl bodies. Toluidine blue. (Brizzee et al., 1975, Plenum Press.) Reprinted with the permission of the publisher.

Golgi complex and smooth surface endoplasmic retiuclum (SER). The neuronal Golgi apparatus in adult mice, as observed at light microscope magnifications, appears as a discrete, reticulated structure composed of coarse threads. In old mice, it has been described as a mass of argentophilic granules of varying shapes and sizes distributed irregularly in the cell (51).

Ultrastructural studies in cerebral cortex have shown that Golgi vesicles as well as those of the SER and RER become dilated with age, as do the cisterns of the RER (50).

Mitochondria. The mitochondria of the nucleus gracilis in aged mice were observed to exhibit a loss of the outer unit membrane, accompanied by vesiculation of cristae and the formation of multivesicular bodies (52). The single unit membrane of the multivesicular body apparently disintegrated, leaving a mass of vesicular material. The author was of the opinion that the latter, through a process of aggregation and joining, gave rise to large reticular masses which were commonly observed in the nucleus gracilis.

Metals and calcifications. Copper content has been observed to increase with age in the mammalian brain (53). Copper granules were most consistently associated with glia which did not manifest TPPase activity in the brain of the aged dog and rhesus monkey (54). Copper has also been localized in the hippocampal fimbria, habenular nucleus and periventricular regions of the hypothalamus in mature and senescent rats (53).

Iron content also increases with age in the human brain (55). Some of the brain cells which contain iron have been identified as oligodendroglia (24). According to Barden (54), there appears to be no correlation between the presence of copper, iron and neuromelanin in any given region of the brain in rats. He concluded that the accumulation of each substance is independent of either of the other two.

Calcium, together with iron, has been identified in the brains of aged horses and cattle, as well as in the human brain (56,57). Bilateral symmetrical calcified deposits have also been observed in the thalamus of old mice. These deposits did not contain iron and were believed to arise in relation to blood vessels (58).

Eosinophilic bodies. The presence of protein-containing eosinophilic bodies in perikarya of thalamic neurons of old mice has been reported by Fraser et al. (59). These elements were characterized by sharply defined contours and were most frequently spherical, though some appeared ovoid, rod- , saucer- , or disc-shaped.

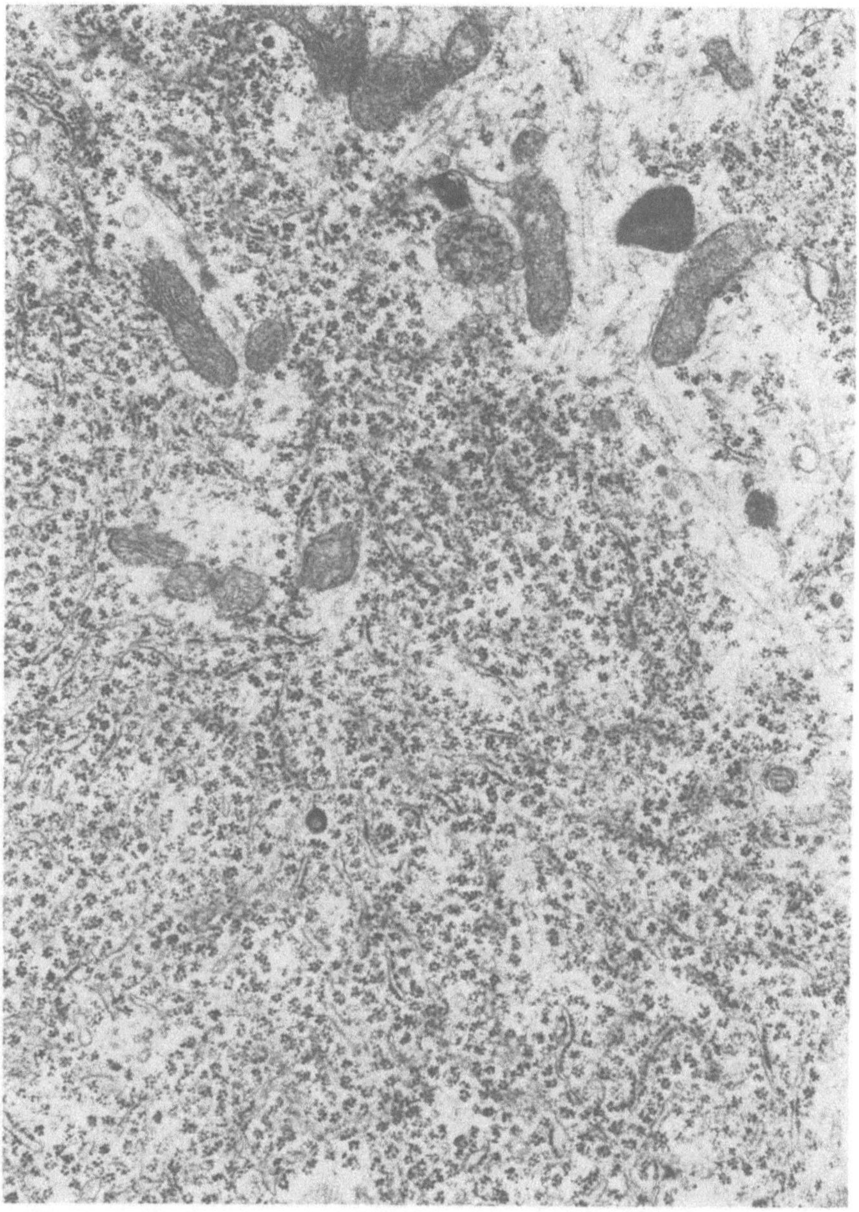

Fig. 6. The rough surface of endoplasmic reticulum (RER) in a neuron of the lateral vestibular nucleus of a 1-month-old albino rat consists of heavy patches of granular cisternae. X 20,500 (Johnson and Miquel, Mech. Ageing Dev. 3:203, 1974). Reprinted with the permission of the publisher and author.

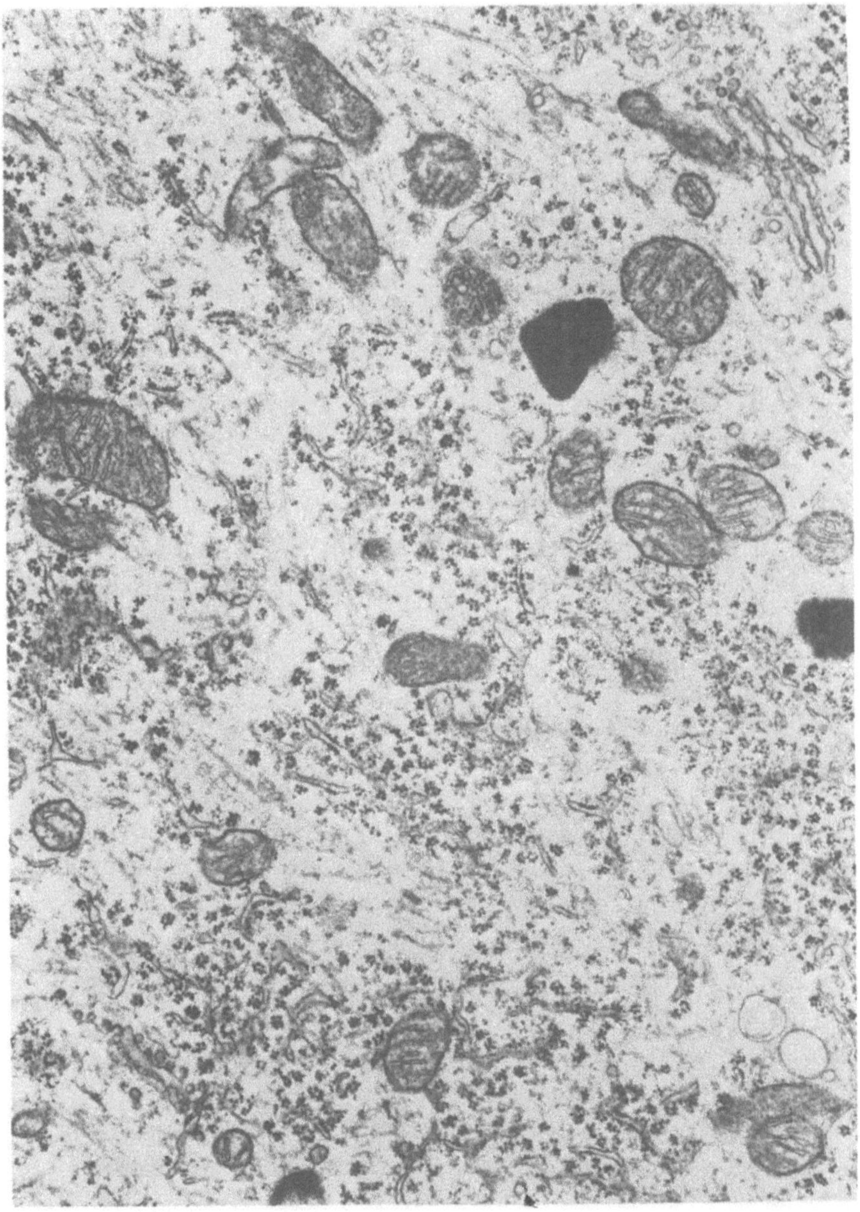

Fig. 7. The rough surface endoplasmic reticulum (RER) in this neuron of the lateral vestibular nucleus in an aged rat exhibits small patches of granular cisternae. X 20,500. (Johnson and Miquel, Mech. Ageing Dev. 3:203, 1974). Reprinted with the permission of the publisher and authors.

Electron micrographs of the eosinophilic bodies revealed arrays of parallel fibrillar crystalline material with a substructure consisting of longitudinal and transverse striations (Fig. 8).

These authors have suggested that the eosinophilic bodies originate from the union of identical macromolecules, and represent an expression of some normal cell activity, accumulating during aging as a normal metabolite or as a result of a reduction in metabolic mechanisms which catalyze their removal. They also suggested that such bodies might arise as a result of reduced cell function with age, unaccompanied by a commensurate reduction in synthesis of the particular macromolecule (59).

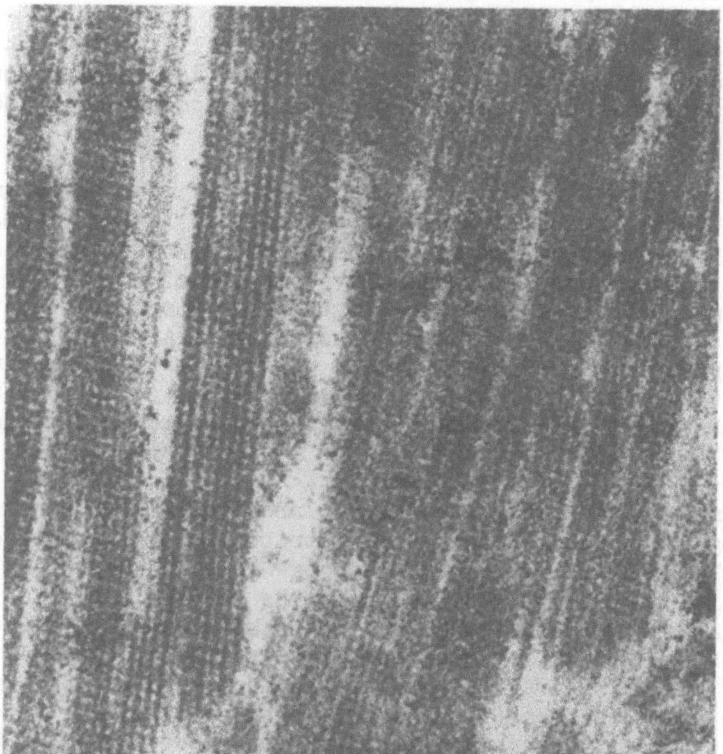

Fig. 8. Electron micrograph of eosinophilic inclusion in a thalamic neuron in an aged mouse, showing transverse and longitudinal striations. (Fraser et al., J. Neurol. Sci. 11:127, 1979). Reproduced with the permission of the publisher and the authors.

Lipofuscin pigment. Hueck (60) was the first to apply the term "lipsofuscin" to the yellow pigment which numerous authors had observed to increase in amount in neurons with age. At light microscope magnifications, this pigment appears to be composed of fine granules (1 to 3 μm in diameter) or clumped masses of variable size. it is easily visualized in PAS, Sudan black, Zielh-Nielson and Nile blue A or B-stained sections. The pigment appears a bright yellow-orange color in adult and aged neurons in blue light fluorescence at an approximate wave-length of 420 μμm, with appropriate filters. In neurons of younger subjects, however, the pigment is a lighter yellow or green color (61,62). The appearance of lipofuscin, as visualized in blue light fluorescence, is shown in neurons of the oculomotor nucleus in young adult, middle-aged, and aged rhesus monkeys in Figure 9A,B,C.

It has been demonstrated in histochemical studies that acid phosphatase, cathepsin type-C esterase, and acid deoxyribonuclease II activity occur at the same sites at which lipofuscin is identified by fluorescence (63).

Ultrastructural studies of liposfuscin pigment have generally shown it to be present in much larger amounts in aged mammalian neurons than in young neurons. The lipofuscin bodies, as seen in electron micrographs, are generally composed of a granular electron dense component and a vacuolar or vesicular electron lucent component (Fig. 10). The entire granule, consisting of a variable number of such components, is ensheathed in a single limiting membrane (64). The vacuolar component has been observed to increase in size with age, with some of the vacuoles attaining a diameter of 1 μm or more (63).

A number of investigators have classified lipofuscin according to morphological types, patterns of distribution or types of components. The classification proposed by Glees and Hasen (65) appears to coincide very closely to the patterns we have observed in our own investigations. These authors divided the lipofuscin patterns into six types, including homogeneous, finely granular, vacuolated, lamellated or banded, coarsely granular, and compound or heterogeneous. From our investigations in rats and rhesus monkeys, it appears that the first three types predominate in young neurons while the last two are commonly observed in aged neurons. The lamellated type was only rarely observed in our preparations, in agreement with the observations of Glees and Hasen (65).

In quantitative studies on regional differences in the accumulation of lipofuscin pigment in rhesus monkeys, it was noted that the nucleus with the highest neuronal pigment content was the inferior olive (61). In marked constrast to that nucleus, the neurons of the medial nucleus of the superior olive exhibited only very fine, widely scattered pigment even in the oldest animals. The

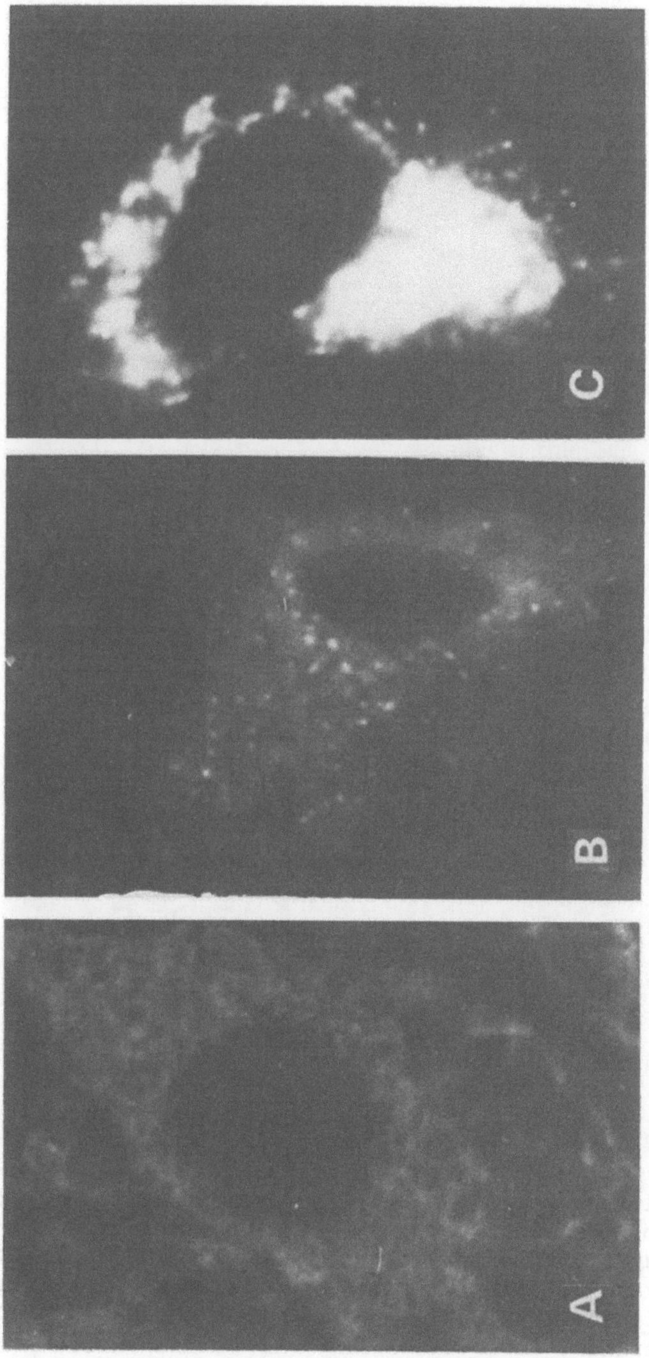

Fig. 9A. Photomicrograph of formalin-fixed unstained section of oculomotor nucleus in newborn rhesus monkey (age 5 days), showing absence of autofluorescent pigment.

B. Photomicrograph of oculomotor neuron of middle-aged rhesus monkey (age about 10 years), showing scattered autofluorescent pigment granules in perikaryon.

C. Photomicrograph of oculomotor neuron in aged rhesus monkey (age estimated to be greater than 22 years), showing heavy accumulation of autofluorescent lipofuscin material in perikaryon.

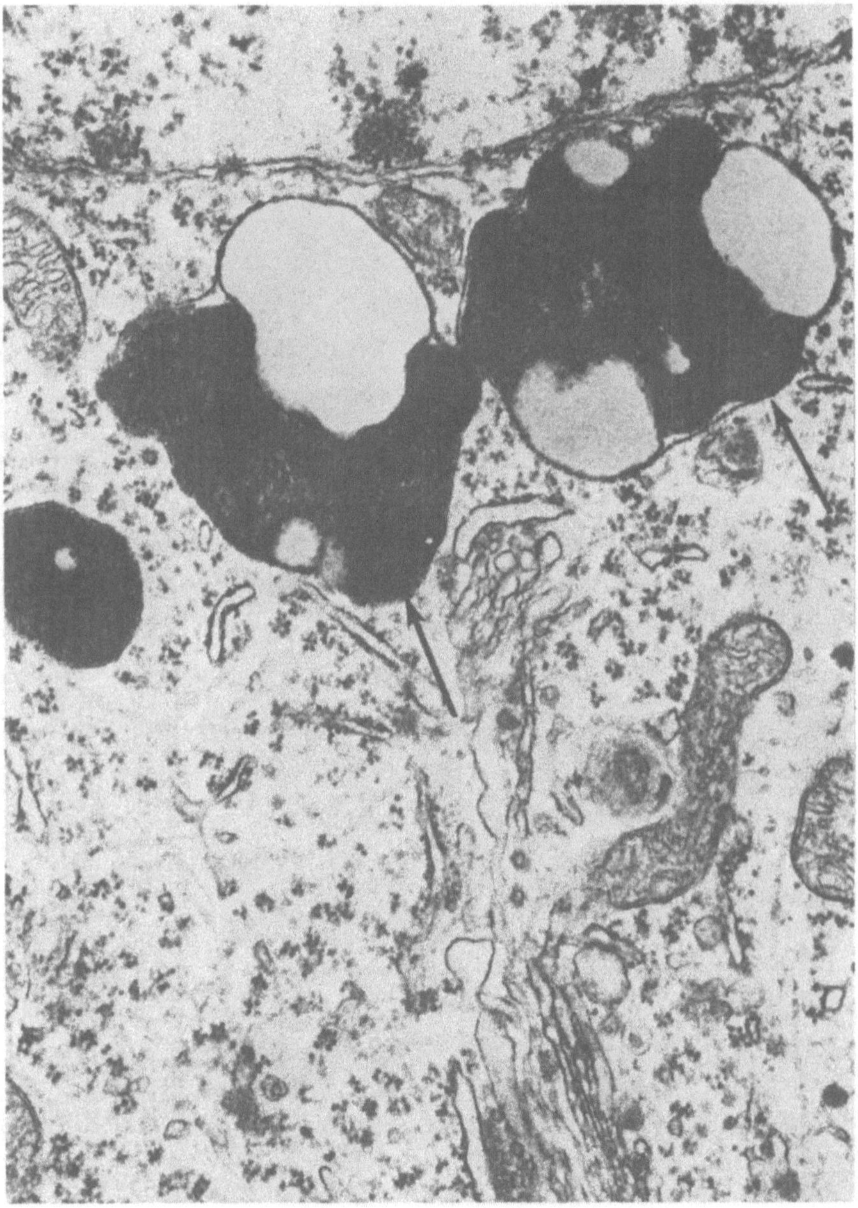

Fig. 10. Electron micrograph of typical lipofuscin body (arrow) in cytoplasm of pyramidal neuron of somatosensory cerebral cortex of aged albino rat, showing granular and vesicular components and limiting membrane. (Brizzee and Cancilla, Gerontologia 18:1, 1972). Reprinted with the permission of the publisher.

relative amounts of lipofuscin pigment in the above nuclei and 15 other CNS structures are shown in a rank order diagram in Figure 11.

Distinct regional differences in the accumulation of lipofuscins have also been observed in glia cells. The glia surrounding the Purkinje neurons of the cerebellum (61,66) and those of the medial nucleus of the superior olive (61) have been shown to exhibit high

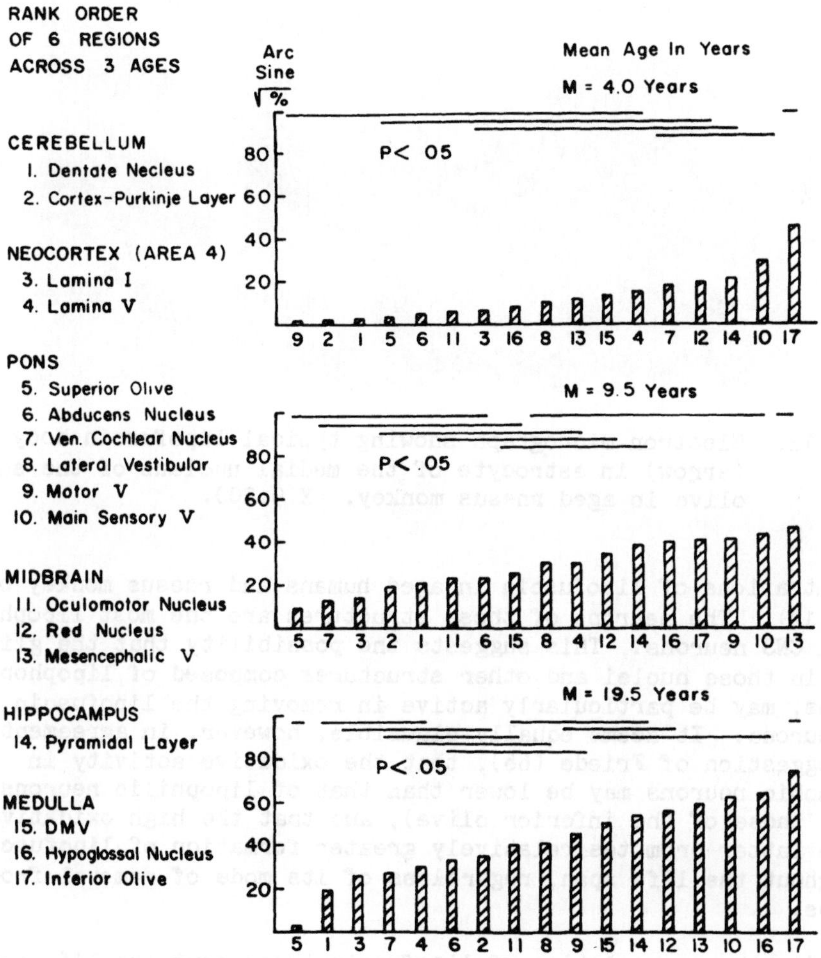

Fig. 11. Differential pattern of accumulation of lipofuscin in 17 areas of the brain, shown at 3 age levels. The horizontal bars at the top of each of the 3 graphs indicate the number of subsets of related data at each age level (Brizzee et al., J. Gerontol. 29:366, 1974).

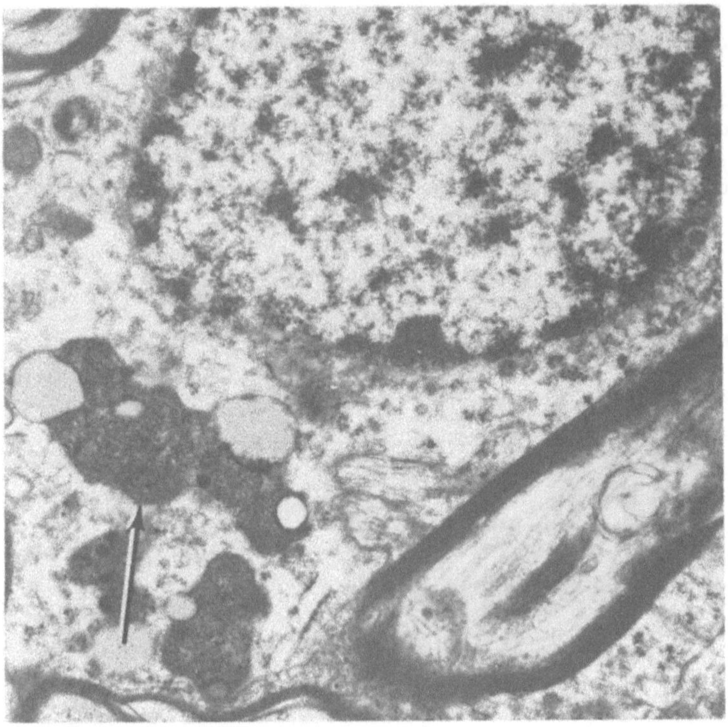

Fig. 12. Electron micrograph showing typical lipofuscin body (arrow) in astrocyte of the medial nucleus of the superior olive in aged rhesus monkey. X 9,200.

concentrations of lipofuscin in aged humans and rhesus monkey brains (Fig. 12). The neurons of these structures are the most lipophobic of all CNS neurons. This suggests the possibility that the glia cells in those nuclei and other structures composed of lipophobic neurons, may be particularly active in removing the lipofuscin from the neurons. It seems equally plausible, however, in agreement with the suggestion of Friede (66), that the oxidative activity in lipophobic neurons may be lower than that of lipophilic neurons (e.g., those of the inferior olive), and that the high oxidative rate in the latter promotes relatively greater formation of lipofuscin throughout the life span, regardless of its mode of removal from neurons.

While the accumulation of lipofuscin throughout the life span obviously occurs at different rates in different regions of the brain, within a given region and type of neuron it appears to increase normally as a linear function (64). It has been shown, however, that under laboratory conditions, the rate of pigment accumulation may be inhibited, and the amount of pigment may be decreased. Injection of centrophenoxine (meclophenoxate, Lucidril), i.p. or i.m. into guinea pigs (80 mg/kg/day) for 4 to 12 weeks resulted in a marked decrease in the amount of lipofuscin in many areas of the CNS (67). In the same studies it was observed that the drug also reduced the activity of succinic dehydrogenase, lactic dehydrogenase, cytochrome oxidase and monoamine oxidase enzymes in the same tissues, and it was concluded that the pigments were eliminated by a possible shunting of glucose metabolism into the pentose cycle. More recently, studies utilizing morphometric techniques have shown that centrophenoxine is effective in reducing the amount of lipofuscin in aged neurons in the rat brain (68).

In view of its widespread phylogenetic ocurrence (69) and its progressive accumulation in organs composed mainly of postmitotic cells, such as the heart (70) and brain (64), lipofuscin deposition with age has been proposed as a basic "law of cellular aging" (71).

Melanin pigment. Cytophotometric studies in the locus coeruleus and substantia nigra in the human brain revealed that melanin granules first appeared in the constituent neurons at birth (49). This pigment then continued to increase in a linear manner until middle age, after which the levels decreased. This decrease in melanin content was thought to be caused by the selective atrophy of the most highly pigmented neurons rather than as a result of a general pigment loss from all such cells.

Neuropil

Axonal and synaptic changes. Alterations in axons characterized by focal swelling and thickening of pericellular baskets of Purkinje neurons have been described in the cerebellum of old human brains (24). Oval or round enlargements (spheroids) of axons in tissues from aging individuals have also been reported (72). Marked variations in size, shape and granularity were observed, and these were especially prevalent in the nucleus gracilis. They have also been observed, though to a lesser degree, in other brain stem structures and basal ganglia.

In aged mice (C57BL/10 up to 32 months of age), myelin sheaths in the pyramidal tracts were reported to be thicker than in young animals (73). Plots of regression curves of ratios between axon circumference and number of myelin lamellae in the sheath revealed a decreasing slope with increasing age, the ratios being linear for all sizes of unmyelinated fibers at each age level. In the same study it was shown that there was a significant decrease in the number of neurofilaments and an increase in the number of microtubules per fiber from 8 to 26 months of age. A statistically significant decrease in mitochondria in axons was observed in the same animals.

Ultrastructural studies in mice revealed neuroaxonal dystrophy (NAD) in the nucleus gracilis in some eight-month animals, and the condition was reported to increase with age. The NAD was characterized by enlarged profiles containing patches of smooth reticular networks and groups of vesicles (52). Degenerative changes in mitochondria were observed, apparently resulting in the formation of multivesicular bodies as intermediate stages, and numerous dense bodies of variable size and configuration were also seen. It was also noted that degenerative changes occurred in axons and synaptic terminals, and by 23 months of age a large number of nerve fibers in the nucleus gracilis had degenerated. The nucleus cuneatus exhibited similar changes, but to a lesser extent.

A decrease in the number of vesicles in boutons of axon terminals in aged rhesus monkeys was reported, although the synaptic clefts were well preserved (83). In the rat hippocampus, axosomatic synapses were observed less frequently in old than young rats (28). Quantitative studies have revealed a decrease in the number of synapses in the molecular layer of the rat dentate gyrus (74,75) and in the human cerebral cortex (76) in the aging brain.

Dendrite changes. In the hippocampus of aged rats, there appeared to be an increase in the incidence of dendritic profiles and dendro-dendritic contacts without intervening glial fibers as compared with those of young adult rats (28). These authors emphasized the possible importance of such data in explaining decremental changes in integration of complex motor skills and decreased responsiveness of motor pathways which occur during old age. They also observed increased numbers of dendritic neurotubules and neurofilaments in aged animals.

Recent morphometric studies in cerebral cortical dendrites in old rats revealed a 35% decrease in the number of dendritic spines, and some of the dendrites appeared aspinous (77). Dendritic diameters also decreased by 12%. In auditory cortex of aged rats, the density of the dendritic arborization was noticeably decreased, but the extent of the arborization did not change (78). Morphological aging changes in dendritic processes, characterized by a loss or distortion of such processes in neurons of human cerebral cortex, have been described by Mann and Yates (48) and Scheibel and Scheibel (43).

In the mouse spinal cord and lower brain stem, Machado-Salas et al. (79) noted that early changes with age included irregular swelling and "lumpiness" of cell bodies and initial portions of dendrites, followed by increasing nodularization of the dendrite tree, and loss of whatever kinds of postsynaptic specializations may have been present in the young adult.

Similar studies of the hypothalamus in aging mice by these workers (80) showed progressive disruption of hypothalamic architecture paralleled by deterioration and loss of dendritic surface. They postulate that the observed dendritic changes in the hypothalamus contribute to the physiological phenomena associated with aging in the decline in the brain-gonadal functions in old individuals.

NEUROFIBRILLARY CHANGES IN AGING

Neurofibrillary tangles constitute a characteristic feature of the cytological changes in the brain in Alzheimer's disease, but are also found, though in lesser numbers, in the human brain in the course of "normal" aging (81). Neurofibrillary tangles are observed predominantly in the frontal and temporal cerebral cortex and hippocampus, but occasionally may be seen in the mesencephalon and rostral rhombencephalon. These elements are observed mainly in the perikaryon, but they may also occur in dendrite and synaptic terminals (81).

At light microscope magnifications, neurofibrillary tangles are characterized by neurofibrils in compact clusters producing abnormal intraneuronal configurations. They are argyrophilic and exhibit birefringence in polarized light. Ultrastructural studies have revealed that the neurofibrillary material consists of masses of modified microtubules. The microtubules measure 200 to 220 Å in width (as compared with normal microtubules of about 240 Å in diameter), and display periodic constrictions every 800 Å. The tubules are actually in the form of paired helical filaments (PHF).

The abnormal tubules seen in the PHF are argentophilic, and are well preserved after direct osmic fixation. Normal neurotubules generally are not observed after osmication, and are not argentophilic (81). PHF have also been observed in neurons of aged rhesus monkeys, but periodicity is somewhat different from that in the human brain (9).

Amyloid and senile plaques

Amyloid is generally described in relation to disease conditions, but it also occurs in "normal" aging. While individual variation in amyloid content in the brain is very great, the amount of this substance in the brain of a given individual tends to increase progressively with age.

In the central nervous system, amyloid in "normal" aging commonly occurs in relation to senile plaques, although this is not the only pattern of distribution. Recent ultrastructural studies have shown that "classical" plaques, as illustated in Figure 13, consist of degenerative neuronal processes, an amyloid core and reactive cells (82). These authors concluded that degenerating neuronal processes constitute the primary source of the plaques. In 50% of "normal"

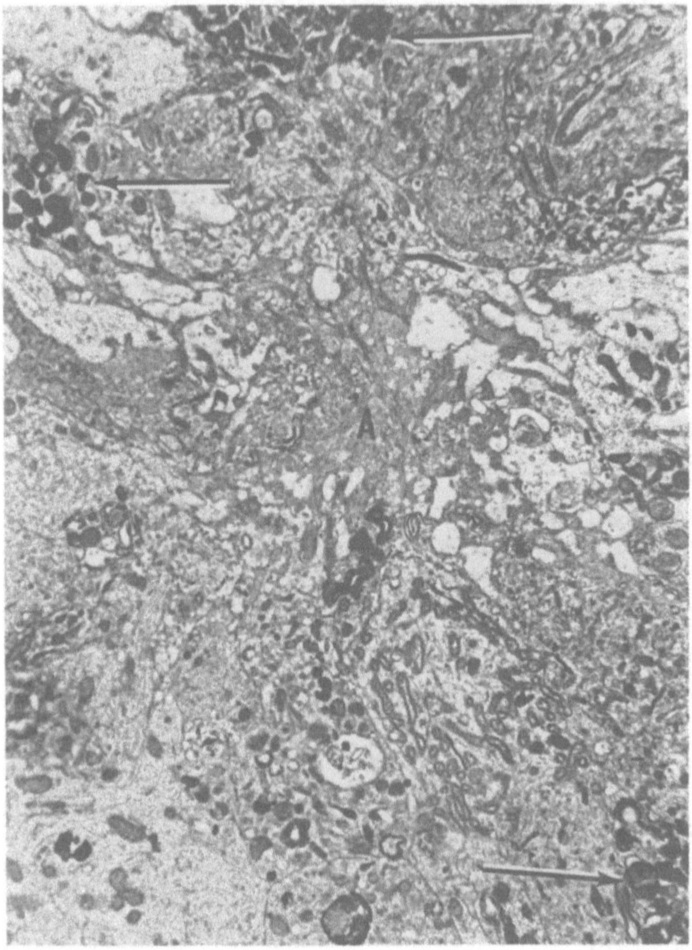

Fig. 13. Senile plague of the "classical" type with central core and amyloid (A) surrounded by clusters of dystrophic neurites (arrows). (Wisniewski et al., J. Neuropath. Exp. Neurol. 32:570, 1973). Reprinted with the permission of the authors and publishers.

aged brains, senile plaques are observed and are reported to increase in numbers with age (72). In studies of large numbers of hospital patients without evidence of dementia, the incidence of plaques was small in middle-aged patients, but increased markedly in older subjects (24,83). Senile plaques are also seen in the CNS of aged mice (38), dogs (84), and monkeys (9).

Neurosecretory neurons

A study of the neurosecretory neurons of the human hypothalamus reported that a marked argentophilia occurred, with an increased density of the neurofibrillary apparatus with age (85,86). Vacuolization of such cells, as well as "retraction" of the cytoplasm, was also described, but there was no evidence of nuclear pyknosis, calcification, pigment accumulation or a decrease in volume of these neurons.

Age changes in glia cells. Aging changes in glia in the brain are reported to be greatest in the ependymal and submeningeal regions, fornix, optic chiasma, mammillary nuclei, and reticular formation, in that order (83).

Ultrastructural studies of age changes in glia in the rat hippocampus have revealed increased oligodendrogial satellitosis, binucleated cells or fusion of oligodendroglia, and invagination of oligodendroglial nuclear membranes with marked marginal condensation of nuclear chromatin (28). Obvious changes in astrocytes were not observed in this study, but numerous lipid vacuoles were seen in microglia.

In the nuclei of Bergmann astrocytes in the cerebellum of chinchillas, it has been shown that nuclear membranes were commonly indented and invaginated, with the tip of each invagination ending near a nucleolus (39). Deep pink PAS-stained bodies of varying shape (irregular rods, bars, spheres, or faceted bodies) were seen within astrocyte nuclei, in 145½-month-old animals.

Degenerative changes have been observed in astrocytes in olfactory bulb tissue of aged human subjects (87). These alterations are characterized by a homogenization of the soma and gradual loss of processes, resulting in a round, homogeneous, dark-staining body with no resemblance to a cell.

REFERENCES

1. A. V. Everitt, and J. A. Burgess, eds., "Hypothalamus, Pituitary and Aging," Charles C. Thomas, New York (1976).
2. T. Hanley, Neuronal "fall-out: in the aging brain: A critical review of the quantitative data, Age and Ageing 3:133 (1974).
3. H. A. Johnson and S. Erner, Neuron survival in the aging mouse, Exp. Gerontol. 7:111 (1972).
4. L. M. Franks, P. D. Wilson, and R. D. Whelan, The effects of age on total DNA and cell number in the mouse brain, Gerontologist 20:21 (1974).
5. H. Brody, Organization of the cerebral cortex. III. A study of aging in the human cerebral cortex, J. Comp. Neurol. 102:511 (1955).

6. E. J. Colon, The elderly brain: A quantitative analysis in the cerebral cortex of two cases, Psychiatria, Neurologia, Neurochirurgia (Amst.) 75:261 (1972).
7. B. G. Shefer, The absolute number of nerve cells in cortical depth in normals and in patients with dementia, Pick's and Alzheimer's disease, Z. Nevropathol. i Psikhiatrii Imen S.S. Korsakova (Moskva) 72:1024 (1972).
8. K. R. Brizzee, J. M. Ordy, J. Hansche, and B. Kaack, Quantitative assessment of changes in neuron and glia cell packing density and lipofuscin accumulation with age in the cerebral cortex of a nonhuman primate (Macaca mulatta), in:"Neurobiology of Aging," R. D. Terry and S. Gershon, eds., Raven Press, New York (1976).
9. H. M. Wisniewski, B. Ghetti, and R. D. Terry, Neuritic (senile) plaques and filamentous changes in aged rhesus monkeys, J. Neuropath. Exp. Neurol. 32:566 (1973).
10. J. M. Ordy, K. R. Brizzee, B. Kaack, and J. Hansche, Age differences in short-term memory and cell loss in the cortex of the rat, Gerontology 24:267 (1978).
11. K. R. Brizzee, N. Sherwood, and P. S. Timiras, A comparison of cell populations at various depth levels in cerebral cortex of young adult and aged Long-Evans rats, J. Gerontol. 23:289 (1968).
12. K. M. Wahal and H. E. Riggs, Changes in the brain associated with senility, AMA Arch. of Neurol. Psychiat. 2:151 (1960).
13. P. S. Timiras and A. Vernadakis, Structural, biochemical and functional aging of the nervous system, in: "Develomental Physiology and Aging," P. S. Timiras, ed., Macmillan Publishing Co., New York (1972).
14. D. W. Vaughan and A. Peters, Neuroglial cells inthe cerebral cortex of rats from young adulthood to old age: An electron microscope study, J. Neurocytol. 3:405 (1974).
15. E. Uemura and H. A. Hartman, Age-related changes in RNA content and volume of the human hypoglossal neuron, Brain Res. Bull. 3:207 (1978).
16. E. Uemura and H. A. Hartman, RNA content and volume of nerve cell bodies in human brain: I. Prefrontal cortex in aging normal and demented patients, J. Neuropath. Exp. Neurol. 37:487 (1978).
17. R. R. Sturrock, Quantitative and morphological changes in neurons and neuroglia in the indusium griseum of aging mice, J. Gerontol. 32:642 (1977).
18. R. R. Sturrock, Changes in neuroglia and myelination in the white matter of aging mice, J. Gerontol. 31:513 (1976).
19. R. S. Ellis, Norms for some structural changes in the human cerebellum from birth to old age, J. Comp. Neurol. 32:1 (1920).
20. T. Inukai, On the loss of Purkinje cells with advancing age, from the cerebellar cortex of the albino rat, J. Comp. Neurol. 45:1 (1928).

21. E. Tarnowska-Dziduszko, Morphological picture of the cerebellum in the course of the aging process, Neuropathol. Pol. 11:199 (1973).
22. T. C. Hall, A. K. H. Miller, and J. A. N. Corsellis, Variations in the human Purkinje cell population according to age and sex, Neuropath. Appl. Neurobiol., 1:267 (1975).
23. K. J. Hempel and M. Namba. Die involution des Supranucleus medialisdorsalis, soie der Lamella medialis und der Lamells interna thalami, J. Hirnforsch. 4:43 (1958).
24. N. Gellerstedt, "Zue kenntuis der Hirveranderungen bei der Normalen Altersunvolution," Almquist and Wiksells Boktryckeri - A -B, Uppsala (1933).
25. O. Bugiani, S. Salvarani, F. Perdelli, G. I. Mancardi, and A. Leonardi, Nerve cell loss with aging in the putamen, Europ. Neurol. 17:286 (1978).
26. K. R. Brizzee and J. M. Ordy, Age pigments, cell loss and hippocampal function, Mech. Ageing Dev., in press (1978).
27. V. F. Shefer, Hippocampal pathology as a possible factor in the pathogenesis of senile dementias, Neuropath. Exp. Neurol. 8:236 (1977).
28. M. Hansan and P. Glees, Ultrastructural age changes in hippocampal neurons, synapses and neuroglia, Exp. Gerontol. 8:75 (1973).
29. P. W. Landfield, G. Rose, L. Sandles, T. C. Wohlstadter, and G. Lynch, Patterns of astroglial hypertrophy and neuronnal degeneration in the hippocampus of aged, memory-deficient rats, J. Gerontol. 228:1335 (1970).
30. B. W. Konigsmark and E. A. Murphy, Neuronal populations in the human brain, Nature 228:1335 (1970).
31. N. Vijayashankar and H. Brody, A Study of aging in the human abducens nucleus, J. Comp. Neurol. 173:433 (1977).
32. P. L. McGeer, E. G. McGeer, and J. S. Suzuki, Aging and extrapyramidal function, Arch. Neurol. 34:33 (1977).
33. H. Brody, An examination of cerebral cortex and brain stem aging, in:"Neurobiology of Aging," R. D. Terry and S. Gershon, eds., Raven Press, New York (1976).
34. R. D. Monagle and H. Brody, The effects of age upon the main nucleus of the inferior olive in the human, J. Comp. Neurol. 155:61 (1974).
35. P. Sandoz, Age-related loss of nerve cells from the human inferior olive and unchanged volume of its grey matter, IRCS J. Med. Sci. 5:376 (1977).
36. E. A. Wright and J. M. Spink, A study of the loss of nerve cells in the central nervous system in relation to age, Gerontolgia (Basel) 3:277 (1959).
37. W. Andrew, and M. A. Bari, Some aspects of age changes in the spinal cord compared with those in other parts of the nervous system, in:"Proceedings of the Fifth International Congress of Neuropathology," Excerpta Medica Fdn., New York, Internat. Cong. Ser. No. 100 (1965).

38. J. Cammermeyer, Cytological manifestations of aging in rabbit and chinchilla brains, J. Geront. 18:41 (1963).
39. K. R. Brizzee, X. Kharetchko, and L. A. Jacobs, Effects of fetal X-irradiation on aging changes in cerebral cortex, in:"Some Aspects of Internal Irradiation," Pergamon Press, New York (1962).
40. K. H. Lin, Y. M. Peng, and M. T. Peng, Changes in the nuclear volume of rat hypothalamic neurons in old age, Neuroendrocrinology 21:247 (1976).
41. I. Klatzo, Uber das verhaltern des nukleolarapparates in den menschlichen pallidumzellen, J. Hirsforsch. 1:47 (1954).
42. F. Sanides, Untersuchumgen uber die histologische struktur des mandelkerngebietes, J. Hirnforsh. 3:56 (1957).
43. K. R. Brizzee, P. Klara, and J. E. Johnson, Changes in microanatomy, neurocytology and fine structure with aging, in:"Neurobiology of Aging: An Interdisciplinary Life Span Approach," J. M. Ordy and K. R. Brizzee, eds., Plenum Press, New York (1975).
44. P. Timiras, Degenerative changes in cells and cell death, in: "Developmental Physiology and Aging," P. S. Timiras, ed., Macmillan Publishing Co., New York (1972).
45. J. E. Johnson and J. Miquel, Fine structural changes in the lateral vestibular nucleus of aging rats, Mech. Ageing Dev. 3:203 (1974).
46. V. Zs-Nagy, C. Bertoni-Freddari, I. Zs-Nagy, C. Pieri, and G. Guili, Alterations in the numerical density of perichronatin granules in different tissues during ageing and cell differentiation, Gerontology 23:267 (1977).
47. D. M. A. Mann and P. O. Yates, Lipofuscin pigments--their relationship to ageing in the human nervous system. I. The lipofuscin content of nerve cells, Brain 97:481 (1974).
48. D. M. A. Mann and P. O. Yates, Lipofuscin pigments--their relationship to ageing in the human nervous system. II. The melanin content of pigmented nerve cells, Brain 97:489 (1974).
49. S. S. Sekhon and D. S. Maxwell, Ultrastructural changes in neurons of the spinal anterior horn of ageing mice with particular reference to the accumulation of lipofuscin pigment, J. Neurocytol. 3:59 (1974).
50. W. Andrew, The Golgi apparatus in the nerve cells of the mouse from youth to senility, Am. J. Anat. 64:351 (1937).
51. J. E. Johnson, W. R. Mehler, and J. Miquel, A fine structural study of degenerative changes in the dorsal column nuclei of aging mice. Lack of protection by vitamine E, J. Gerontol. 30:395 (1975).
52. N. Kaneta, Histochemical studies on the diencephalon of senescent rats, Tohoku J. Exp. Med. 90:249 (1966).
53. H. Barden, The histochemical distribution and localization of copper, iron, neuromelanin and lysosomal enzyme activity in the brain of aging rhesus monkey and the dog, J. Neuropath. Exp. Neurol. 30:650 (1971).

54. B. Hallgren and P. Sourander, The effect of age on the nonhaemin iron in the human brain, J. Neurochem. 3:41 (1958).
55. E. W. Hurst, Calcification of the brains of Equidae and bovidae, Am J. Path. 10:795 (1934).
56. G. Strassman, Iron and calcium deposits in the brain: Their pathologic significance, J. Neuropath. Exp. Neurol. 8:428 (1977).
57. H. Fraser, Bilateral thalamic calcification in aging mice, J. Path. Bact. 96:220 (1968).
58. H. Fraser, W. Smith, and E. W. Gray, Ultrastructural morphology of cytoplasmic inclusions within neurons of ageing mice, J. Neurol Sci. 11:123 (1970).
59. W. Hueck, Pigmenstudien, Beitrag. Path. Anat. 54:68 (1912).
60. K. R. Brizzee, J. M. Ordy, and B. Kaack, Early appearance and regional differences in intraneuronal and extraneuronal lipofuscin accumulation with age in the brain of a nonhuman primate, J. Gerontol. 29:366 (1974).
61. K. Nandy, Properties of neuronal lipofuscin pigment in mice, Acta Neuropath. (Berl.) 19:25 (1971).
62. T. Samorajski, J. R. Keefe, and J. M. Ordy, Intracellular localization of lipofuscin age pigments in the nervous system, J. Gerontol. 19:262 (1964).
63. K. R. Brizzee, and F. A. Johnson, Depth distribution of lipofuscin pigment in cerebral cortex of rat, Acta Neuropathol. 16:205 (1970).
64. P. Glees and M. Hasan, Lipofuscin in neuronal aging and diseases, Norm. Pathol. Anat. (Stuttg.) 32:1 (1933).
65. R. L. Friede, The relation of formation of lipofuscin to the distribution of oxidative enzymes in the human brain, Acta Neuropath. (Berl) 2:113 (1962).
66. K. Nandy, Further studies on the effects of centrophenoxine on the lipofuscin pigment in the neurons of senile guinea pigs, J. Gerontol. 23:83 (1968).
67. S. Riga and D. Riga, Effects of centrophenoxine on lipofuscin pigments on the nervous system of old rats, Brain Res. 72:265 (1974).
68. A. D. Dayan, Comparative neuropathology of ageing--studies on the brains of 47 species of vertebrates, Brain 94:31 (1971).
69. B. L. Strehler, D. D. Mark, A. S. Mildvan, and M. V. Gee, Rate and magnitude of age pigment accumulation in the human myocardium, J. Gerontol. 14:430 (1959).
70. B. L. Strehler and C. H. Barrows, Senescence: Cell biological aspects of aging, in: "Cell Differentiation," O. A. Schjeide and J. DeVellis, eds., Van Nostrand, New York (1970).
71. J. H. Sung, Neuroaxonal dystrophy in aging, in:"Proc. 5th Int. Congr. Neuropathol., Zurich," Excerpta Medica Fdn, New York, Interat. Contr. Ser. No. 100 (1966).
72. J. Samorajski, R. L. Friede, and J. M. Ordy, Age differences in the ultrastructure of axons in the pyramidal tract of the mouse, J. Gerontol. 26:542 (1971).

73. W. Bondareff, and Y. Geinisman, Loss of synapses in the dentate gyrus of the senescent rat, Am. J. Anat. 145:129 (1976).
74. Y. Geinisman and W. Bondareff, Decrease in the number of synapses in the senescent brain: A quantitative EM analysis of the dentate gyrus molecular layer in the rat, Meh. Ageing Dev. 5:11 (1976).
75. B. G. Cragg, The density of synapses and neurons in normal, mentally defective and ageing human brains, Brain 98:81 (1975).
76. M. L. Feldman, Degenerative changes in aging dendrites, Gerontolgist 14:34 (1974).
77. D. W. Vaughan, Age-related deterioration of pyramidal cell basal dendrites in rat auditory cortex, J. Comp. Neurol. 171:601 (1977).
78. M. E. Scheibel and A. B. Scheibel, Structural changes in the aging brain, in: "Aging," vol. 1, H. Brody, D. Harman, and J. M. Ordy, eds., Raven Press, New York (1975).
79. J. Machado-Salas, M. E. Scheibel, and A. B. Scheibel, Neuronal changes in the aging mouse. Spinal cord and lower brain stem, Exp. Neurol. 54:504 (1977a).
80. J. Machado-Salas, M. E. Scheibel, and A. B. Scheibel, Morphologic changes in the hypothalamus of the old mouse, Exp. Neurol. 57:102 (1977b).
81. H. M. Wisniewski and R. D. Terry, Morphology of the aging brain, human and animal, Progr. Brain Res. 40:167 (1973).
82. R. D. Terry and M. Wisniewski, Some structural and chemical aspects of the aging nervous system. Proc. IVth European Symposium on Basic Research in Gerontology, Scand. J. Clin. Lab. Invest. 34:(Suppl. 141)13 (1974).
83. B. E. Tomlinson, Morphological brain changes in non-demented old people, in:"Aging of the Central Nervous System. Biological and Psychological Aspects, H. H. van Praeg and A. F. Kalverboer, eds., DeErven F. Bohm, N.V. Hoarlem (1972).
84. A. Wisniewski, A. B. Johnson, C. S. Raine, W. J. Kay, and R. D. Terry, Senile plaques and cerebral amyloidosis in aged dogs. A histochemical and ultrastructural study, Lab. Invest. 23:287 (1970).
85. J. E. Azcoaga, Modificaciones gliales del hipotalamo senil, Archivos de Histologia Normal y Pathologica 8:278 (1963).
86. J. E. Azcoaga, Senilidad de las neuronas de los nucleos magnocellulares del hipotalamo, Archivo de Histologia Normal y Pathologica (Buenos Aires) 9:40 (1965).
87. L. Liss and F. Gomez, The nature of senile changes of the human olfactory bulb and tract, AMA Aidi 67:167 (1958).

HYPERTENSION, VASCULATURE AND AGING

Akira Ooshima and Yukio Yamori

Department of Pathology
Shimane Medical University
Izumo 693, Japan

INTRODUCTION

Essential hypertension develops with age, and its complication, arteriosclerosis, seems to be an accelerated form of aging process in blood vessels. With advancing age, the blood vessels lose elasticity and become stiff. This may be due in part to an increase in vascular connective tissue components. Special attention will be given in this report to the cardiovascular connective tissue and especially to the fibrils of collagen, which is known to be the major protein of connective tissue. The experiments were undertaken to elucidate an interrelationship between hypertension and vascular collagen metabolism. This report is a summary of experiments conducted during the past several years.

METHODS

Two different types of hypertensive animals were used as experimental animals. Hypertension was induced in a group of uninephrectomized, 8-week-old, male Wistar rats by twice-weekly subcutaneous injections of deoxycorticosterone acetate (DOCA) (5 mg/rat) and maintenance on 1% NaCl. The other hypertensive model was spontaneously hypertensive male rat (SHR) developed by Okamota and Aoki (1). As a control for SHR, genetically related male Wistar-Kyoto rats were used. All the animals were fed on regular stock chow diet and given either tap water or 1% NaCl throughout experiments.

The availability of methods in our laboratory for measuring a number of biochemical markers of collagen metabolism made it possible to determine the effects of hypertension on vascular collagen synthesis. Activities of prolyl hydroxylase and lysyl oxidase were

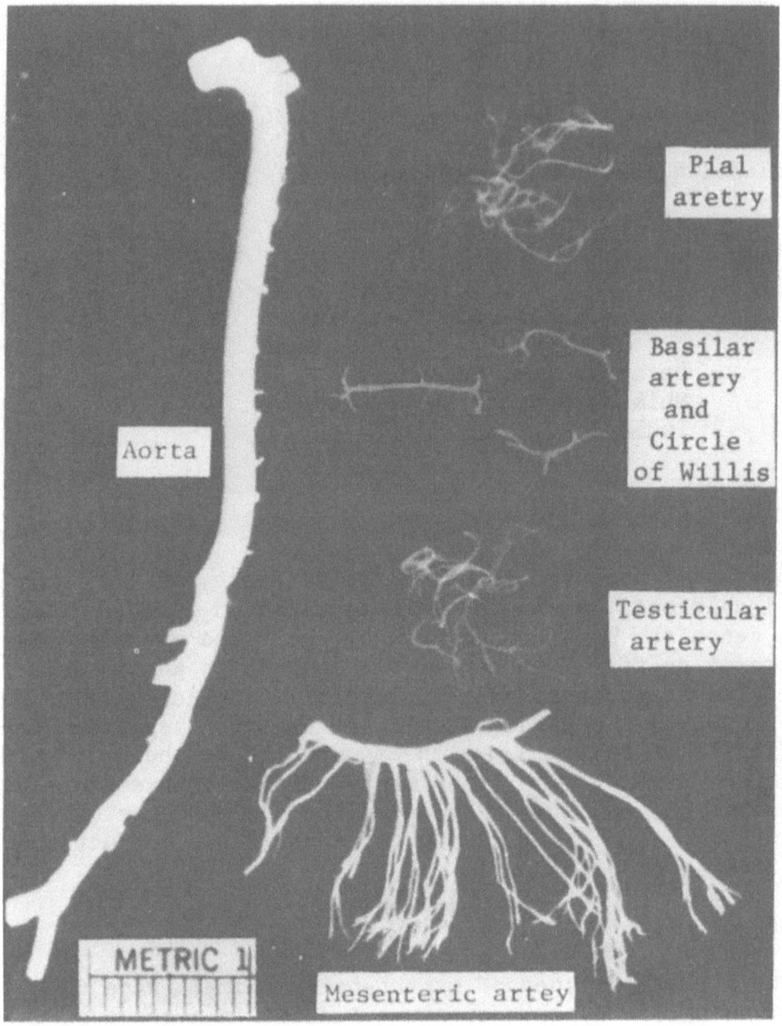

Fig. 1 The preparation of blood vessels used for assay. Samples are taken from a 4-month-old, male rat.

measured by the tritium release assays of Hutton et al. (2) and Seigel et al. (3), respectively. Incorporation of labeled proline into collagen was measured as described elsewhere (4). The amount of net collagen deposition was determined by hydroxyproline assay (5). Protein concentration was determined by the method of Lowry et al. (6), with bovine serum albumin as the standard. DNA was determined by the method of Burton (7). Blood vessels were isolated and prepared for assay as previously reported (4) (Fig. 1). Brain microvessels were neatly isolated without loss of metabolic activity

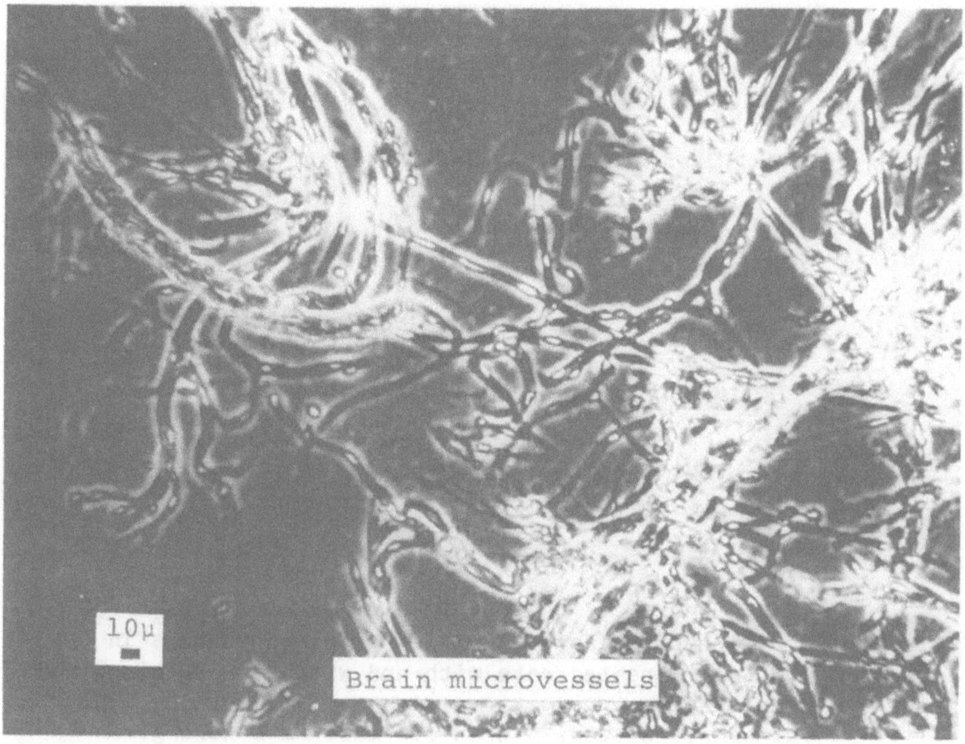

Fig. 2. A portion of brain microvessels from a 4-month-old, male rat is shown in phase contrast microphotograph.

by a modification (8) of the method of Brendel et al. (9) (Fig. 2). For the immunohistochemical demonstration of prolyl hydroxylase, the immunoperoxidase method, using monospecific antibody against this enzyme prepared from newborn rat skins, was utilized (10,11).

RESULTS

Initial experiments were conducted with deoxycorticosterone acetate (DOCA)-salt hypertensive rats, which developed severe hypertension within 4 to 6 weeks. As shown in Figure 3, prolyl hydroxylase activities in DOCA-salt hypertensive rats was increased as compared to normotensive controls in blood vessels of different diameters. The other two indicators of collagen biosynthesis, ^{14}C-proline incorporation into collagen and net deposition of collagen in the tissues, were also shown to be elevated in DOCA-salt hypertensive rats (not shown). To determine whether the increase in collagen biosynthetic activity was related to the hypertension or to the DOCA-salt treatment itself, the antihypertensive agent, reserpine (0.75 mg/kg, i.p.), was administered to a subgroup of the experimental

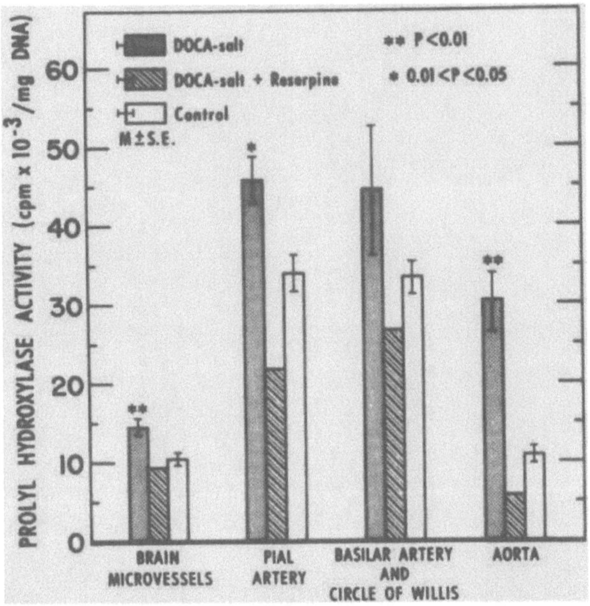

Fig. 3. Prolyl hydroxylase activities of blood vessels in DOCA-salt treated rats with and without reserpine, and normotensive controls.
Uninephrectomized, 8-week-old male rats were given deoxycorticosterone acetate (DOCA) (5 mg/rat) twice-weekly and maintained on 1% NaCl. Concomitant with DOCA-salt treatment, reserpine (0.75 mg/kg, i.p.) was administered daily by intraperitoneal injection for 4 to 6 weeks. Final blood pressures were DOCA-salt treated hypertensive rats, 210 ± 2 mmHg. From Ooshima et al. (8).

animals at the time of initiation of DOCA-salt treatment. Administration of reserpine prevented or reversed the increase in vascular collagen biosynthesis comcomitant with the reduction of blood pressure (Fig. 3).

The effects of hypertension on vascular collagen biosynthesis were also investigated in spontaneously hypertensive rats (SHR) (Fig. 4). The blood pressure of SHR was greatly elevated over that of controls. Two results were obtained by the prolyl hydroxylase levels. First, the level of prolyl hydroxylase fell with age. The second, and more important, was that the SHR consistently showed higher enzyme activity when compared with normotensive controls. In addition to these results, it was observed that when SHR yielded severe arterial damage (such as periarteritis nodosa of mesenteric artery, which is often observed in severe and prolonged hypertension) the level of prolyl hyroxylase activity rose markedly. Since there

BLOOD PRESSURE (mm Hg)

Rats	50 days	120 days	240 days	365 days
SHR	148 ± 2.0*	203 ± 4.9*	204 ± 5.8*	212 ± 7.0*
Control	118 ± 1.5	121 ± 3.6	122 ± 1.3	126 ± 4.0

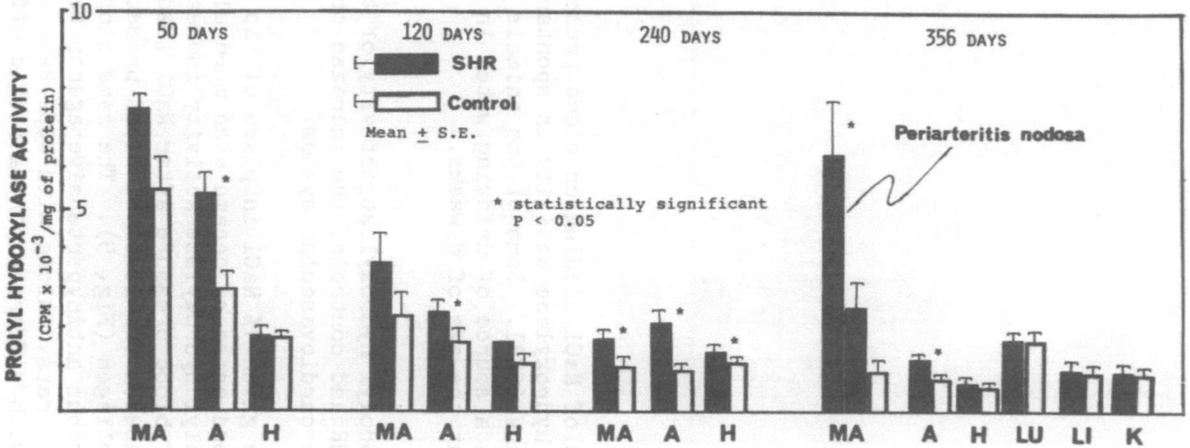

Fig. 4. Variations in cardiovascular prolyl hydroxylase activity with age in spontaneously hypertensive rats (SHR). MA, mesenteric artery; A, aorta; H, heart; Lu, lung; Li, liver; K, kidney. From Ooshima et al. (4).

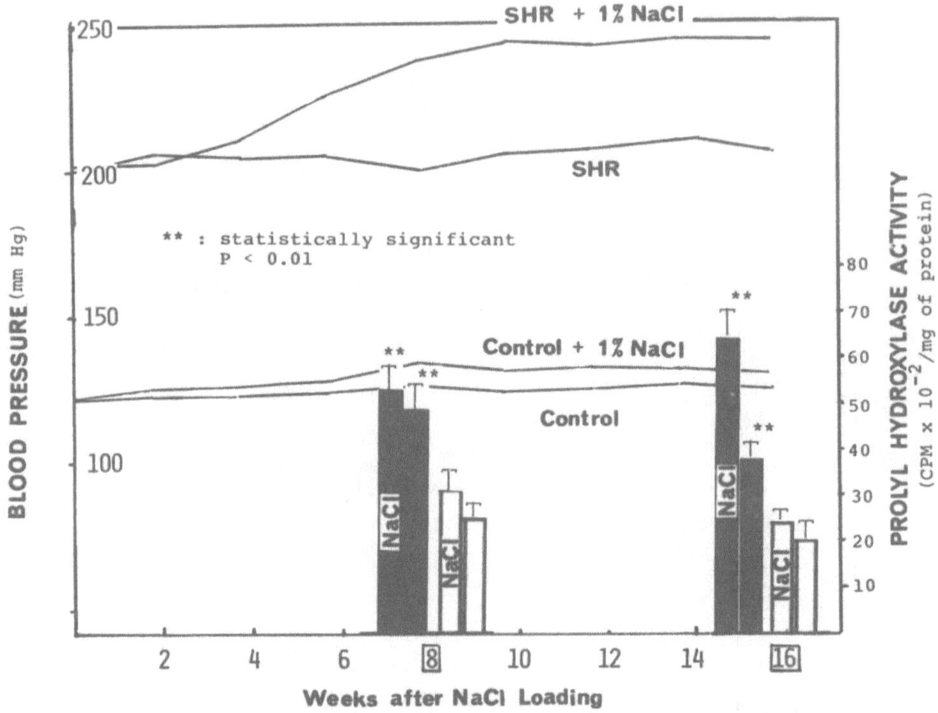

Fig. 5. Effects of NaCl loading on blood pressure and vascular prolyl hydroxylase activity in spontaneously hypertensive rats (SHR). Some of the animals were given 1% NaCl as a source of drinking water in place of tap water at the age of 8 weeks.

is no difference in prolyl hydroxylase activity of the lung, liver and kidney between SHR and controls, the increase observed here is very specific for the cardiovascular system.

When the SHR were given 1% NaCl in place of tap water at the age of 8 weeks, their blood pressure became even more elevated. The level of vascular prolyl hydroxylase activity increased concomitant with the elevation of blood pressure after NaCl loading, suggesting a close relationship between the level of blood pressure and the synthesis of vascular collagen (Fig. 5). The same close relationship was observed when various antihypertensive agents were injected into DOCA-salt hypertensive rats. Along with DOCA-salt treatment, antihypertensive agents with different pharmacologic effects (reserpine 0.75 mg/kg, chlorothiazide 10 mg/kg, hydralazine 5 mg/kg, α-methyl DOPA 40 mg/kg, phentolamine 5 mg/kg, propranolol 5 mg/kg) were administered intraperitoneally on a daily basis. Figure 6 shows that the development of hypertension in these animals was suppressed by the

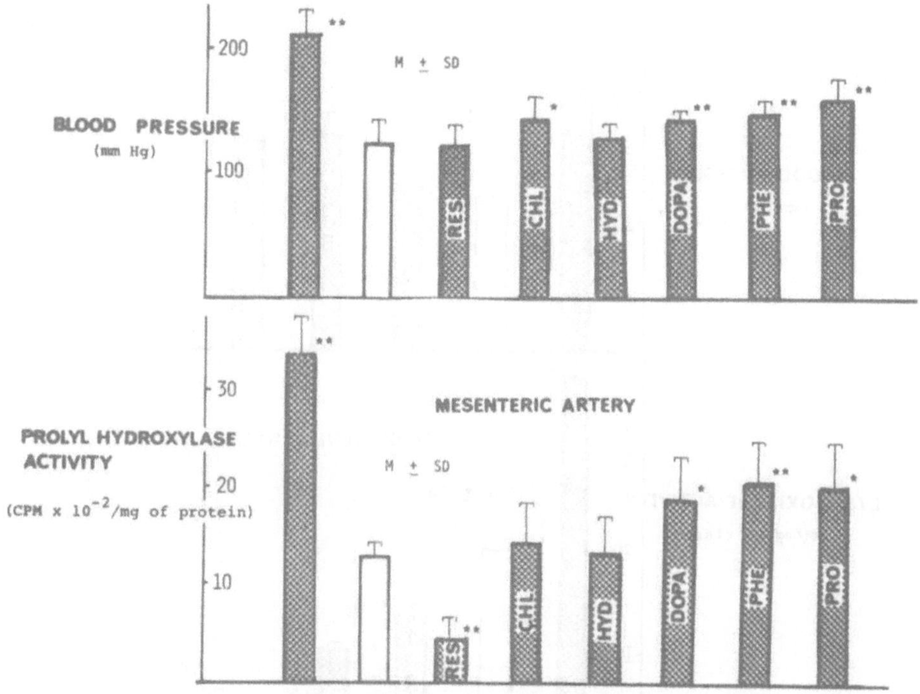

Fig. 6. Effects of various antihypertensive agents on vascular prolyl hydroxylase activity and blood pressure in DOCA-salt treated rats. Hypertension was induced by DOCA-salt treatment for 4 weeks. Refer to Fig. 3. Concomitant with the DOCA-salt treatment, various antihypertensive agents (RES, reserpine 0.75 mg/kg; CHL, chlorothiazide 10 mg/kg; HYD, hydralazine 5 mg/kg; DOPA, α-methyl DOPA 40 mg/kg; PHE, phentolamine 5 mg/kg; PRO, propranolol 5 mg/kg) were injected daily for 4 weeks intraperitoneally.
*,**, Statistically significant compared to control:
*, $0.01 < P < 0.05$; **, $P < 0.01$.

administration of antihypertensive agents, and that the level of prolyl hydroxylase activity was decreased as compared to those of non-treated DOCA-salt hypertensive rats.

In Figure 7, vascular lysyl oxidase activity and the effects of lathyrogens, β-aminopropionitrile and D-penicillamine on blood pressure and vascular collagen deposition are presented. Lysyl oxidase activity of blood vessels in DOCA-salt hypertensive rats was increased as compared to that of controls. The daily injection of reserpine 0.75 mg/kg, β-aminopropionitrile 150 mg/kg or D-penicil lamine 150 mg/kg, i.p, decreased lysyl oxidase activity. Concomitant

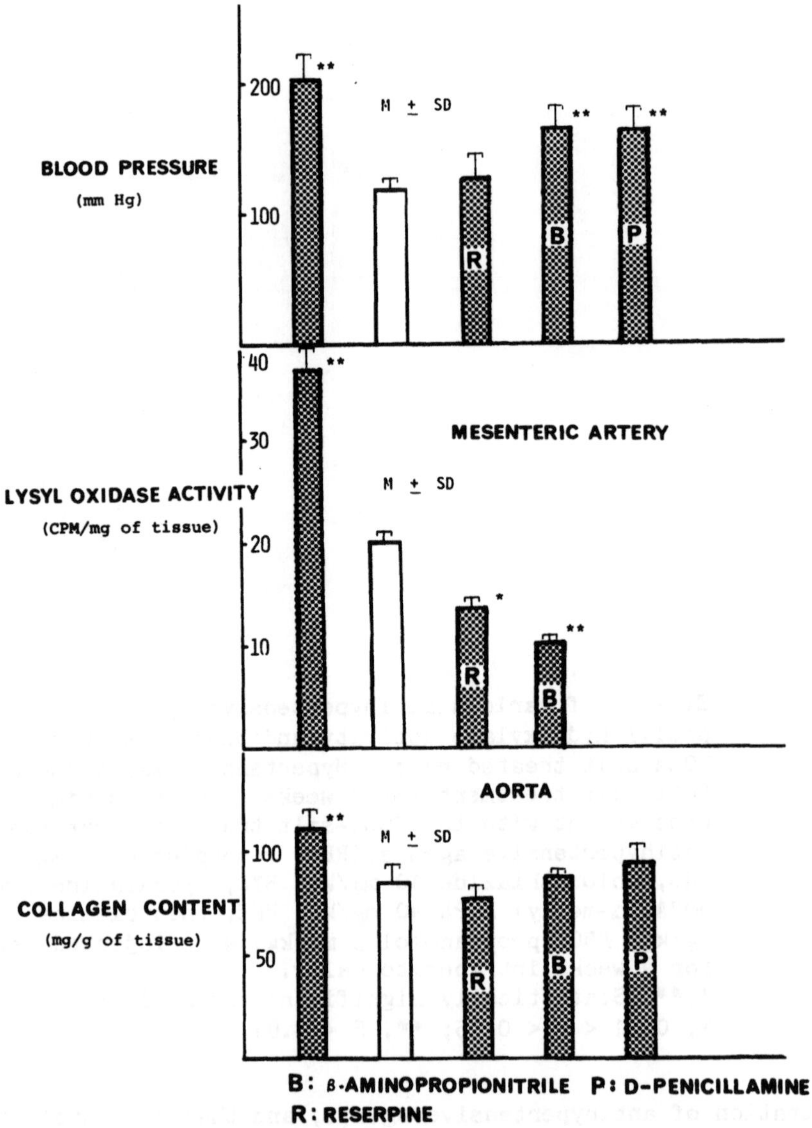

Fig. 7. Effects of lathyrogen on blood pressure, vascular lysyl oxidase activity and collagen content in DOCA-salt treated rats. Hypertension was induced by DOCA-salt treatment for 4 weeks. Refer to Fig. 3. Concomitant with the DOCA-salt treatment, reserpine (R) 0.75 mg/kg, β-aminopropionitrile (B) 150 mg/kg or D-penicillamine (P) 150 mg/kg was administered daily for 4 weeks by intraperitoneal injection. From Ooshima and Midorikawa (16).
*,**, statistically significant compared to control.
*, $0.01 < P < 0.05$, **, $P < 0.01$.

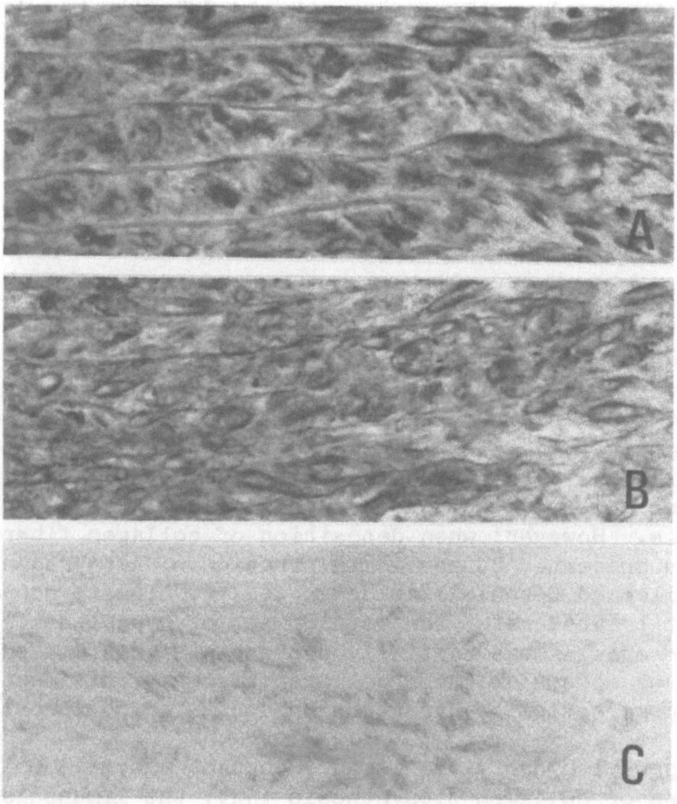

Fig. 8. Immunohistochemical localization of prolyl hydroxylase in aortas of 4-month-old spontaneously hypertensive rats (SHR) (A) and age-matched normotensive rats (B). Note more intense immunostaining in SHR (A) as compared to normotensive rats (B). No specific staining is seen in control section reacted with preimmune serum (C). x 200. See reference (11) in detail.

with the reduction of the enzyme activity, the increase in vascular collagen deposition was prevented. Histopathologically, DOCA-salt animals treated with lathyrogens showed a lower incidence of vascular damage and arteriosclerosis as compared to non-treated DOCA-salt DOCA-salt hypertensive rats. It is of interest that along with the reduction of these parameters, the development of high blood pressure was partially prevented.

The last part of the experiments focused on identifying the collagen-producing cells in the cardiovascular tissues by an immunohistochemical localization of prolyl hydroxylase using monospecific antibody against this enzyme (10,11). As shown in Figure 8, aortic medial smooth muscle cells in 4-month-old SHR (A) showed more intense immunoreaction as compared to age-matched normotensive controls (B). Control sections treated with preimmune serum did not show a non-specific reaction (C). The same was true in mesenteric artery and other blood vessels (not shown). It was of interest that brain microvessels from SHR yielded more intense immunostaining when compared to those from normotensive controls (11).

DISCUSSION

It has been demonstrated, by using various biochemical markers, that hypertension does induce an increased biosynthesis of collagen in blood vessels. When hypertensive rats were treated with anti-hypertensive agents, the increase in vascular collagen synthesis reverted to normal values, indicating that the vascular collagen synthetic activity is closely related to the level of blood pressure. It is likely that blood vessels produce collagen in response to hypertension, which acts as a physical insult or injury to the vessel walls. However, when deposition of collagen fibers in blood vessels was prevented by the administration of lathyrogens, β-aminopropionitrile and D-penicillamine in deoxycorticosterone acetate (DOCA)-salt treated rats, the development of hypertension and arteriosclerotic changes was partially prevented. This may suggest that the increased accumulation of collagen also has an effect of initiation and progression of hypertension and arteriosclerosis.

Since prolyl hydroxylase is an important enzyme involved in an initial step of collagen biosynthesis (12), the immunohistochemical demonstration of this enzyme is assumed to be a sensitive indicator for cellular fibrogenetic activity in cardiovascular tissues. Using the immunoperoxidase method, it was demonstrated that medial smooth muscle cells yielded the most prominent immunostaining in the vascular wall. The immunoreaction for prolyl hydroxylase was more intense in SHR as compared to normotensive controls. This result supports previous findings by other workers, who showed that medial smooth muscle cells in culture actually produce connective tissue components, including collagen (13,14,15), and may play a principal role in the pathogenesis of vascular diseases, particularly atherosclerosis.

SUMMARY

Essential hypertension is the most common disease which develops with advancing age, and its complication, arteriosclerosis, seems to be an exaggerated form of aging process in the mesenchymal tissues. Our present investigation demonstrated that deposition of collagen fibers in vessel wall may represent one aspect of the aging phenomenon occurring in normal vasculature.

ACKNOWLEDGEMENT

The authors wish to express their gratitude to Miss M. Kameda for her excellent assistance with this manuscript.

REFERENCES

1. K. Okamoto and K. Aoki, Development of a strain of spontaneously hypertensive rats, Jap. Circ. J. 27:282 (1963).
2. J. J. Hutton Jr., A. L. Tappel, and S. Udenfriend, A rapid assay for collagen proline hydroxylase, Anal. Biochem. 16:384 (1966).
3. R. C. Giegel and G. R. Martin, Collagen cross-linking. Enzymatic synthesis of lysine-derived aldehydes and the production of cross-linked components, J. Biol. Chem. 245:1653 (1970).
4. A. Ooshima, G. C. Fuller, G. J. Cardinale, S. Spector, and S. Udenfriend, Increased collagen synthesis in blood vessels of hypertensive rats and its reversal by antihypertensive agents, Proc. Natl. Acad. Sci. USA 71:3019 (1974).
5. K. I. Kivirriko, O. Laitinen, and D. J. Prockop, Modification of a specific assay for hydroxyproline in urine, Anal. Biochem. 19:249 (1967).
6. O. H. Lowry, N. J. Rosebrough, A. L. Farr, and R. J. Randall, Protein measurement with the Folin phenol reagent, J. Biol. Chem. 193, 265 (1951).
7 K. Burton, A study of the conditions and mechanism of the diphenylamine reaction for the colorimetric estimation of deoxyribonucleic acid, Biochem. J. 62:315 (1956).
8. A. Ooshima, G. C. Fuller, G. J. Cardinale, S. Spector, and S. Udenfriend, Collagen biosynthesis in blood vessels of brain and other tissues of the hypertensive rat, Science 190:898 (1975).
9. K. Brendel, E. Meezan, and E. C. Carlson, Isolated brain microvessels: A purified, metabolically active preparation from bovine cerebral cortex, Science 185:953 (1974).
10. A. Ooshima, Immunohistochemical localization of prolyl hydroxylase in rat tissues, J. Histochem. Cytochem. 25:1297 (1977).
11. A. Ooshima, Localization of prolyl hydroxylase by the immunoperoxidase method in cardiovascular tissues of hypertensive rats, Jap. Circ. J. 42:971 (1978).
12. G. J. Cardinale and S. Udenfriend, Prolyl hydroxylase, Adv. Enzymol. 41:245 (1974).
13. R. Ross and S. J. Klebanoff, The smooth muscle cell. I. In vitro synthesis of connective tissue proteins, J. Cell Biol. 50:159 (1971).
14. R. Ross, The smooth muscle cell. II. Growth of smooth muscle in culture and formation of elastic fibers, J. Cell Biol. 50:172 (1971).

15. R. Ross and J. A. Glomset, The pathogenesis of arteriosclerosis, New Engl. J. Med. 295:369 (1976).
16. A. Ooshima, and O. Midorikawa, Increased lysyl oxidase activity in blood vessels of hypertensive rats and effect of β-aminopropionitrile on arteriosclerosis, Jap. Circ. J. 41:1337 (1977).

AGING OF *IN VIVO* CARTILAGE CELL

Mitsuo Igarashi and Yasufumi Hayashi

Department of Orthopedic Surgery
Tokyo Metropolitan Geriatric Hospital
Sakae-cho 35-2, Itabashi-ku, Tokyo
Japan

INTRODUCTION

A characteristic of cartilage cells is that, *in vivo*, small numbers of cartilage cells are present in a large volume of matrix composed of such substances as collagen, glycosaminoglycan, and glycoprotein. So, the metabolic behavior of *in vivo* cartilage cells, especially of *in vivo* aged cartilage cells, can be investigated by studying the nature of the products of cartilage cells, such as the biochemical and morphological natures of the matrix Only molecular studies on cartilage collagen that accounts for 60 to 70% of the organic matrix of cartilage can show the change of metabolic behavior of cartilage cells associated with aging.

Therefore, the changes in cartilage collagen of aged, fibrillated, and osteoarthritic cartilage were investigated in order to distinguish the effect of physiological versus pathological aging on the behavior or metabolism of *in vivo* cartilage cells.

MATERIALS AND METHODS

Samples of cartilage were obtained from 7 normal adults, 6 aged individuals, 7 patients with osteoarthritis, and 6 with rheumatoid arthritis. The samples were obtained at autopsy or on surgical treatment for total joint replacement. Age of donor and site from which sample materials were taken are summarized in Table 1. Samples of cartilage were carefully cut away to avoid contamination with subchondral bone, perichondrium or fibrous tissue. They were examined histologically to classify the pathological findings of hyaline cartilage and also to eliminate any possible contamination

Table 1. Materials of Articular Cartilage

	Number	Age (Mean)	Location
Young and adult	7	13 - 33 (23.9)	Shoulder j., 2 Knee j., 1 Ankle j., 4
Aged	6	72 - 82 (79.2)	Hip j., 6
Osteoarthritic	7	52 - 80 (73.3)	Hip j., 7
Rheum. Arthritic	6	51 - 84 (66.3)	Knee j., 6

with subchondral bone and fibrous tissue. Pieces of the hyaline cartilage embedded in paraffin were stained with hematoxyline and eosine, and toluidine blue.

Pepsin-soluble collagen and pepsin-insoluble collagen were obtained from different parts of normal and pathological cartilage by the method of Miller (1). A portion of the pepsin-insoluble collagen was reduced _in vitro_ with sodium borohydride as described by Tanzer (2). Insoluble collagen, both reduced and untreated (not reduced) _in vitro_, was hydrolyzed. Quantitative analysis of aldimine cross-links were performed by the method of Masuda (3). A portion of the soluble collagen was cleaved with cyanogen bromide, and the collagen types were analyzed by calculation from the disc electrophoretic pattern of CNBr peptides (4).

Pepsin-insoluble collagen was extracted with 50% phenol to check the strength of hydrophobic bonds between collagen molecules. The procedure is summarized in Figure 1. This technique was originally devised for the separation of connectin, elastic protein in muscle fiber (5).

RESULTS

Solubilities of collagens from articular cartilage and fibrocartilage of the meniscus of the knee joint with pepsin at 40°C for 48 hours are shown in Figure 2. The solubility of collagen is calculated from the ratio of dry weight of solubilized collagen to original collagen before pepsin digestion. Although 7 to 70% of the collagen

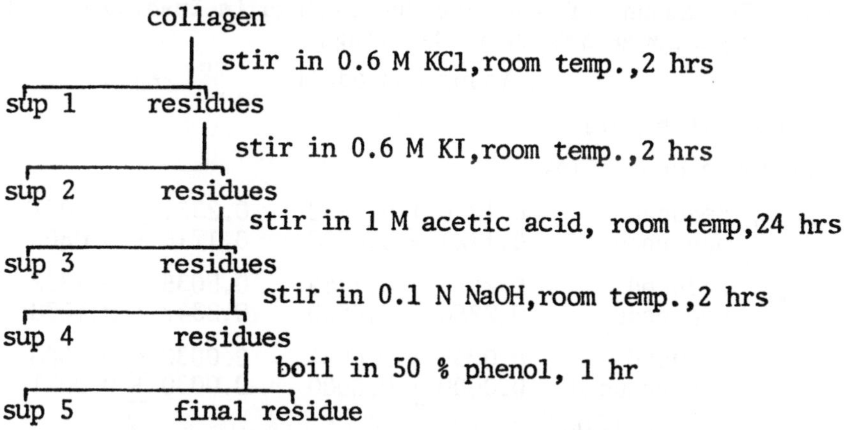

Fig. 1. Procedure of phenol extraction to check the strength of the hydrophobic bond between collagen molecules.

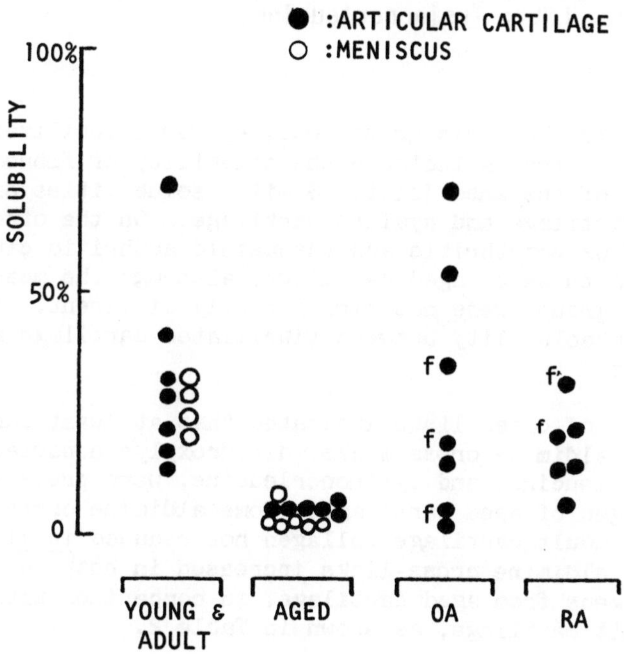

Fig. 2. Solubility of collagens from articular cartilages and menisci following pepsin digestion (calculated from the ratio of dry weight of solubilized collagen to original collagen before digestion). OA, osteoarthritis; RA, rheumatoid arthritis; F, fibrillated cartilage.

Table 2. The Amount of Aldimine Cross-Links in Insoluble Collagen from Human Articular Cartilage

		Young and adult	aged
Number of sample		7	6
aldimine cross-links			
DHLNL	reduced	0.1810 ± 0.0832	0.2321 ± 0.1071
	non-reduced	0.1121 ± 0.0708	0.1716 ± 0.0603
HLNL	reduced	0.2554 ± 0.1769	0.5035 ± 0.2322
	non-reduced	0.2256 ± 0.0560	0.3343 ± 0.1078
LNL	reduced	0.0095 ± 0.0054	0.0030 ± 0.0008
	non-reduced	0.0000 ± 0.0000	0.0030 ± 0.0021
sum of cross-links			
	reduced	0.4459 ± 0.2323	0.7386 ± 0.4555
	non-reduced	0.3377 ± 0.2034	0.5089 ± 0.2876

Each cross-links is calculated from the color yield of lysine and expressed as mean of residues ± standard error per 1,000 amino acid residues.
DHLNL ; dihydroxylysinonorleucine, HLNL ; hydroxylysinonorleucine, LNL ; lysinonorleucine.

was solubilized in the adult group, only 4% was solubilized in the aged group. Open circles indicate the solubility of fibrocartilage of the meniscus of the knee joint. Similar solubilities can be seen for both fibrocartilage and hyaline cartilage. On the other hand, solubilities of osteoarthritic and rheumatoid arthritic cartilage were higher than those of aged cartilage, although the mean ages of the three donor groups were not significantly different. There was no difference in solubility between fibrillated cartilage and the other cartilages.

The analysis of cross-links indicated that at least three different kinds of aldimine cross-links, dihydroxylysinonorleucine, hydroxylysinonorleucine, and lysinonorleucine, were present in the insoluble collagen of aged cartilage. Some aldimine cross-links are present even in adult cartilage collagen not reduced in vitro. The total number of aldimine cross-links increased in both reduced and untreated collagens from aged cartilage, in comparison with those from normal adult cartilage, as shown in Table 2.

Figure 3 shows the extractibility of insoluble collagen of various tissues from aged donors using neutral salt, weak acid, weak alkaline solution, and 50% phenol to study the strength of hydrophobic bonds. Extractability is calculated from the dry weight of each extract per that of the original collagen. In comparison with skin

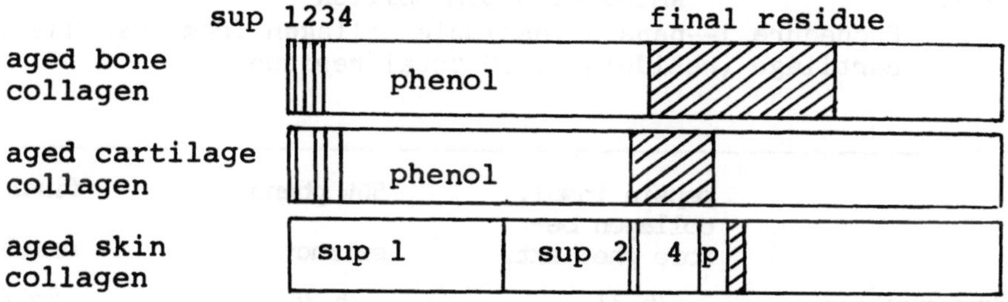

Fig. 3. Extractability of pepsin insoluble collagens (dry weight of each extract per original collagen). Sup 1, extract of 0.6 M KCl; sup 2, extract of 0.6 M KI; sup 3, extract of 1 M acetic acid; sup 4, extract of 0.1 N NaOH solution, phenol or p, extract of 50% phenol.

collagen, a large portion of cartilage collagen was found in the phenol extract, and a final residue remained which was not extracted by any of the procedures. These results suggested that aged cartilage collagen contained a large number of hydrophobic bonds soluble only in phenol. As shown in Table 3, the amino acid composition of both extracts and final residues were unchanged from those of the original collagen before the extraction.

A large nunber of aldimine cross-links were lost in each step of the extraction procedure, and only a small number of aldimine cross-links were present in the final residue (Table 4). This shows that hydrophobic bonds are as important as aldimine cross-links for the stability of aged cartilage collagen.

The disc electrophoretic patterns and their densitograms of CNBr (cyanogen bromide) peptides of authentic type I collagen, normal aged cartilage collagen, rheumatoid arthritic cartilage collagen, and authentic type II collagen are shown in Figures 4 and 5, respectively. The characteristic α2CB3,5 peak of type I collagen is present and is shown as a black peak in Figure 5 A. The characteristic α1(II)CB10 peak of type II collagen is present, and is shown as a shaded peak in Figure 5, D. The characteristic peak of type I collagen, α2CB3,5, can be seen in the middle two densitograms of Figure 5, which show the cyanogen bromide peptides of normal aged and rheumatoid arthritic cartilage collagens. The ratio of type I collagen to type I plus type II collagens can be calculated from the ratio of the density of the α2CB3,5 peak to that of the α1(II)CB10 peak.

On microscopic examination, all the cartilage studied was found to be composed of hyaline cartilage uncontaminated with fibrocartilage, fibrous tissue, and bone. With toluidine blue staining, a change of metachromasia was seen in the osteoarthritic cartilage, especially in the fibrillated and osteophytic cartilage (Fig. 6).

Table 3. AMINO ACID COMPOSITION
Procedure 1--pepsin insoluble collagen from aged human cartilage (residues/1,000 total residues)

	pepsin insol. collagen before phe. ext.	50% phenol extract	final residue
Hydroxyproline	76.27	76.98	96.75
Aspartic acid	50.45	48.10	45.10
Threonine	24.15	23.89	18.68
Serine	30.98	23.50	22.75
Glutamic acid	94.14	94.56	84.23
Proline	105.08	98.27	112.01
Glycine	327.35	356.40	364.89
Alanine	93.93	93.92	90.16
Valine	25.04	23.60	19.81
Methionine	9.21	8.70	8.29
Isoleucine	11.99	14.12	11.43
Leucine	33.39	30.77	28.32
Tyrosine	7.81	6.17	3.70
Phenylalanine	19.19	21.22	17.42
Histidine	5.03	4.60	2.89
Hydroxylysine	12.47	12.73	13.18
Lysine	21.06	19.11	16.41
Arginine	52.45	46.60	43.91

To observe the relation between the type of collagen and the classified lesions of pathological cartilage, the type of collagen in the remaining hyaline areas was compared with those in fibrillated and osteophytic areas (Fig. 7). Although cartilage from the remaining hyaline areas contained only type II collagen, hyaline cartilages from fibrillated and osteophytic areas contained two types of collagen giving various ratios. The ratio of type I collagen to type I plus type II collagens in fibrillated cartilage was not lower than that found in the other pathological cartilage. The ratio of type I collagen to type I plus type II collagens is correlated with the severity of degenerative changes in pathological cartilage, and is not correlated with aging.

DISCUSSION

It was concluded from these results that the pepsin solubility decreased and the number of aldimine cross-links increased in the cartilage from aged donors; and the types of collagen present also changed in aged cartilage.

Table 4.

The Amount of Aldimine Cross-links
Aged human cartilage collagen (pepsin insol.)

aldimine cross-links	pep.insol. coll.before phe. ext.	usp 1 (KCl)	sup 2-4	sup 5 (phenol)	final residue
DHLNL	0.000	0.000	-------	0.359	0.000
HLNL	0.470	1.650	-------	0.762	0.084
LNL	0.000	0.000	-------	0.000	0.000
total (res./1,000 amino acid residues)	0.470	1.650		1.121	0.084
percentage to original collagen (A)	100 %	3 %	3 %	41 %	15 %
total aldimine cross-links $\times \frac{A}{100}$	0.470	0.050	-------	0.460	0.013

With respect to glycosaminoglycan, the amount of chondroitin sulfate present does not change significantly following maturation, but the amount does decrease during the developmental period (6).

Using the fixed charge density method to estimate the total glycosaminoglycan content in tissue, the amount of glycosaminoglycan in normal cartilage does not change with age, but the amount decreases in fibrillated cartilage in a process unrelated to that of aging (7). In the cartilage of pig knee joint, the percentage or uronic acid and the ratio of molar galactosamine to glucosamine does not change between 3 and 5 years of age, although the percentage and ratio are very different prior to maturity, in the developmental period up to 25 weeks of age. Age has not been found to influence the concentration, nor the chain length, of chronodroitin sulfate (8).

Cellularity of human articular cartilage in the femoral condyle does not change after 20 years of age, although many differences can be seen between newborn and adult cartilages (9). Cartilage cells of normal appearance do not change their number of nuclei during aging, but the number decreases in cells of the superficial layer of fibrillated cartilage (10). The cell size of cartilage, rate of cell division, oxygen utilization, total amount of expressible fluid content, and extractable lipid are unaffected by aging.

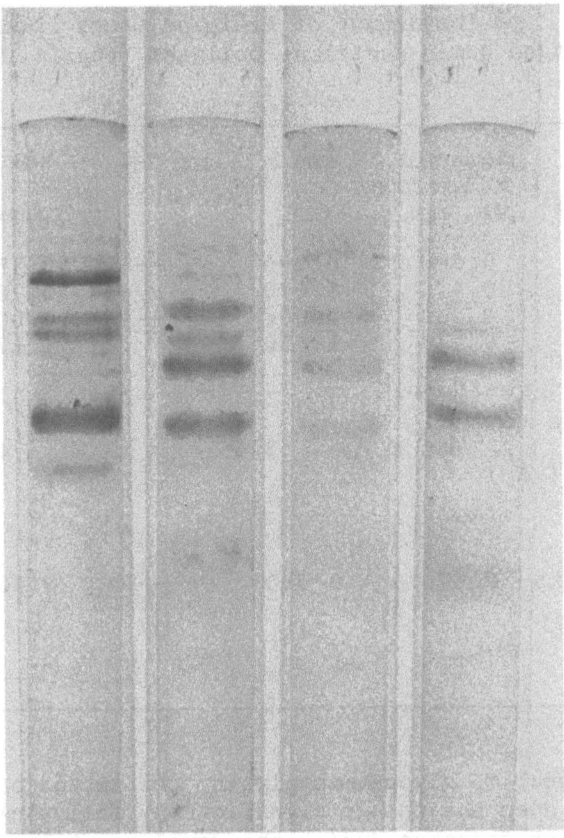

Fig. 4. Disc electrophoretic pattern of cyanogen bromide peptides of authentic type 1 collagen in the left gel, normal aged cartilage in the second gel, rheumatoid arthritic cartilage collagen in the third gel, and authentic type 2 collagen in the right-most gel.

It is very interesting to find out whether these various changes of the matrix of articular cartilage result from the change of the matrix of cartilage cells in vivo associated with aging. Figure 8 summarized our hypothesis.

First, the decrease of solubility is not influenced directly by in vivo cartilage cells, but is influenced by the amounts of glycosaminoglycan surrounding the cartilage collagen, the numbers of aldimine cross-links and of hydrophobic bonds. The strength and the amount of hydrophobic bonds depend on the alignment and tertiary structure of collagen molecules in the extracellular environment. The quantitative and qualitative changes of glycosaminoglycan cannot be seen in aged cartilage of normal appearance.

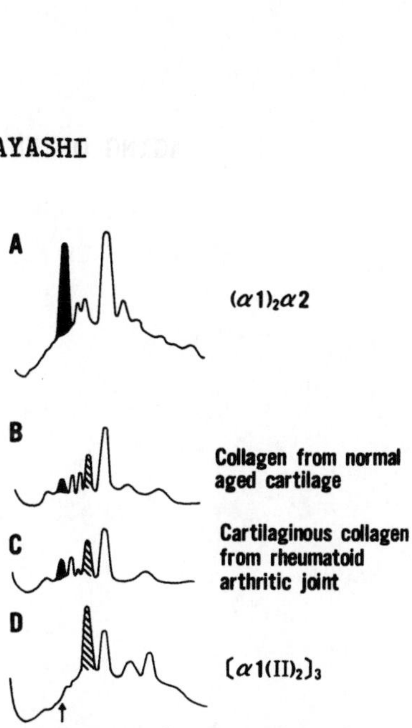

Fig. 5. Densitogram of disc electrophoretic bands shown in Figure 7. Characteristis of type 1 collagen are the presence of α2CB3,5 peak, as shown as black peak in A. Characteristic peak of type 2 collagen is α1(II)CB10, as shown as shadow peak in D. Characteristic peak of type 1 collagen, namely α2CB3,5, can be detected in the middle two figures of normal aged and rheumatoid arthritic cartilage collagens.

Second, the number of aldimine cross-links is influenced by the activity of lysyl oxidase and extracellular formation of Schiff's base to derive ε-amino groups and aldehyde groups, derivatives of lysine and hydroxylysine in collagen molecular sequences.

Third, the type of collagen is influenced by the gene expression of cartilage cells. Type I collagen which is not included in normal cartilage is synthesized in aged cartilage and pathological cartilage from disease processes associated with aging. In these last two types of cartilage, chondrocytes change their gene expression. This change is not irreversible, however, because in cartilage cells of a pathological area, syntheses of both type I and type II collagens were observed at the same time by immunofluorescent study. It is also recognized that the change of collagen type is reversible and is influenced by the amount of environmental calcium ions in an in vitro study of a cell culture. Therefore, the change of collagen type is due to changes in the environment surrounding cartilage cells rather than to the aging phenomena intrinsic to the cells (11,12).

Although we cannot recognize the irreversible changes in articular cartilage cells, various biochemical changes of collagen occur in

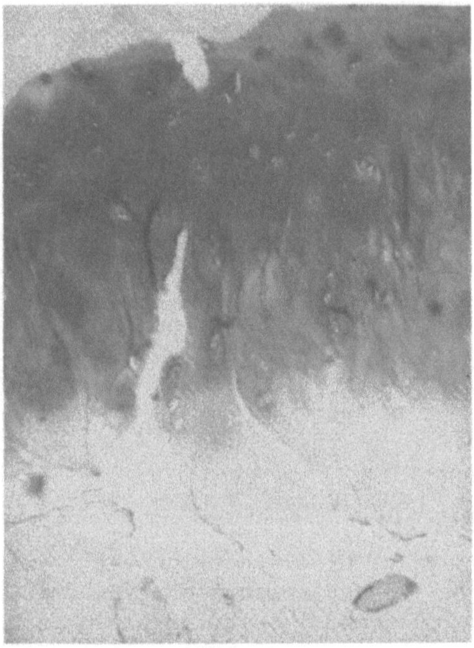

Fig. 6. Histological finding of fibrillated cartilage with toluidine blue staining. Change of metachromasia is recognizable. (x 100).

the cartilage matrix associated with aging once maturation has occurred. The role of a cartilage cell in the joint is to maintain the constancy of the cartilage acquired during the maturation period thoughout the whole life. Our investigation of collagen indicated, however, a disturbance of constancy in articular cartilage following maturation. Also, in advanced stages of aging, normal articular cartilage becomes osteoarthritic. From this, we question the occurrence of physiological aging in articular cartilage.

SUMMARY

It can be seen from our results that, in aged cartilage: (1) pepsin solubility of collagen increases; (2) the number of aldimine cross-links of insoluble collagen increases; and (3) the type of collagen changes.

Quantitative and qualitative changes of glycosaminoglycan cannot be recognized, and cellularity does not change after 20 years of age, or maturation. Only molecular research on cartilage collagen, which accounts for 60 to 70% of the organic matrix in cartilage, can show the changes in metabolic behavior of cartilage cells that are associated with aging.

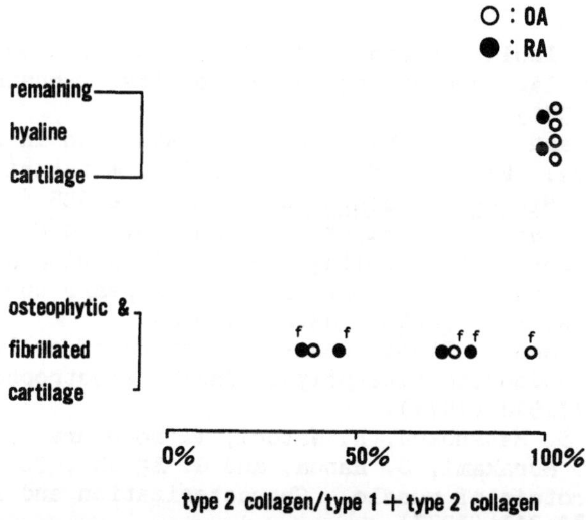

PERCENTAGE OF TYPE 2 COLLAGEN IN SOLUBLE COLLAGENS FROM VARIOUS ARTICULAR CARTILAGES

Fig. 7. Relation between the type of collagen and the classified lesions of pathological cartilages. "f" indicates fibrillated cartilage. Cartilage of remaining area contains only type 2 collagen, but hyaline cartilages of fibrillated and osteophytic areas contain two types of collagens in various ratios.

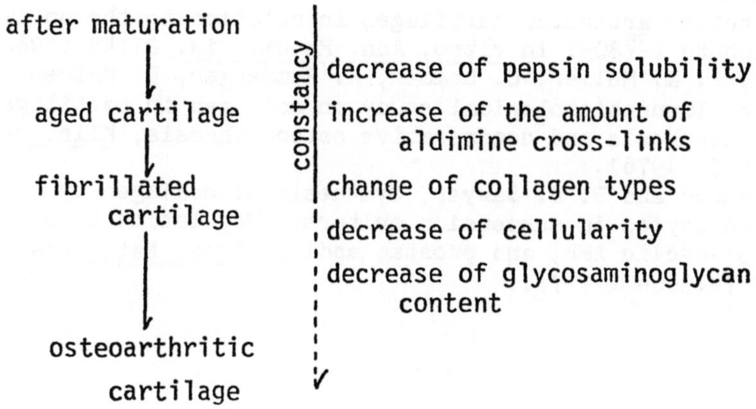

Fig. 8. Changes of cartilage associated with aging.

REFERENCES

1. E. J. Miller, Isolation and characterization of a collagen from chick cartilage containing three identical α-chain, Biochem. 10:1652 (1971).
2. M. L. Tanzer and G. Meckanic, Collagen reduction in sodium borohydride: Effects of reconstruction, maturation and lathyrism, Biochem. Biophys. Res. Comm. 32:885 (1968).
3. M. Masuda, S. Karube, Y. Hayashi, H. Shindo, and M. Igarashi, Direct measurement of collagen cross-links with automatic amino acid analyzer - Identification of peaks due to cross-links, FEBS Letters 63:245 (1976).
4. H. Furthmayer and R. Timpl, Characterization of collagen peptides by sodium dodecylsulfate-polyacrylamide electrophoresis, Anal. Biochem. 41:510 (1971).
5. K. Maruyama, S. Matsubara, R. Natori, Y. Nonomura, S. Kimura, K. Ohashi, F. Murakami, S. Handa, and G. Eguchi, Connectin, an elastic protein of muscle - Characterization and function, J. Biochem. 82:317 (1977).
6. R. Kyselka, Biochemical alteration of hip joint cartilage in aged subject, Z. Alternsforsch. 20:279 (1967).
7. C. Ficat and A. Maroudas, Cartilage of the patella. Topographical variation of glycosaminoglycan content in normal and fibrillated tissue, Ann. Rheum. Dis. 34:515 (1975).
8. C. A. McDevitt, Biochemistry of articular cartilage. Nature of proteoglycans and collagen of articular cartilage and their role in aging and in osteoarthrosis, Ann. Rheum. Dis. 32:364 (1973).
9. R. A. Stockwell, The cell density of human articular and costal cartilage, J. Anat. 101:753 (1967).
10. G. Meachims and D. H. Collins, Cell count of normal and osteoarthritic articular cartilages in relation to the uptake of sulphate ($^{35}SO_4$) in vitro, Ann. Rheum. Dis. 21:45 (1962).
11. S. Gay, P. K. Muller, C. Lemmen, K. Remberger, K. Matzen, and K. Kuhn, Immunohistological study on collagen in cartilage-bone metamorphosis and degenerative osteoarthrosis, Klin. Wschr. 54:969 (1976).
12. K. Deshmukh and B. D. Sawyer, Synthesis of collagen by chondrocytes in suspension culture: Modulation by calcium, 3':5'-cyclic AMP, and prostaglandins, Proc. Natl. Acad. Sci. USA 74:3864 (1977).

AGING AND CHANGES IN GENETIC INFORMATION*

R. W. Hart+ and S. P. Modak‡

+Professor of Radiology, Pharmacology and Preventive Medicine, The Ohio State University College of Medicine 410 W. 10th Ave., Columbus, Ohio 43210, USA

‡Visiting Professor in Radiology

INTRODUCTION

Although all placental mammals are characterized by similar morphological, physiological, and biochemical parameters, they differ from one another in maximum achievable life span by approximately fifty-fold (1,2). Even within closely associated families of recent evolutionary occurrence, such as the primates and Myomorph rodents, e.g., Mus musculus and Peromyscus leucopus, life spans vary by more than twenty fold (3) and three fold (4), respectively. Thus, it appears that whatever governs the life span of a species must be able to be modified rapidly. This imposes strong constraints on the possible genetic mechanisms for the evolution of longevity-assurance systems (4). Two ways by which rapid evolution of longevity could occur, and yet be consistent with basic molecular genetics, would be either via modification of already existing genetic information (species differences in longevity reflecting differences in the turning off of longevity-assurance systems during fetal development), or through slight but significant changes in a number of interlocking processes governing phenotypic expression. Either or both of these mechanisms might explain the rapid evolution of life span within species without necessitating the concurrent input of new genes.

Physiological data further supports the contention that DNA is a primary target and that the rate of accumulation of various forms of

*This work was supported by National Cancer Institute Contract No. Nol-CB-84226.

genetic damage may be a governing factor in longevity. When different mammalian species are compared on a fraction of maximum life span basis, most age-related changes observed appear to occur at similar times (5). Likewise, the decline in "normal" physiological and biochemical processes occurs at equivalent rates when maximum life span within the placental mammals is normalized (6,7). The time of onset of various degenerative diseases and loss of immune function and wound-healing capacity also progress at similar rates in different mammalian species (8,9,7,4). These facts further emphasize a commonality of target between species and differences in the rate of loss of genomic fidelity.

The ability of an organism to maintain the stability of its unit components determines its functional capacity. The higher the differentiated state of a system, the greater the amount of stability required to maintain that state as a function of time. Stability can be achieved by prevention, repair or redundancy. Instability occurs when damage or noise is introduced into a system, where it remains and may be expressed. In addition to external agents which produce DNA damage, various internal processes also induce such damage. For example, approximately 1,000 lesions occur per day per cell as a result of apurinic sites induced at a 37°C body temperature. Thus, while the number of internal and external DNA damaging events to which animals are exposed is relatively constant, maximum achievable life span among mammalian species is not. This suggests that if the causal factor in aging is the expression or rate of accumulation of DNA damage, then among different species there must exist different degrees: 1) to which the DNA is protected from damaging agents and 2) for the removal of the damaged portions of DNA and of the expression of damaged regions of the genome. The net effect of the combination of these processes will be dependent on the absolute residual level of unrepaired DNA damage and on its expression.

PROCESSES RELATED TO THE CONSERVATION OF DNA STABILITY

Metabolite Induction and Removal

DNA damage arises partly as a result of the interaction of exogenously or endogenously generated free radicals and electrophilic molecules with cellular DNA. Differences appear to exist with regard to cell-mediated carcinogen activation among cultivated fibroblasts derived from different species. An inverse correlation between species life span and the capacity of cultured fibroblasts to activate the potent chemical carcinogen 7,12-dimethylbenz(a)anthracene (DMBA) to its mutagenic form has been observed (10). Subsequent studies by this group further confirmed this observation with several independently isolated fibroblast strains from these same six species, and also showed an excellent inverse correlation between species life span and the rate and extent to which the metabolites of the polycyclic aromatic hydrocarbon (PAH) DMBA bind to DNA (11). The difference in extent of binding of DMBA to cellular DNA in these species was over thirty-fold, with rat binding approximately 130 pmoles DMBA/mg DNA, rabbit 55 pmoles DMBA/mg DNA, and man less than 10 pmoles DMBA/mg DNA. It is not known whether other cell types or tissues follow a similar pattern. Nor is it known whether a similar life span correlation holds for metabolic activation and metabolite-binding of other chemical carcinogens.

It has been proposed that the metabolites resulting from intracellular oxidation of DMBA are derived from epoxide intermediates, and that these epoxides are the electrophilic species responsible for the DNA-damaging properties of DMBA (12). These epoxides are formed by microsomal oxidation of DMBA and benzo(a)pyrene (BP) as well as other PAH (13). The major metabolic products of BP oxidations are transdihydrodiols, phenols, and glutathione conjugates (13). For PAH-containing exocylic methyl functions (e.g., DMBA), the situation is considerably more complex, since these compounds form metabolites from both ring oxidations and methyl hydroxylation (Fig. 1). Cultured cells metabolize both DNA-damaging and non-DNA-damaging PAH at roughly equal rates (14). However, human cells generally oxidize PAH at a slower rate than rodent cells (15,16).

It has been established that the process of epoxide formation is initiated by the action of the aryl hydrocarbon hydroxylase (AHH) enzyme system found in the microsomal membrane (17). The AHH system requires NADPH and oxygen, and contains the cytochromes P448 and P450 (18). AHH enzyme systems are present in the microsomes of most tissues that have been studied, but are generally found at the highest concentration in hepatic cells (18). This general nature of the AHH system may reflect its wide range of functions, including oxidation of a wide variety of xenobiotic substances in both rodent (19) and human (20) cells *in vitro*. Whitlock and Gelboin (21) have shown that both RNA and protein synthesis are required for AHH induction. There exists, however, evidence demonstrating induction of AHH by PAH in the presence of inhibitors of protein synthesis (22). Similarly, studies on the genetics of AHH inducibility have led to contradictory results. Nebert at al. (23) have shown that the gene required for AHH inducibility segregates as a simple autosomal dominant trait, and that inducibility is an all-or-none phenomenon in all tissues of the organism. Kouri et al. (24) also found that AHH inducibility in two strains of mice, C57Bl/6 and DBA/6, behaved as a simple autosomal trait, but only hepatic levels were measured. Weibel et al. (25), on the other hand, observed that in some strains of mice the liver AHH is not inducible via PAH, while the AHH levels in target tissues of the same animal (i.e., lung, skin, small intestine and kidney) were inducible. Additionally, studies comparing mice with a high (AKR) vs. low (AF) incidence of leukemia for AHH induction via 3-methyl cholanthrene (3MC) also indicate a genetic system more complicated than a single Mendelian one (26).

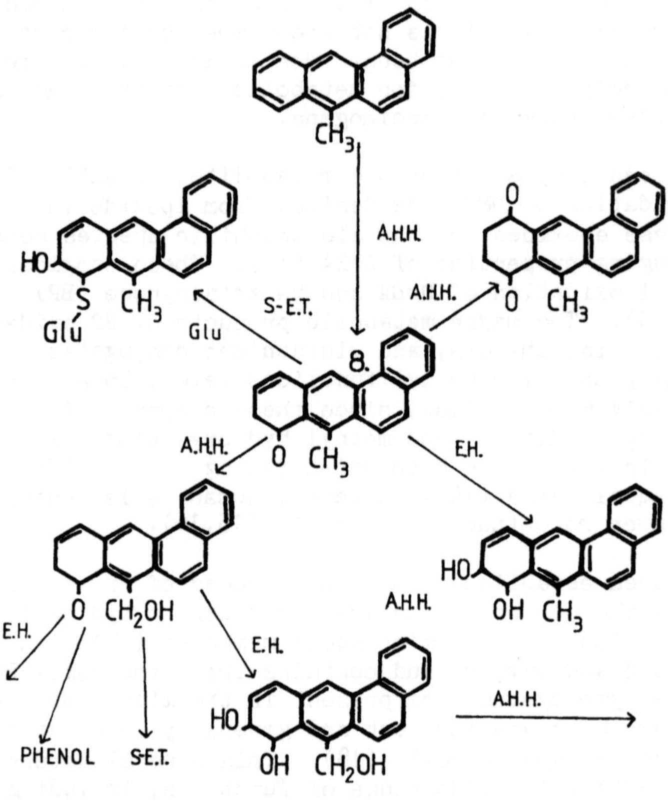

Fig. 1. Some examples of the possible metabolic pathways for oxidation of 7-methylbenz(a)anthracene.

Kellerman et al. (20) have measured the 3MC induction in mitogen-stimulated lymphocytes from man. They found the lymphocytes fell into two to three groups (27): low (1.8-fold), medium (2.5-fold), and high (5.6-fold). Their subsequent studies on families and identical twins suggest that AHH inducibility in humans is under genetic control. Similarly, aging rates in man also appear to be the same in identical, but not fraternal, twins (28).

Since the capacity to perform metabolic activation correlates well in an inverse fashion with species maximum achievable life span, it would be interesting to determine if cells or animals treated with PAH demonstrate any life span shortening effect minus tumor induction; whether non-DNA damaging analogs of these agents (i.e., DMBA vs. 2F-DMBA) induce similar or different effects on life span; and if blocking of AHH activation retards any life span shortening effects observed. All of the experiments listed are feasible, since:

a) doses of carcinogens can be controlled so as to achieve anywhere between 10 and 90 percent killing from carcinogen-induced tumors, with the remaining fraction of survivors being monitored as to variation in life span against controls; b) a series of DMBA analogs with varying abilities to damage cellular DNA are available; and c) inhibitors of AHH-catalyzed conversion of BP and DMBA to water-soluble derivatives are available.

Other factors affecting the extent of damage to cellular DNA by DNA-damaging agents include the ability of other cellular components to scavenge free radicals (e.g., vitamin E), break down nucleophilic molecules (e.g., epoxide hydrase and superoxide dismutase), absorb their deleterious interactions (e.g., attacks on membrane, protein, and RNA rather than DNA), and modify their metabolism and rate of removal. While the modes of action of certain of these phenomena are well understood, their roles in aging are not. Ascribing any particular role for any of these events has an underlying pitfall: i.e., since several events exist, the modification of any single event would be expected only to modify those facets of aging related to that event or form of DNA damage, rather than all facets of aging.

The Induction of DNA Damage and Its Removal

Among the longevity-assurance genes, there are probably several sets of genes responsible for both preservation of DNA damage and control of the repair of such damage (29,4). For example, there are at least four general categories of DNA repair: excision, strand break, postreplication, and photoreactivation (30). Each of these may have several subcategories. Of the various forms of DNA repair, only large patch excision repair has been widely examined relative to longevity (30).

Excision or prereplication repair of UV-induced damage has been measured in a number of different species (31) by a number of different techniques (32,33). Although these techniques measured different parameters, they all seem to give similar estimates of excision repair (29). These earlier studies tended to indicate that human cells (34) and cow cells (35) were very efficient at dimer excision (a direct measure of DNA damage and repair), while those from the hamster (36) showed less excision repair than those from cow or human, but more than cells from the mouse (36). A subsequent study, attempting to minimize different variables between laboratories and cell strains, used primary cell cultures derived from the same anatomical location of animals that had completed the same proportion of the species' maximal life span. This study showed an excellent correlation between both the rate and extent of unscheduled DNA synthesis induced by ultraviolet radiation, as measured by autoradiography, and the life span of seven species drawn from five orders of mammals (29).

A subsequent study examined this correlation in a well-defined comparative system consisting of two Myomorph rodent species, Mus musculus and Peromycus leucopus, which are similar in size, organ weight, and gestation time, but which differ in life span by a factor of 2.5 (4). Agreement was observed between the life spans and the extend of UV-induced unscheduled DNA synthesis for primary fibroblast cell cultures derived from these two species. A determination of patch size (size of the repaired regions) following exposure of the cells to UV light agreed with the aforecited unscheduled DNA synthesis data, thereby confirming a genuine difference in excision repair between two species. These studies indicated that the previous results could not be accounted for by differences in the size of radio-labeled patches. Furthermore, no significant differences in either the amount of DNA per cell or in the rate and extent single-strand break repair following exposure of these cells to X-rays were observed between these two species (4).

A still more recent study using primate fibroblast cell cultures again supports the aforementioned correlation between unscheduled DNA synthesis, as determined by autoradiography, and species life span for UV-induced damage (37). In this study, eleven fibroblast cell cultures derived from punch biopsies of similar-aged primates were shipped blind and coded. These samples were exposed under identical conditions to identical fluences of ultraviolet light, and the extent of unscheduled DNA synthesis measured. The results were then exchanged for the code, and the data calculated. Again a direct correlation between extent of unscheduled DNA synthesis and species life span was observed, with longer-lived species being capable of approximately eight times more repair than shorter-lived species. Additionally, using the assay for endonuclease-sensitive sites, it now appears that UV-endo-sensitive sites are removed at approximately equal rates in all primate cell lines under low-salt conditions, and that in all cases additional sites can be demonstrated after treatment with high-salt. Experiments are now in progress to determine whether there exists species-dependent differences in chromatin structure in relation to the accessibility of damaged sites. Recently, studies which were performed under similar conditions on inbred rodent strains exhibiting approximately a three-fold difference in life span have suggested that this correlation holds between strains of the same species (38). Such studies have not yet been performed with any chemical agent. However, there do exist certain reports relevant to the discussion of this question. For example, as seen in Table 1, it has been observed that the hamster cell line BHK21/C13, which is excision positive for UV-induced cyclobutane-type pyrimidine dimers, is more proficient in removal of DNA adducts induced by benzo(a)pyrene from its DNA than the mouse cell line C57Bl over the same time period following exposure to the same concentration of BP (39). In these studies, the initial number of DN-BP adducts induced were approximately equal in each cell type. Additionally, Smith-Sonneborn (40) has recently used photoreactivation

Table 1. Data on Removal of Chemical Carcinogens. These data are based on actual measurment of lost chemical adducts by chromatographic procedures, and do not reflect mere loss of specific activity from DNA.

Carcinogen	Cell-Type	Strain	Dimer Excision	Treatment Conc. (uM)	% Removal	Time of Removal	Reference
4NQO	E. Coli	H/r30	+	400	80	60 min.	Ikenaga et al., 1975
"	"	Hs30R	-	400	0	60 min.	"
"	mouse	A31-714	?	4	70	24 hr.	"
"	human	FL	+	4	60	24 hr.	"
"	human	XP	-	4	20	24 hr.	"
7BrMBA	hamster	V-79	+	0.1-0.2	50	30 hr.	Dipple and Roberts, 1977
"	human	HeLa	+	0.1-0.2	50	30 hr.	"
"	human	lympho-cytes	+	1	15-17	12 hr.	"
"	human	lympho-cytes	+	5	15-19	6 hr.	"
"	human	lympho-cytes	-	5	1.4-2	6 hr.	"
"	E. Coli	WP2	+	38.5	70	30 min.	Venitt and Tarmy, 1972
"	E. Coli	WP2uvrA⁻	-	38.5	10	2 hr.	"
"	E. Coli	WP2(uvrA⁻ (exrA⁻)	-	38.5	0	2 hr.	"
BP	hamster	BHK21/C13	+	1.3	27.7	24 hr.	Cerutti et al., 1977
"	mouse	C57Bl	+	1.3	15.1	24 hr.	"

(the specific and direct monomerization of UV-induced cyclobutane-type pyrimidine dimers) as an exquisite tool to demonstrate that the life span shortening effects of UV-light in the clonal Paramecium aging model system can be reversed. She speculates that, since the treatment of UV-irradiated cells with photoreactivating light not only overcomes the life span shortening effects of UV, but extends life span significantly, this observation may result from the action of a nondamage-specific repair recognition system in Paramecium which is free to operate upon non-UV-induced damage in cellular DNA following photoreactivation. Interestingly, in single cell systems there is precedent for such enzymes.

On the other hand, the Chinese hamster V-79 cell line appears to be as repair-proficient for similar concentrations of 7-bromoethylbenz(a)anthracene-induced DNA damage as is the human cell line HeLa, both removing approximately 50 percent of the total number of DN-chemical complexes within 24 hours (41). Additionally, the rodent cell line A31-714 appears to remove the DNA damage induced by 4-nitroquinoline-1-oxide (4NQO) at approximately the same rate and to the same extent as human fetal lung cells in vitro (42). This latter observation is especially interesting in light of the fact that 4NQO is a classical UV-mimicking agent which produces DNA damage that is not repaired in excision-defective strains of xeroderma pigmentosum (42). Another possibly relevant observation is the study of Ben-Ishai and Peleg (43), who showed that cell cultures taken from mouse embryos between day 5 and day 19 of gestation have a high level of UV-induced excision repair which subsequently is turned off just prior to birth.

It is important to note that while these studies are intriguing, they nevertheless represent studies performed with model agents. They measure the repair of only a small number of the potential forms of DNA damage as carried out by only a few of the various types of excision repair over limited time frames, and use restricted methodologies under in vitro cell culture conditions. Any general extrapolation from these data to a process such as aging would be premature, if not naive. Any alteration in the structure of DNA would be expected to lead to alteration in cellular function and the ability of a system to respond to various external and internal stress factors. Since there exist numerous forms of DNA damage and repair system, it is a reasonable expectation that neither a single type of DNA damage nor a lack of any individual type of repair would mimic the aging process in all aspects. However, one would expect that individuals exhibiting such defects would mimic, in some form or the other, certain facets of premature aging. Indeed, this seems to be the case for selected human repair defective syndromes, such as xeroderma pigmentosum, ataxia telangectasia, progeria, Down's syndrome, Fanconi's anemia, etc. (44). Likewise, since no single agent induces all forms of DNA damage uniformly and proportionately to what might be expected to occur naturally, it would not be expected that any single agent would bring forth uniformly and proportionately all facets of aging. Again, this expectation is consistent with the known facts (45).

Chromatin Structure and Its Possible Role in the Control of Genome Integrity

A number of studies on terminally differentiated and aging post-mitotic cells (46-56) have shown that DNA in these cells progressively accumulate strand breaks. Evidence has been presented recently that in terminally differentiating postmitotic lens fibers, single-strand breaks affect DNA in the region between nucleosomes, and are converted to double-strand breaks giving rise to a multimeric series of low M_w DNA fragments resembling those produced by Ca^{++}-dependent nuclease-catalyzed digestion of chromatin (57).

From earlier studies, it was hypothesized (51) that the progressive accumulation of damage in DNA in terminally differentiating and aging postmitotic cells is probably related to a defective DNA repair machinery. Considerable evidence now exists that in terminally differentiating and aging cells, excision-repair and strand-break rejoining does indeed become defective (54,58-67). Cellular DNA does not exist as a naked molecule, but rather in the form of a complex with histone and nonhistone protein (68). The DNA-histone complex forms a flexible string of closely packed beads of chromatin subunits, also called 'nubodies' or 'nucleosomes' (69,70), each containing a stretch of DNA (71,72) varying in length between species (73,74). These nucleosomes contain two molecules each of H2A, H2B, H3 and H4 (75,76) to form the "core particle" (77,78), which contains 165-212 base pairs of DNA, with 25-72 base pairs in the spacer or linker region outside the core particle (79,80). Histone H1 is associated with the spacer region (81-83).

It is generally assumed that the distribution of damaged sites in DNA produced by ionizing radiation or UV is random. While this may hold true for naked DNA, there is as yet no evidence on the validity of the above assumption for chromatin-associated DNA. Wilkins and Hart (84) found that a significant portion of pyrimidine dimers induced by UV is masked in nuclei and can be made fully accessible _in vitro_ to UV-endonuclease by high-salt treatment, thereby showing for the first time preferential DNA repair. Treatment of mouse mammary cells with methyl methane-sulfonate and subsequent analysis of the site of damage and repair in chromatin suggest that either damaged sites are non-uniformly distributed, or that the repaired regions are distributed non-randomly relatively to the nucleosomes (85). In UV-irradiated human fibroblasts, the initial repair replication seems to occur preferentially in the linker region (86); nothing is known, however, concerning the frequency of occurrence of pyrimidine dimers in DNA associated with chromatin subunits. The above studies thus indicate that at least the accessibility of the damaged site in DNA is controlled by the chromatin organization, but say little about the precise structural parameter involved. A classical case demonstrating the complexity of this issue is found in V-79 cells, in which 85-90% of UV-induced dimers remain unexcised after six hours (87), although only 20% of the chromatin-DNA is associated with staphylococcal nuclease-resistant nucleosome core particles (Modak, D'Ambrosio, and Hart, unpublished data). Thus, any model conferring upon the chromatin subunits the role of controlling the accessibility of damaged sites to repair enzymes seems naive unless it takes into account histone-histone, histone-DNA, and nonhistone-DNA interactions. Perhaps the most overwhelming consideration is that DNA repair enzymes represent large complexes and must require at least a temporary weakening of the DNA-histone complex, if not its complete disassociation or displacement in order to render accessible the template DNA. Thus, while the existing data (85-87) emphasize the importance of the chromatin organization, a direct extrapolation of results on excision repair in purified DNA may be misleading at this time. In any case, the template-active and repair-active fractions of chromatin seem to be structurally distinct from the inactive regions (84-86,88-91).

In attempts to investigate causes for the aging process, several authors have analyzed the thermal melting behavior (92-96) and the template activity for exogenous RNA polymerase (92,95,97,98) of chromatin in aging tissues, but their results do not always agree. Chromatin Tm increases as a function of age in bovine thymus and rat liver (92,95). Similarly, it has been found that the chromatin template activity for exogenous RNA polymerase decreases with age (92,95,98). Complexity measurements suggest that the number of different types of RNA sequences expressed in mouse tissues decreases with age (99). Taken together, these studies indicate that the chromatin structure undergoes discrete changes during the aging process. Relevant to this, the DNA repeat size remains unchanged as a function of time, although in old mice (28-33 months) a considerable heterogeneity appears in the digestion products with staphylococcal nuclease. Additionally, the proportion of staphylococcal nuclease-sensitive fraction in mouse liver chromatin decreases from 50% (1.75-18 months of age) to 38% at 28-33 months of age, so that the actual proportion of DNA organized into chromatin subunits increases from 70% at 18 months to 90% in very late age. Although these differences suggest that the histone:DNA ratio should increase, this has not been found to be the case (98). Alternate explanations include the possibility that there exists a free pool of histones in mouse liver cells, or that at early and mid-ages half-nucleosome-like structures similar to those suggested by Weintraub et al. (89) may exist containing DNA which is fully sensitive to staphyloccocal nuclease. In the latter case, the half-nucleosome pairs may reassociate to form full nucleosomes, thus rendering resistance to DNA from the staphylococcal nuclease. So far, it has not been possible to ascertain whether non-histone protein confers a nuclease-resistant property upon chromatin-DNA, but this possibility cannot be excluded at present. Non-histone proteins play an important role in regulation of gene expression (68), but nothing is known of their involvement in age-dependent genome inactivation.

Medvedev et al. (100,101) have recently found that histone H1 is modifed in old cells. Two-dimensional electrophoretic analysis of histones from mouse liver chromatin suggests that significant histone modification may appear at 28-33 months of age. Histone modifications can be expected to affect the conformation of chromatin, e.g., an increased charge on H1 would result in condensation of the chromatin, while appearance of H4 with greater charge would tend to increase histone:histone interactions, while at the same time decreasing DNA:histone interactions. Thus, at present the evidence is suggestive of significant changes in the chromatin structure as a function of age. Detailed analyses are necessary, using a variety of organ systems and comparative-evolutionary model systems, in order to comprehend the molecular basis of changes in DNA:histone and histone:histone interactions on one hand and increased concentration of nucleosomes on the other. Such studies should shed light on the possible cell cycle-, differentiation-, and age-specific modulation of the stability and mobility of histone octamers along DNA in a manner relevant to the understanding of the accessibility of nucleosome-bound sites in DNA to the damaging agents and repair enzyme on the one hand and to DNA and RNA polymerases on the other.

CONCLUSION

Mammalian DNA *in vivo* can be damaged by normal body temperature (102), X-rays, ultraviolet light, metabolites, free radicals, and numerous chemical agents. Such damage, if not repaired, will lead to alterations in various physiological functions. Accumulation of DNA damage will result in accumulated changes in the information flow and content of the genetic material. Four ways in which fidelity of information flow can be maintained are: 1) prevention of the induction of DNA damage; 2) repair of the resulting damage; 3) redundancy of information content; and 4) repression of damaged regions. Studies bearing on the first three of these indicate that: 1) fibroblasts derived from longer-lived species are less able to metabolically activate certain chemical agents to their nucleophilic forms than those derived from shorter-lived species; 2) fibroblasts derived from longer-lived species generally are better able to excise UV-induced DNA damage than those derived from shorter-lived species and 3) redundancy of information content appears to play a minor role in maintenence of DNA information flow. Little is presently known about the role of chromatin in either the interference of DNA repair processes or control of the expression of altered regions of the DNA.

While a paucity of data exists regarding the role of DNA damage in aging, it is a reasonable assumption that it will alter the flow of information with a resultant decreased ability of the cell to respond to either exogenously or endogenously generated stress. Longevity assurance mechanisms which might serve to regulate the rate of accumulation of such damage have been outlined above. Since: 1) no human syndrome totally mimics the aging process, and yet many, if not most, repair-defective syndromes exhibit certain facets of premature aging, and 2) no known DNA-damaging agent brings forth in time uniformly and proportionately all aspects of aging, but, for those agents thus far studied, each appears to accelerate certain aspects of aging, it therefore would appear that the total repair capacity of a system for all forms of genetic damage must be studied in order to strictly determine the role of DNA damage in the aging process. Further, due to the complexity of the aging process and the role of various cell-cell and tissue-tissue interactions, it would appear that these processes would be best evaluated in vivo. Further, since each of these interlocking longevity assurance systems (each composed of multiple steps and sub-systems) is directly involved in maintaining the fidelity of the information content within the cell, then each must therefore be evaluated separately and in concert with one another in order to determine their overall importance in longevity.

REFERENCES

1. A. Comfort, in:"Ageing, The Biology of Senescence," Holt, Rinehart and Wilson, New York (1964).
2. W. Andrew, in:"The Fine Structure and Histochemical Changes in Ageing," Academic Press, New York (1968).
3. R. G. Cutler, Exp. Gerontol. 10:37 (1975).
4. G. A. Sacher and R. W. Hart, in:"Genetic Effects of Aging," D. Bergsma and D. Harrison, eds., Alan R. Liss, New York (1978).
5. P. Burch, in:"The Fine Structure and Histochemical Changes in Ageing," Academic Press, New York (1968).
6. C. Finch, in:"Animal Models for Biomedical Research IV", Nat. Acad. Sci. USA, Wash., D.C. (1971).
7. N. Shock, Ann. Rev. Physiol. 23:97 (1961).
8. A. Engel and R. Larsson, in:"Cancer and Aging," Norcliska Bakhandelns Forlag, Stockholm (1978).
9. T. Makinodan, E. Perkins, and M. Chen, Adv. Gerontol. Res. 3:171 (1971).
10. A. G. Schwartz, Exp. Cell Res. 94:445 (1975).
11. A. G. Schwartz and C. J. Moore, Exp. Cell Res. 109:448 (1977).
12. E. Boyland, Biochem. Soc. Symp. 5:40 (1950).
13. P. Sims and P. L. Grover, Adv. Cancer Res. 20:165 (1975).
14. M. E. Duncan and P. Brookes, Int. J. Cancer 4:813 (1970).
15. E. Huberman, J. K. Selkirk, and C. Heidelberger, Cancer Res. 31:2161 (1971).
16. M. E. Duncan and P. Brookes, Int. J. Cancer 9:349 (1972).
17. A. H. Conney, Science 178:576 (1972).
18. H. V. Gelboin, F. J. Weibel, and H. Kinoshita, in:"Chemical Carcinogenesis," P. O. P. T'so and J. A. DiPaolo, eds., Marcel Dekker, New York (1974).
19. D. W. Nebert and H. V. Gelboin, Arch. Biochem. Biophys. 134:76 (1969).
20. G. Kellerman, E. Cantrell, C. R. Shaw, Cancer Res. 33:1654 (1973).
21. J. P. Whitlock and H. V. Gelboin, J. Radiol. Chem. 249:2616 (1974).
22. J. P. Whitlock, and H. V. Gelboin, J. Biol. Chem. 248:6114 (1973).
23. D. W. Nebert, W. F. Benedict, J. E. Gielen, F. Oesch, and J. W. Daly, Mol. Pharmacol. 8:374 (1972).

24. R. E. Kouri, H. Ratrie, and C. E. Whitmore, J. Natl. Cancer Inst. 51:197 (1973).
25. F. J. Weibel, J. C. Leutz, and H. V. Belboin, Arch. Biochem. Biophys. 154:292 (1973).
26. K. Burki, A. G. Liebelt, and E. Bresnick, J. Natl. Cancer Inst. 50:369 (1973).
27. G. Kellerman, C. R. Shaw, M. Lugten-Kellerman, N. Engl. J. Med. 289:934 (1973).
28. A. Comfort, in:"Ageing, the Biology of Senescence," Holt, Rinehart and Wilson, New York (1964).
29. R. W. Hart, and R. B. Setlow, Proc. Natl. Acad. Sci. USA 71:2169 (1974).
30. D. E. Brash and R. W. Hart, J. Environ. Pathol. Toxicol. 2:79 (1978).
31. H. F. Stich and R. H. C. San, Proc. Soc. Exp. Biol. Med. 142:155 (1973).
32. J. E. Cleaver, in:"Methods in Cancer Research," vol. 9, H. Busch, ed., Academic Press, New York (1975).
33. R. W. Hart and J. E. Trosko, Interdisc. Top. Gerontol. 9:134 (1976).
34. J. E. Cleaver and J. E. Trosko, Photochem. Photobiol. 11:547 (1970).
35. J. E. Cleaver, Nature 270:451 (1977).
36. R. B. Setlow, J. D. Regan, and W. L. Carrier, Biophys. Soc. Abstr. 12:19a (1972).
37. K. Hall, C. Albrightson, and R. W. Hart, XIth Internat. Cong. Gerontol., Tokyo, Japan (1978).
38. V. Paffenholz, Mech. Ageing Dev. 7:131 (1978).
39. P. Cerutti, K. Shinohara, and J. Remsen, J. Toxicol. Environ. Health 2:1375 (1977).
40. J. Smith-Sonneborn, personal communications (1978).
41. A. Dipple and J. J. Roberts, Biochemistry 16:1499 (1977).
42. M. Ikenaga, Y. Ishii, M. Toda, T. Kakunaga, H. Takebe, and S. Kondo, in:"Molecular Mechanisms for Repair of DNA," P. C. Hanawalt and R. B. Setlow, eds., Plenum Press, New York (1975).
43. R. Ben-Ishai, and I. Peleg, in:"Molecular Mechanisms for Repair of DNA, P. C. Hanwalt and R. B. Setlow, Plenum Press, New York (1975).
44. R. W. Hart, S. D'Ambrosio, K. J. Ng, and S. P. Modak, Mech. Ageing Dev. 9:203 (1978).
45. R. W. Hart, K. Y. Hall, and F. B. Daniel, Photochem. Photobiol. 28:131 (1978).
46. S. P. Modak and F. J. Bollum, Exp. Cell Res. 62:421 (1970).
47. S. P. Modak and F. J. Bollum, Exp. Cell Res. 75:307 (1972).
48. S. P. Modak and G. B. Price, Exp. Cell Res. 65:289 (1971).
49. G. B. Price, S. P. Modak, and T. Makinodan, Science 190:917 (1971).
50. H. R. Massie, M. B. Baird, and R. J. Nicolosi, Arch. Biochem. Biophys. 153:736 (1972).

51. S. P. Modak, in:"Cell Differentiation," R. Harris, P. Allen, and D. Viza, eds., Munksgaard Publications, Copenhagen (1972).
52. S. P. Modak and H. Traurig, Cell Differentiation 1:351 (1972).
53. J. Piatigorsky, S. S. Rothschild, and L. M. Milstone, Dev. Biol. 34:334 (1973).
54. P. Karran and M. G. Ormerod, Biochim. Biophys. Acta 299:54 (1973).
55. K. J. Wheeler and J. T. Lett, Proc. Natl. Acad. Sci. USA 71:1962 (1974).
56. M. F. Counis, E. Chaudun, and Y. Courtois, Dev. Biol. 57:47 (1977).
57. D. W. Appleby and S. P. Modak, Proc. Natl. Acad. Sci. USA 74:5579 (1977).
58. S. Goldstein, N. Engl. J. Med. 285:1120 (1971).
59. G. M. Hahn, D. King, and S. J. Yang, Nature 230:242 (1971).
60. F. E. Stockdale, Science 171:1145 (1971).
61. F. E. Stockdale and M. C. O'Neil, J. Cell Biol. 52:589 (1972).
62. R. W. Hart and R. B. Setlow, Mech. Ageing Dev. 5:67 (1976).
63. M. R. Mattern and P. Cerutti, Biochim. Biophys. Acta 395:48 (1975).
65. G. E. Milo and R. W. Hart, Arch. Biochem. Biophys. 176:324 (1976).
66. A. C. Chen, S. K. C. Ng, and I. G. Walker, J. Cell Biol. 70:685 (1976).
67. J. Treton, S. P. Modak, and Y. Courtois, manuscript in preparation (1978).
68. A. Ruiz-Carillo, L. J. Wangh, and V. G. Allfrey, Science 190:117 (1975).
69. A. Olins and D. E. Olins, Science 183:330 (1974).
70. P. Oudet, M. Gross-Bellard, and P. Chambon, Cell 4:281 (1975).
71. D. R. Hewish and L. A. Burgoyne, Biochem. Biophys. Res. Comm. 52:504 (1973).
72. M. Noll, Nature 251:249 (1974).
74. E. M. Bradbury, in:"The Organization of Expression of Ekaryotic Genome," E. M. Bradbury and K. Javaherian, eds., Academic Press, New York (1977).
75. R. D. Kornberg, Science 184:868 (1974).
76. R. D. Kornberg and J. O. Thomas, Science 184:865 (1974).
77. B. Sollner-Webb and G. Felsenfeld, Biochemistry 14:2915 (1975).
78. R. Axel, H. Cedar, and G. Felsenfeld, Proc. Natl. Acad. Sci. USA 70:2921 (1975).
79. J. O. Thomas, in:"The Organization and Expression of Eukaryotic Genome," E. M. Bradbury and K. Javaherian, eds. Academic Press, New York (1977).
80. N. R. Morris, Cell 9:627 (1976).
81. B. R. Shaw, T. M. Herman, R. T. Kovacic, G. S. Beaudreau, and K. E. van Holde, Proc. Natl. Acad. Sci. USA 73:505 (1976).
82. A. J. Varshavsky, V. V. Bakayev, and G. P. Georgiev, Nucleic Acids Res. 3:477 (1976).
83. J. P. Whitlock and R. T. Simpson, Biochemistry 15:3307 (1976).

84. R. J. Wilkins and R. W. Hart, Nature 247:35 (1976).
85. W. J. Bodell, Nucleic Acids Res. 4:2619 (1977).
88. W. Andrew, in:"The Fine Structure and Histochemical Changes in Ageing," Academic Press, New York (1968).
89. H. Weintraub, A. Worcel, and B. Alberts, Cell 9:409 (1978).
90. A. Garel and R. Axel, Proc. Natl. Acad. Sci. USA 73:3966 (1976).
91. H. Weintraub and M. Groudine, Science 193:848 (1976).
92. M. J. Pythilla and F. G. Sherman, Biochem. Biophys. Res. Comm. 31:340 (1968).
93. D. I. Kurtz and F. M. Sinex, Biochim. Biophys. Acta 145:840 (1967).
94. H. P. von Hahn, Gerontologia 16:116 (1970).
95. S. M. Zhelabovskaya and G. D. Berdyshev, Exp. Gerontol. 7:313 (1972).
96. D. I. Kurtz, A. P. Russel, and F. M. Sinex, Mech. Ageing Dev. 3:37 (1974).
97. H. Y. Samis and V. J. Wulff, Exp. Gerontol. 4:111 (1969).
98. B. T. Hill, Gerontologia 22:111 (1976).
99. R. G. Cutler, Proc. Natl. Acad. Sci. USA 72:4664 (1975).
100. Zh. A. Medvedev, M. N. Medvedeva, and L. I. Huschtscha Gerontology 23:334 (1977).
101. Zh. A. Medvedev, M. N. Medvedeva, and L. Robson, Gerontology 24:286 (1978).
102. T. Lindahl and S. Ljungquist, in:"Molecular Mechanisms for Repair of DNA," P. C. Hanawalt and R. B. Setlow, eds., Plenum Press, New York (1975).

EVIDENCE AGAINST SOMATIC MUTATION AS A MECHANISM OF CLONAL SENESCENCE

George M. Martin, Holger Hoehn and Eileen M. Bryant

Division of Genetic Pathology
Center for Inherited Diseases
and Institute on Aging
University of Washington
Seattle, Washington 98195

SUMMARY

In order to carry out complementation tests of the somatic cell mutational theory of clonal senescence, methods were developed for the isolation of proliferating hybrid and parental tetraploid human cells which would not depend upon biochemical selection. Crosses between short-lived strains resulted in short-lived offspring and crosses between long-lived parents tended to be long-lived, in experiments involving skin fibroblast-like cells. Crosses between strains of contrasting longevities gave growth potentials approximately intermediate to those of the parentals.

Crosses were also carried out between euploid fibroblast-like cells and two other distinctive euploid cell types ("E," or epitheloid and "AF," or aminiotic fluid cells, both derived from second trimester aminotic fluid) (Hoehn et al., 1974), and both having replicative life spans which are much more limited than the fibroblast-like skin cell ("F" cells). Compared to F x F tetraploids, F x AF and F x E hybrids had lesser growth rates, but were superior to those of parental AF and E cells.

The results are interpreted as evidence in favor of a programmed mechanism for clonal senescence and against somatic cell mutation, at least for the case of mutations involving single copy DNA.

INTRODUCTION

It has been well established that normal diploid human somatic cells have limited replicative life spans in culture (for reviews, see 1,2). There is controversy concerning the probable mechanisms of such in vitro clonal senescence. Some investigators favor a genetic program related to cell differentiation, while others emphasize protein synthesis error catastrophe theories and somatic cell mutation (1,2).

We thought it useful to carry our complementation tests of the somatic cell mutation theory in hybrids synthesized between different strains. We reasoned that if such mutations were in fact random, predominantly recessive and involved (among other types of DNA) single copy DNA, crosses between strains with different prior in vivo and in vitro histories would be likely to demonstrate significant enhancements of their growth potentials because of the mutual complementation of defective genes significant for mitotic cell cycle function. The results failed to show evidence of such complementation.

This paper summarizes research which has been presented in more detail elsewhere (3,4).

METHODS

The papers by Hoehn et al. (3) and Bryant et al. (4) should be consulted for methodological details. The cell strains were derived from various human donors, via skin biopsy or from second trimester amniotic fluid. In the determination of replicative life spans, cultures were teminated when counts were equal or less than the input inoculum of 5×10^4 cells (weekly passages in 25 cm^2 plastic flasks). Cell fusions were carried out with a modification of the polyethylene glycol-dimethysulfoxide technique of Norwood et al. (5). Putative tetraploid clones were harvested after dilute plating, on the basis of morphology. Tetraploidy was confirmed cytogenetically and by the use of flow microfluorescence. Hybrid tetraploids were distinguished from parental tetraploids by electrophoretic detection of a heterodimer of glucose-6-dehydrogenase (G6PD), the parental strains having been chosen on the basis of contrasting G6PD types (A and B).

RESULTS

The first point to make is that at least a proportion of parental and hybrid clones was chromosomally stable throughout their replicative life spans. Those clones which were mixoploid (diploid + tetraploid) could well have resulted from inter-clonal contamination. Such cytogenetic stability is in contrast to what is observed with the more conventional hybrids between parents, one of which is aneuploid.

Figure 1 summarizes the longevities of parental diploid (A), parental tetraploid (B) and hybrid tetraploid (C) colonies derived

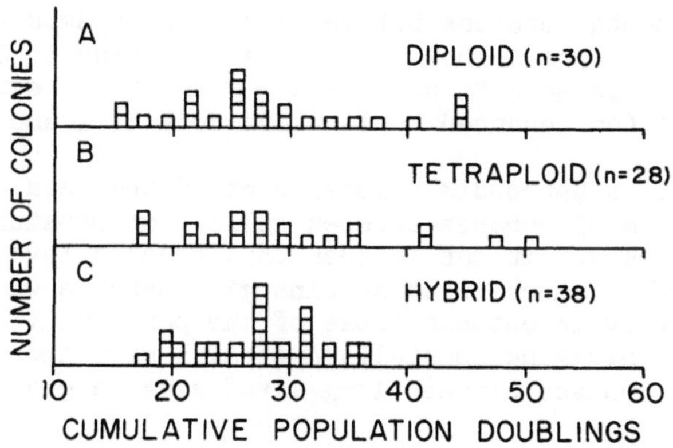

Fig. 1. Comparison of clonal longevities: (A) parental diploids; (B) tetraploids of single G6PD phenotype; (C) hybrid tetraploids. Reproduced from Hoehn et al. (1978) with permission of publisher.

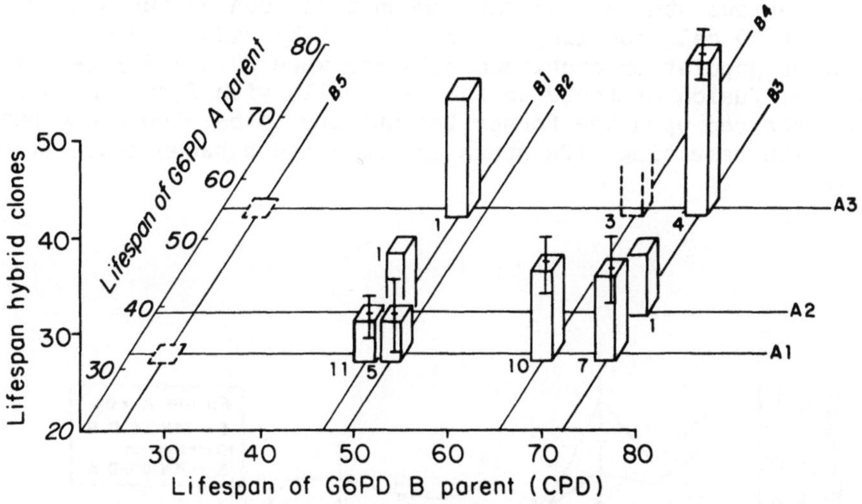

Fig. 2. Life span of hybrid clones as a function of growth potential of G6PD A and G6PD B parental mass cultures. Each vertical tower represents mean (± standard deviation) life span of the number of hybrid isolates indicated by arabic numerals at the base of each tower. The incomplete tower (dashed outline) of cross A3 x B4 indicates loss of isolates due to culture mishap. The flat squares with dashed outline refer to attempts to obtain hybrids with an extremely short-lived strain (B5) derived from a patient with Werner syndrome (Bryant et al., 1978). Reproduced from Hoehn et al. (1978) with permission of publisher.

from 12 experimental crosses between 7 different skin fibroblast strains. The histograms show that the modal value is quite comparable between the three sets of clones. There is no evidence of a complementation for enhanced replicative potential among the hybrids.

In Figure 2, a three-dimensional plot of the data of Figure 1 shows the results of crosses between cells from strains with contrasting life spans. It can be seen that crosses involving long-lived strains with short-lived strains give hybrids whose life spans fall approximately in between those of the parental lines. In contrast, crosses involving short-lived strains give short-lived hybrids, while crosses between long-lived strains give long-lived hybrids.

In Figure 3, the growth rates of groups of hybrid tetraploid fibroblast clones are compared with parental tetraploids. In keeping with the longevity data, the growth rates of the hybrids are intermediate to those of the parents.

"E" type cells rarely, if ever, can be cloned after trypsinization. Previous studies (6) have shown that such cultures grow for only about 10 cell doublings. For 9 F x E hybrids, the mean cumulative population doublings acheived were 20.5 ± 2.3 (s.d.). Therefore, fusion of these epithelioid cells with fibroblast-like cells conferred upon the former the ability to be cloned and passaged, with resulting life spans intermediate between those of the parents.

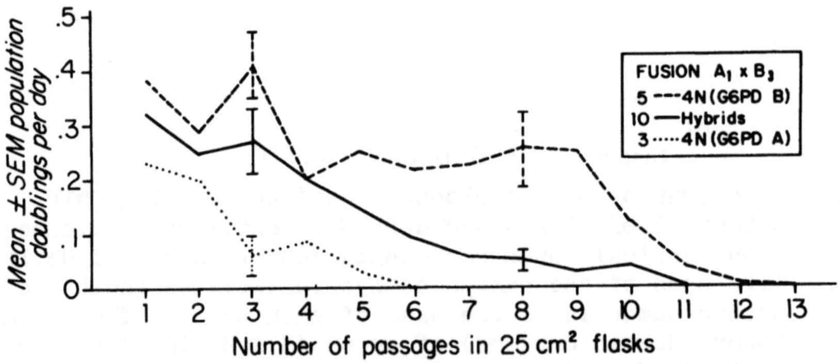

Fig. 3. Mean growth rates of isolates obtained from crosses between hybrids and parental skin fibroblast cultures. The error bars represent standard errors at selected points. Reproduced from Hoehn et al. (1978) with permission of publisher.

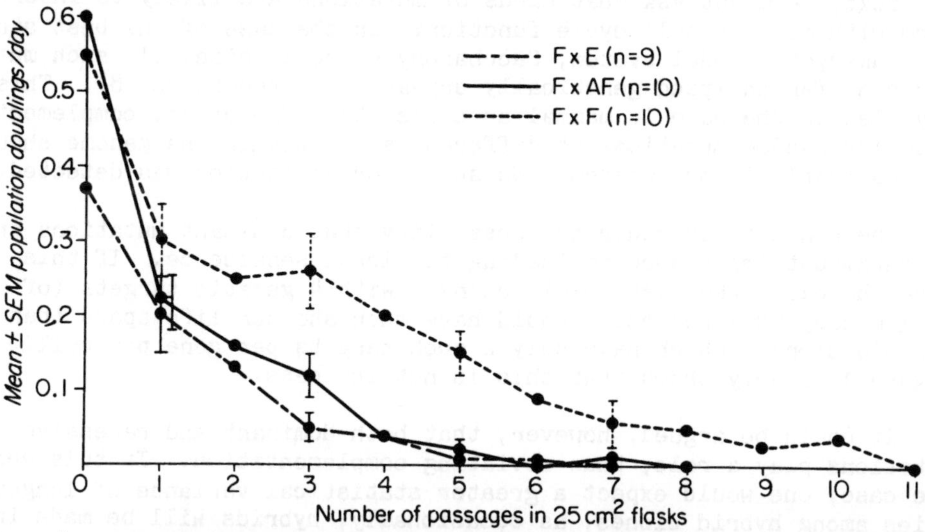

Fig. 4. Growth histories of serially passaged hybrid isolates from F x E, F x AF, and a control F x F fusion. SEM, standard error of mean. Reproduced from Bryant et al. (1978) with permission of publisher.

The life spans of ten hybrid clones derived from crosses between F and AF cells were also investigated. Once again, they gave results (22.5 ± 7.6 cumulative population doublings) approximately intermediate between those of the two parents.

Figure 4 shows that the growth curves of the F x E and F x AF hybrid tetraploids were consistently less than those of F x F tetraploids over a series of passages.

DISCUSSION

The first question that one must deal with in the interpretation of the results is the extent to which the life spans of individual clones from a mass culture reflect the life spans of the mass cultures. It is well established that there is a great deal of variation with respect to the growth potentials of such clones (7,8). In the present experiments, however, the methods were such that only the best growing clones could be studied, since only these provided enough growth for the initial isolation and passaging. This automatically eliminated a great deal of the variance. Furthermore, we could experimentally demonstrate that a sample of 22 parental tetraploid clones from 5 strains showed a high correlation (r = 0.89) of their replicative life spans with those of their respective parental mass cultures (3).

Next, we might ask what kinds of mutations are likely to interfere with mitotic cell cycle function? In the case of the best studied eukaryotic model system, Saccharomyces cerevesiae, all such mutations so far analyzed genetically appear to be recessive (8). This may also be the case in mammalian cells (9). Therefore, complementation for random mutations at different sites within the genome should be observable in our system. No such complementation was detected.

One can also consider the possiblity that dominant mutations are of paramount importance in leading to clonal senescence. If this were the case, then tetraploid clones, with 4 genetic targets (of single copy DNA) per cell should have much shorter life spans than diploid clones, which have only 2 such targets per gene per cell. Figure 1 clearly shows that this is not the case.

It could be argued, however, that both dominant and recessive mutations play a role, thus obviating complementation. If this were the case, one would expect a greater statistical variance of longevities among hybrid clones, as occasionally, hybrids will be made in which there is a predominance of dominant mutations, giving very short life spans--or, alternatively, hybrids will be made in which there is a predominance of recessive mutations, giving complementation and enhanced life spans. (The effects of such dominant or recessive mutant alleles need not be lethal, but could act to slow the cell cycle, with the cumulative effects of many such mutations eventually leading to cessation of replication.) Although the total number of hybrids examined is limited, Figure 1 shows no such evidence of an increased variance of longevities; if anything, there is <u>less</u> variance among hybrids than among the tetraploid parentals.

Finally, one might argue that the mutations which are of importance are not those involving single copy DNA, but rather those that involve repetitive genes, such as those which code for ribosomal RNA and the various species of transfer RNA. DeMars (10) and Ohno (11) have reasoned that selection against mutations in single copy genes would lead to rapid elimination of the cells bearing such mutations, whereas mutations in reiterated genes could gradually accumulate, having the effect of a type of delayed dominance. DeMars and Ohno essentially invoke the Orgel hypothesis of protein synthesis error-catastrophe (12) to explain such delayed dominance. However, there are strong arguments why this may not be a valid general mechanism of clonal senesence (3).

In conclusion, we believe that the experiments we have cited count as strong evidence against somatic mutational theories of clonal senescene, certainly as it involves single copy DNA, although, as originally pointed out by Littlefield (13), one could not rule out a situation in which there were very large numbers of somatic mutations, such that complementation was not effective.

REFERENCES

1. G. M. Martin, Cellular aging--clonal senescence, Amer. J. Path. 89:484 (1977).
2. T. H. Norwood, Somatic cell genetics in the analysis of in vitro senescence, in:"Genetics of Aging," E. L. Schneider, ed., Plenum Press, New York (1978).
3. H. Hoehn, E. M. Bryant, and G. M. Martin, The replicative life spans of euploid hybrids derived from short-lived and long-lived human skin fibroblast cultures, Cytogenet. Cell Genet., 21:282 (1978).
4. E. M. Bryant, E. Crouch, P. Bornstein, G. M. Martin, P. Johnston, and H. Hoehn, Regulation of growth and gene activity in euploid hybrids between human neonatal fibroblasts and epithelioid amniotic fluid cells, Am. J. Hum. Genet., 30:392 (1978).
5. T. H. Norwood, C. J. Zeigler, and G. M. Martin, Dimethyl sulfoxide enhances polyethylene glycol mediated somatic cell fusion, Somat. Cell Genet. 2:263 (1976).
6 H. Hoehn, E. Bryant, L. Karp, and G. M. Martin, Cultivated cells from diagnostic amniocentesis in second trimester pregnancies. I. Clonal morphology and growth potential, Ped. Res. 8:746 (1974).
7. J. R. Smith and L. Hayflick, Variation in the life span of clones derived from human diploid cell strains, J. Cell Biol. 62:48 (1974).
8. L. H. Hartwell, Sequential function of gene products relative to DNA synthesis in the yeast cell cycle, J. Mol. Biol. 104:803 (1976).
9. R. M. Liskay and H. K. Meiss, Complementation between two temperature-sensitive mammalian cell mutants, each defective in G_1 phase of the cell cycle, Somat. Cell Genet. 3:343 (1977).
10. R. DeMars, Somatic cell mutations and cellular senescence, in: "Senescence Dominant or Recessive in Somatic Cell Crosses?" W. W. Nichols and D. G. Murphy, eds, Plenum Press, New York (1977).
11. S. Ohno and Y. Nagai, Genes in multiple copies as the primary cause of aging, in: "Genetic Effects on Aging, Birth Defects, Orig. Art. Series," Vol. XIV, Alan R. Liss, New York (1978).
12. L. E. Orgel, The maintenance of the accuracy of protein synthesis and its relevance to aging, Proc. Natl. Acad. Sci. USA 49:517 (1963).
13. J. W. Littlefield, Attempted hybridizations with senescent human fibroblasts, J. Cell Physiol. 82:129 (1973).

EPIDERMAL CARCINOGENESIS IN YOUNG AND AGING ANIMALS

P. Ebbesen

Department of Tumor Virus Research
Institute of Medical Microbiology
22 Juliane Maries vej
DK-2100 Copenhagen, Denmark

Spontaneous epidermal carcinomas show an age (t) related incidence (I) conforming to the following expression:

$$I = ct^b$$

(c and b are constants) (1). As an explanation of these age incidence curves, the local multistep mutation hypothesis (2) is widely, but not universally, accepted.

When it comes to epidermal carcinomas known to be elicited by external factors in adult humans, most studies indicate that the risk of cancer increases with the age of the first exposure (3-6), but that there are important exceptions (6,7).

Experimental studies on epidermal carcinogenesis in young adult and so-called old animals are numerous. However, in nearly all cases, young animals are compared with what should be called middle-aged animals--e.g., mice 14 months of age. About 80 per cent of a cohort of untreated animals will still be alive at 14 months, and this is comparable to a cohort of Danes of around 50 years of age. When such young and middle-aged animals are treated with skin paintings or irradiation, tumor incidence usually is unaffected by age (8).

However, if we turn to senescent animals, those left when 50 per cent have died (comparable to a 70-year-old cohort of humans), very little has been done in the way of studying epithelial carcinogenesis.

With mice, we have found senescent skin to be more susceptible to chemical carcinogen than middle-aged or young skin. Work in progress indicates the same to be the case when β-irradiation is used for tumor induction. By grafting skin from old donors to young recipients, we demonstrated that this increase in susceptiblity with advanced age also occurs when old skin is located on young syngeneic recipients. It therefore appears to be due to a local, autonomous aging process (9). This was further confirmed by the finding that skin of the same age grafted to young and old recipients remained equally susceptible (10).

What are the local, autonomous processes responsible for the increased susceptiblity of senescent skin? We do not know. One possibility is a spontaneous, stepwise alteration of normal cells, creating so-called variant cells which might need only a little further pushing to become malignant cells. This assumption would be in line with present knowledge about the persistent effect of carcinogen-initiators (11), and with the multistep hypothesis for spontaneous cancer development. There is, furthermore, in vivo evidence for the existence of such variant cells (12-14), and for variant cells being very susceptible to carcinogens (15). The apparent reversibility of in vivo malignancy, in certain cases (16,17), makes one wonder whether there exists a dynamic equilibrium between normal and cancer-like cells which shifts towards the abnormal, carcinogen-sensitive cells with aging, rather than a series of mutational events.

An alternative, or additional, explanation for the enhanced susceptiblity to carcinogen of senescent skin is some change in the intercellular regulatory mechanisms postulated to exist by Weiss and Kavanau (18).

We studied the effect on skin of young mice of a 30-50,000 MW extract of skin from old and young mice. Our finding was that while extract of young skin when injected intraperitoneally into young mice strongly inhibited mitosis of skin epithelial cells, extract of old skin, whether from an old mouse or a skin graft from an old donor on a young recipient, had hardly any inhibitory effect on young mice (19). In recently completed experiments, we found, furthermore, that the epithelial cells of middle-aged skin also react to intraperitoneal injection of extract from young skin with mitotic arrest. In contrast, senescent skin grafted on middle-aged recipients reacted with enhancement of the mitotic rate. And what was more surprising, this proliferative response to the extracts was also seen in the skin of middle-aged mice when the animals were carrying syngeneic grafts from senescent donors. Thus, extract of a young skin is likely to contain both a mitogen inhibitor and a mitogen stimulator; which one is dominating may depend on the age of the skin on which the test has been made (20). It may be pertinent to this that tumor cells growing in vivo (21) and in vitro (22) may lack mitotic inhibitor, and that injection of skin extract into carcinogen-treated skin may inhibit tumor development (23).

Summing up: 1) there is an enhanced susceptibility to carcinogen in senescent mouse skin which we believe should cause deliberations about safety regulations for humans; 2) both accumulation of variant cell and/or change in a local mitosis regulatory system should serve as working hypothesis for further studies.

REFERENCES

1. J. A. H. Lee, P. G. Chin, W. A. Kukull, R. S. Tompkins, and A. F. Wetherall, J. Natl. Cancer Inst. 57:753 (1976).
2. C. A. Nordling, Brit. J. Cancer 7:68 (1953)
3. R. A. M. Case, M. E. Hosker, D. B. McDonald, and J. T. Pearson, Brit. J. Industr. Med. 11:75 (1954).
4. R. E. W. Fisher, in:"Twelfth International Congress on Occupational Health," V. Kirjapaino, ed., Helsinski (1958).
5. J. F. Know, S. Holmes, R. Doll, and I. D. Hill, Brit. J. Industr. Med 25:293 (1968).
6. R. Doll, L. Morgan, and F. E. Speizer, Brit. J. Cancer 24:623 (1970).
7. D. H. McGregor, C. E. Land, K. Chorik, S. Tovokn, P. I. Liv, T. Wakabayashi, and G. W. Beebe, J. Natl. Cancer Inst 59:799 (1977).
8. R. Peto, F. J. C. Roe, P. N. Lee, L. Levy, and J. Clack, Brit. J. Cancer 32:411 (1975).
9. P. Ebbesen, Science 183:217 (1974).
10. P. Ebbesen, J. Natl. Cancer Inst. 58:1057 (1977).
11. I. Berenblum and P. Shubik, Brit. J. Cancer 3:383 (1949).
12. R. T. Prehn, Adv. Cancer Res. 23:203 (1976).
13. T.-W. Tao and M. M. Burger, Nature 270:437 (1977).
14. N. Haran-Ghera, J. Natl. Cancer Inst. 60:707 (1978).
15. P. M. Naha and M. Ashworth, Brit. J. Cancer 30:448 (1974).
16. G. B. Pierce, Amer. J. Pathol. 77:103 (1974).
17. M. C. Revilla, M. T. Gonzalez, M. Z. Balderas, and G. Romero, Nature 272:454 (1978).
18. P. Weiss and J. L. Kavanau, J. Gen Physiol. 41:1 (1957).
19. L. Olsson and P. Ebbesen, Exp. Gerontol. 12:59 (1977).
20. P. Ebbesen, L. Olsson, and C. Due, Exp. Gerontol. 13:365 (1978).
21. W. S. Bullough and J. U. R. Deol, Brit. J. Derm. 92:417 (1975).
22. P. Ebbesen and L. Olsson, in:"Antiviral Mechanisms in the Control of Neoplasia," P. Chandra, ed., NATO Advanced Study Center, Corfu, March 5-11, 1978.
23. S. A. Winkel and S. L. Smith, Nature 260:48 (1976).

TRANSLATIONAL ACTIVITY AND FIDELITY OF PURIFIED RIBOSOMES FROM AGING MOUSE LIVERS

Nozumi Mori, Den'ichi Mizuno, and Sataro Goto

Faculty of Pharmaceutical Sciences
University of Tokyo
Hongo, Bunko-ku, Tokyo, Japan

INTRODUCTION

Since early years of modern molecular biology, it has been suggested that there must be some functional changes in the flow of genetic information which are almost universal to any type of cells, and hence very likely to be a general cause of functional deterioration during the aging of animals (1,2). In fact, various aspects of transcription and translation have been studied in relation to both the aging of tissues in vivo and cells in culture (3,4).

Production and accumulation of defective proteins during aging appears to be of a rather general nature, and post-translational modifications have been suggested to be a major cause of protein alterations (5,6). In studies on viral infections, Pithe et al. (7) could not find the production of defective viral proteins by senescent fibroblasts in culture. However, it is not certain whether the frequency of translational error changes in tissues of old animals where post mitotic cells predominate.

We have previously reported that 18S ribosome RNA accumulates, relative to 28S ribosmal RNA, in the cytoplasm of some tissues during the aging of mice (8). This observation was confirmed by an experiment in which a greater accumulation of free small subunits was present in the cytoplasm, relative to that of large subunits (9). These observations raised the question as to whether or not there are any functional changes in ribosomes in aging tissues.

Table 1. Requirements for the Incorporation of Phenylalanine and Leucine in the Translation in Vitro (Mori et al., 1979).

Omission	^{14}C-Phenylalanine incorporated		^{3}H-Leucine incorprated	
	cpm	%control	cpm	%control
None	1245	100	5591	100
Ribosome	79	6	739	13
Factors	28	2	764	14
Poly(U)	63	5	1149	21
t-RNA	151	12	1327	24
$Mg(CH_3COO)_2$	45	4	723	13
Energy mixture	35	3	608	11

RESULTS AND DISCUSSION

Translational Activity of Purified Ribosomes

It is generally accepted that protein synthesis in vivo declines with age in amimals. Since Mainwaring (10) reported an age-associated decrease in the activity of translation in a cell-free system derived from mouse livers of various ages, several reports have appeared in which translational activity of microsomes or polysomes of tissues during aging have been shown to decline (11,12). However, the components of protein synthetic machinery that are responsible for this decrease in activity have not been identified in these studies.

We therefore examined whether the ribosome itself is responsible for the decrease (9). Ribosomes from mouse livers of various ages were purified by treatment with puromycin and a high salt medium. This type of purification has not been done in previous studies by other investigators (10,11,12). In each such experiment, ribosomes were prepared from each of three young and three old mice in parallel to minimize the possibility of artifacts being introduced by the preparation process. Ribosomes thus obtained were shown to be free from mRNA, peptidyl tRNA and factors necessary for translation, as shown in Table 1. Translational activity for these purified ribosomes was determined for poly(U)-dependent incorporation of phenylalanine, in the presence of aminoacyl tRNA synthetases and translational factors obtained from rabbit reticulocyte ribsomes as well as tRNAs prepared from young mouse livers. As shown in Table 2, translational efficiency of the ribosomes was usually lower in older animals, confirming reports by other investigators who have used more crude ribosome preparations (10,11,12). It should be noted that variation in this activity in old animals is much greater than that in young animals. This may indicate that variation at the translational level is a reflection of the variation of physiological age among old individuals. Since, in our study, components other than purified ribosomes were common in all assays, we may conclude that the decline in the activity of protein synthesis as animals age could be explained at least in part by the decreased activity of the ribosome itself. However, other components, such as tRNA, aminoacyl tRNA synthetases and translational factors, may also be responsible for the decline.

Coding Fidelity of Purified Ribosomes

The extent of mis-translation (i.e., mis-charging and mis-coding) may be increased by alterations in aminoacyl tRNA synthetases, tRNA, ribosomes and/or translational factors. Among these possibilities, we have examined whether there is any change in the level of mis-coding due to ribsomes during aging. As shown in Table 1, poly(U)-dependent incorporation of radioactive leucine, in the presence of sufficient amounts of non-radioactive phenylalanine, was dependent on components essential to translation. It was thus demonstrated that leucine was mis-incorporated into polypeptides, using a protein synthetic apparatus dependent on poly(U) that does not code for leucine. The level of mis-coding was defined as the molar ratio of leucine to phenylalanine incorporated in the standard assay system. Results of two sets of experiment are shown in Table 2. These data indicate that mis-coding was on the order of 10^{-3} under standard experimental conditions. We next examined the coding fidelity at various concentrations of magnesium ion, which is known to affect the activity and fidelity of translation *in vitro* (13,14). The incorporation of phenylalanine and leucine occurred at different optimal concentrations of the ion, and were independent of age. Thus, the level of coding fidelity of old ribosomes was essentially the same as that of young ribosomes. These findings do not necessarily exclude the possibility that changes occur in the fidelity of coding with age, because the fidelity *in vivo* should be much higher than that observed in the *in vitro* experiment where synthetic polymers were employed as a template. This point should be examined in more detail, using mRNA, which has natural initiation and termination codons.

The error frequency in translation during aging observed *in vitro* by other investigators (15,16), as well as by us, is summarized in Table 3. In all cases, the error was measured as the frequency of mis-incorporation of leucine in place of phenylalanine in a system for poly(U)-directed polypeptide synthesis. The results are not consistent with each other in either the level of error or the magnitude of the change with age. This could be due to differences in the assay system used, which may be critical for the fidelity of translation *in vitro*.

CONCLUSION

Functional alterations of purified ribosomes from mouse liver

Table 2. Summary of the Efficiency and the Coding Fidelity of Translation _in Vitro_ of Mouse Liver Ribosomes as Determined by Poly(U) Dependent Assay System.

Amount of amino acid incorporated is expressed as pmoles per A260 unit of ribosome per 40 min. Infidelity level is the molar ratio of leucine to phenylalanine incorporated. av. ± S.D.: average ± standard deviation. (Mori et al., 1979)

	age of mouse	phenylalanine incorporated	av. ± S.D.	leucine incorporated	infidelity level ($\times 10^{-3}$)	av. ± S.D.
Exp.1	Young 2 mon.	9.8		0.108	11.9	
	2 mon.	13.5	11.6 ± 1.9	0.124	9.3	9.8 ± 1.9
	2 mon.	11.5		0.093	8.1	
	Old 21 mon.	6.4		0.411	62.5	
	22 mon.	10.2	6.8 ± 3.3	0.096	9.4	18.5 ± 21.6
	22 mon.	3.7		0.037	9.9	
Exp.2	Young 2 mon.	14.8		0.087	5.8	
	2 mon.	15.6	14.3 ± 1.6	0.096	6.1	5.7 ± 0.4
	2 mon.	12.5		0.066	5.3	
	Old 15 mon.	8.5		0.026	3.1	
	19 mon.	11.1	11.9 ± 3.9	0.037	3.3	4.9 ± 1.4
	19 mon.	16.1		0.100	6.3	

Table 3. Fidelity of Translation in vitro as Determined by Poly (U) Dependent Phenylalanine or Leucine Incorporation. The level of error is shown as molar ratio of leucine to phenylalanine incorporated (x 10^{-3}).

animal and tissue (age)	system	level of error	reference
mouse liver (2 mon. vs. 31 mon.)	microsome chick embryo factors E.coli amino acyl tRNA 4 mM Mg++	100 vs. 70	Kurtz,1975
rat liver (3 mon. vs. 12 mon.)	ribosome corresponding pH 5 fraction 10 mM Mg++	0.2 vs. 0.6	Mariotti and Ruscitto,1977
mouse liver (2 mon. vs. 22 mon.)	ribosome mouse tRNA rabbit reticulocyte factors 10 mM Mg++	7 vs. 6	Mori et al,1979

were examined in relation to the age of the experimental animals. This study suggests that an age-associated decline in protein synthetic activity can be ascribed, at least in part, to the ribosome itself. The coding fidelity of ribosomes does not change with age in our poly(U)-dependent assay system.

Obviously, additional studies are required, using natural mRNA as a template, to further define age-associated alterations of components in each step of translation.

REFERENCES

1. Z. A. Medvedev, Ageing at the molecular level, in:"Biolgical Aspects of Ageing," N. W. Shock, ed., Columbia University Press, New York (1962).
2. L. E. Orgel, The maintencance of the accuracy of protein synthesis and its relevance to ageing, Proc. Nat. Acad. Sci. U.S.A. 49:517 (1963).
3. R. G. Cutler, in:"Interdisciplinary Topics in Gerontology," H. P. von Hahn, ed., Vol. 9 and 10, S. Karger, Basel (1976).
4. F. M. Sinex, The molecular genetics of aging, in:"Handbook of the Biology of Aging," C. E. Finch and L. Hayflick, eds., Van Nostrand Reinhold Co., New York (1977).
5. D. Gershon, Current status of age altered enzymes: Alternative mechanisms, Mech. Ageing Dev. 9:189 (1979).
6. M Rothstein, The formation of altered enzymes in aging animals, Mech. Ageing Dev. 9:197 (1979).

7. J. Pitha, E. Stork, and E. Wimmer, Protein synthesis during aging of human cells in culture, Exp. Cell Res. 94:310 (1975).
8. N. Mori, D. Mizuno, and S. Goto, Increase in the ratio of 18S RNA to 28S RNA in the cytoplasm of mouse tissues during ageing, Mech. Ageing Dev. 8:285 (1978).
9. N. Mori, D. Mizuno, and S. Goto, Conservation of ribosomal fidelity during ageing, Mech. Ageing Dev. 10:379 (1979).
10. W. I. P. Mainwaring, The effect of age on protein synthesis in mouse liver, Biochem. J. 113:869 (1969).
11. G. W. Britton and F. G. Sherman, Altered regulation of protein synthesis during aging as determined by in vitro ribosomal assays, Exp. Gerontol. 10:67 (1975).
12. D. K. Layman, G. A. Ricca, and A. Richardson, The effect of age on protein synthesis and ribosome aggregation to messenger RNA in rat liver, Arch. Biochem. Biophys. 173:246 (1976).
13. J. M. Gilbert and W. F. Anderson, Cell-free hemoglobin synthesis. II. Characterization of the transfer ribonucleic acid-dependent assay system. J. Biol. Chem. 245:2342 (1970).
14. M. R. Capecchi, Polarity in vitro, J. Mol. Biol. 30:213 (1967).
15. D. I. Kurtz, The effect of ageing on in vitro fidelity of translation in mouse liver, Biochim Biophys. Acta 407:479 (1975).
16. D. Mariotti and R. Ruscitto, Age-related changes of accuracy and efficiency of protein synthesis machinery in rat, Biochim. Biophys. Acta 475:96 (1977).

INTERACTION OF HORMONES WITH RECEPTORS AND ALTERATIONS OF THESE PROCESSES WITH AGE

George Roth

Gerontology Research Center
Baltimore, Maryland

INTRODUCTION

We have been studying alterations in hormone action during the aging process. If one looks in the literature at studies of hormonal responses during aging, it becomes readily apparent that many responses at both the physiological and biochemical levels have been observed to change (for reviews, see refs. 1 and 2). In many cases, the changes are in a negative direction: decreased responsiveness or decreased sensitivity to various hormones. In some cases, however, there is no change; and in a few situations there may actually be increases in sensitivity. However, the large majority of changes for many different hormones, target cells, and tissues are post-maturational reductions in responsivenss.

In order to better understand the mechanisms involved in such changes, we are using the knowledge gained by endocrinologists, biochemists, and molecular biologists, who have elucidated the mechanisms of the hormone action at the cellular or molecular levels, independent of aging. These are rather complex processes, with many molecular events occurring between the time that the hormone reaches the cell and the time that the final biological effect is elicited. We can make some generalizations, however, especially in the case of the initial event--attachment of hormones to specific cellular receptors. These receptors can be located on the cell surface, as is the case of the catecholamines, glucagon, or insulin. Alternatively, receptors can be located inside the cell, as is the case with the steroid and thyroid hormones. Subsequent to this initial interaction, many other biochemical events occur. There are age changes in many of these intercellular events, but for the purposes of this paper, I am going to limit discussion to the interactions of hormones with receptors, and to how these processes change during aging.

HISTORICAL BACKGROUND

I want to briefly review some of the studies of hormone receptors during the aging process. I have grouped these studies of changes in hormone receptors during aging into four categories. The first of these are those studies that show hormone receptor concentrations which decrease during senescence (Table 1). (References to all the cases cited in Tables 1-4 can be found in reference 2). In essentially all the studies mentioned here, the changes in receptors that occur are in the apparent concentration of quantity of the receptors, rather than in the binding affinity or in the tightness of the fit. Those hormone receptors which are present in old cells and tissues are just as capable of binding the hormone as are those present in the young tissues.

The first group of hormones listed here (in Table 1) are the steroids. Studies have taken place using many tissues. Also shown are some correlations between biological responsiveness and changes in receptor concentrations that have been carried out in some of these tissues. The reader will notice some apparent conflicts, contradictions or discrepancies in Tables 1-4. This is typical of aging research in general. Possible reasons for these particular disagreements have been discussed elsewhere (2). Changes have also been reported for some hormone receptors that are located on the cell surface, such as those for insulin, the adrenergic agents, acetylcholine, gonadotropin, and dopamine.

In the case of some hormone receptor changes which occur during senescence, changes are progressive over the entire life span. It is interesting to note that if one compares the relative decreases in different species with different maximal or different mean life spans (for example, in two rat strains, in the rabbit or in the human) that the relative uptake or binding loss is, in many cases, fairly comparably expressed as a function of the percentage of the life span completed (Fig. 1). So, this may indicate that there is some genetic specificity and that the changes that occur are not simply thermodynamic, but do have something to do with the life span of the species.

Some receptors have been reported to change only during early adulthood or else have not been examined during the latter phase of the life span (Table 2). Again, many different tissues, species, and hormones have been studied.

Table 3 shows some receptor studies in which no changes have been reported. A few of these are similar to some of the systems in which changes have been reported. As mentioned above, possible reasons for

Table 1. Decreases in Hormone Receptor Concentrations During Senescence

Hormone Receptor	Tissue or Cell	Species	Concomitantly Reduced Biological Response
Corticosteroid)	Splenic lymphocytes	Rat	Inhibition of uridine uptake
	Cerebral Cortex	Rat	
	Cortical Neurons	Rat	
	Skeletal Muscle	Rat	
	Adipose Tissue	Rat	
	Adipocytes	Rat	Inhibition of glucose oxidation
	Liver	Human	
	Skin Fibroblasts (WI-38)	Human	Prolongation of *in vitro* life span
Androgen)	Liver	Rat	Induction of α2μ globulin
	Ventral Prostate	Rat	Maintainance of cell content
	Lateral Prostate	Rat	
	Hypothalamus	Rat	
	Pituitary	Rat	
	Testes	Rat	
Estrogen)	Uterus	Rat	Induction of phospho-fructokinase
	Uterus	Mouse	
	Brain	Rat	Induction of acetylcholin-esterase
Insulin)	Skin Fibroblasts	Human	Stimulation of glucose uptake
β-adrenergic)	Lymphocytes	Human	
	Adipocytes	Rat	Lipolysis
	Cerebellum	Rat	
	Corpus Striatum	Rat	
Acetylcholine)	Cerebral Cortex	Rat	
	Cerebellar Cortex	Rat	
Gonadotropin)	Testes	Rat	
Dopamine)	Corpus Striatum	Rat	Induction of turning behavior
Low Density Lipoprotein)	Lung Fibroblasts (WI-38)	Human	

these discrepancies have been discussed elsewhere. Table 4 shows some actual increases in receptor levels during senescence. Thus, a whole spectrum of observations exists: decreases during the entire life span, decreases early in the life span, no change, and actual increases.

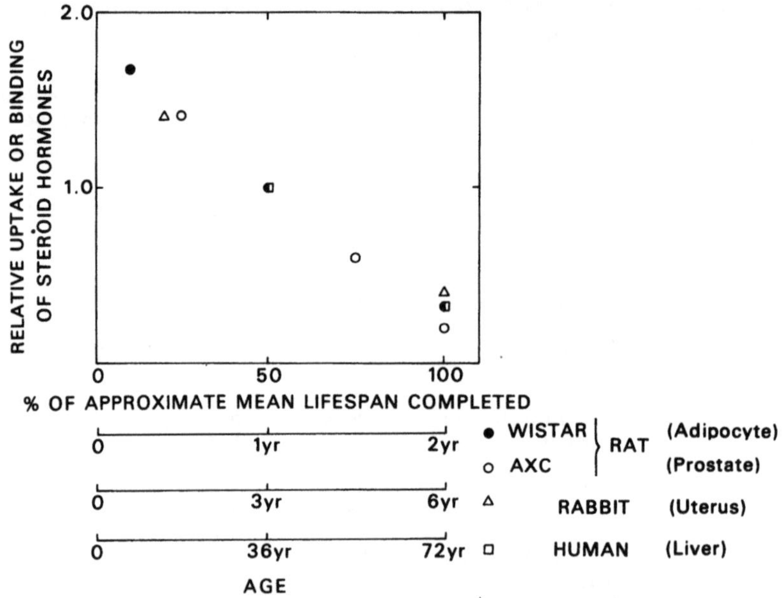

Fig. 1. Representative age changes in steroid hormone uptake or binding in different species. Receptor concentrations or uptake rates for steroid hormones were compared in different genotypes. Values obtained for the 50% point of mean life span were arbitrarily classified as 1.0. Data are adapted from studies cited in ref. 2.

At this point, I would like to focus on one or two studies in which we have been involved. One of them deals with the membrane-associated hormone receptors and the other with intercellular receptors. Many investigators have reported that the ability of adenylate cyclases in various brain regions to respond to dopamine changes with increasing age (see ref. 1). The maximal response seems to be progressively reduced with increasing age in most studies. Several species have now been examined with respect to dopaminergic stimulation of adenylate cyclase in the corpus striatum. These include mice, rats and rabbits.

METHODS AND RESULTS

In collaboration with our behavioral group at the Gerontology Research Center, we examined the concentration of dopaminergic receptors in the corpus striatum region of the brain, as well as some dopaminergic behavioral modifications (3). We used ^{3}H-haloperidol as the ligand for receptor binding studies. At the time the work was done (several years ago), many groups were using this compound, which is a potent dopaminergic antagonist. More recently, spiroperidol, a much more specific ligand, has been employed. The data were analyzed

Table 2. Decreases in Hormone Receptor Concentrations During Early Adulthood

Hormone Receptor	Tissue or Cell	Species	Concomitantly Reduced Biological Response
Corticosteroid)	Liver	Rat	
	Thymus	Rat	
Androgen)	Cerebral Cortex	Rat	
Insulin)	Liver	Rat	
β-andrenergic	Erythrocyte	Rat	Stimulation of adenylate cyclase
	Pineal	Rat	
Glucagon)	Adipocyte	Rat	Stimulation of lipolysis
Prolactin)	Prostate	Rat	
	Seminal Vesicles	Rat	
Thyroid)	Cerebral Hemisphesis	Rat	

Table 3. Unaltered Hormone Receptor Concentrations During Adulthood

Hormone Receptor	Tissue or Cell	Species
Corticosteroid)	Liver	Rat
	Liver	Mouse
	Cerebral Cortex	Mouse
	Hypothalamus	Mouse
	Hippocampus	Mouse
Androgen)	Anterior Prostate	Rat
	Dorsal Prostate	Rat
	Seminal Vesicles	Rat
	Prostate	Dog
Insulin)	Liver	Mouse
	Heart	Mouse
β-adrenergic)	Cerebral Cortex	Rat
Low Density Lipoprotein)	Skin Fibroblasts	Human
Growth Hormone)	Liver	Mouse

Table 4. Increases in Hormone Receptor Concentrations During Senescence

Hormone Receptor	Tissue or Cell	Species
Androgen)	Seminal Vesicles	Rat
Estrogen)	Seminal Vesicles	Rat
Insulin)	Skin Fibroblasts	Human
Epidermal Growth Factor)	Lung Fibroblasts (WI-38)	Human

by the method of Scatchard (4), plotting the bound over free hormone concentration as a function of the bound concentration (Fig. 2). These were experiments in which crude membrane preparations were incubated with various concentrations of ^{3}H-ligand. Non-specific binding was determined by competition with excess unlabeled dopamine. From such analysis, one can see that the concentration of receptors (as taken from the intercept on the abscissa) is reduced about 35% between 6 months to 25 months of age. Wistar rats from the Gerontology Research Center were used in these experiments. The slopes of the two lines are not significantly different, indicating no change in binding affinity. When data were obtained from six experiments using these two age groups, no change in binding efficiency, but a significant 40% reduction in the concentration of the receptors, was detected. This is roughly comparable to the reduction in the ability of dopamine to stimulate adenylate cyclase. More recently, confirming data have been obtained from the laboratory of Finch using mice (5) and Makman using rabbits (6). Both groups have employed the newer tritiated dopaminergic antagonist, spiroperidol.

Under these conditions, one observes much less non-specific binding, and is able to generate more precise data. Data from all three laboratories are basically in agreement that this particular receptor is lost with age. The loss is probably closely related to the loss in ability to stimulate adenylate cyclase, as reported by many investigators

Now, I would like to deal with the system on which we are spending more of our time. This is the rat epididymal fat pad adipocyte and the effect of glucocorticoid hormones, which work through intracellular receptor systems. Two rat strains have been employed, the CD Sprague-Dawley from Charles River Breeding

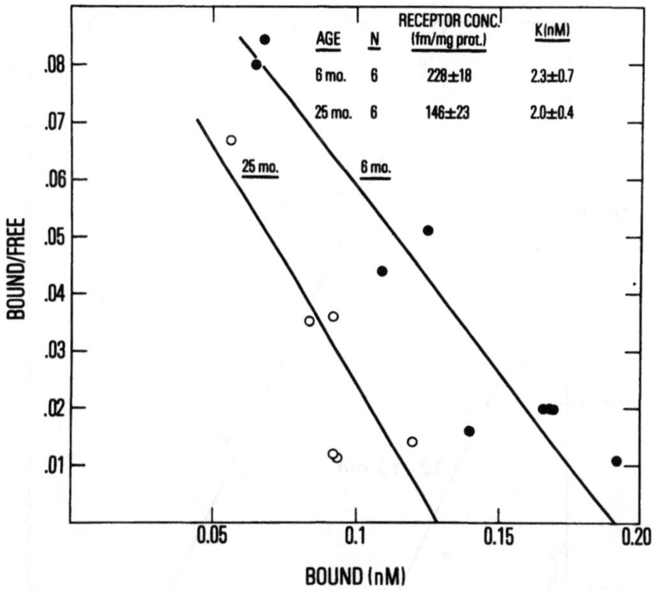

Fig. 2. Scatchard analysis of ^{3}H-haloperidol specific binding to crude membranes of rat corpus striatum. Binding studies were performed as described in ref. 3. Statistics from 6 individual experiments are pictured in the inset.

Laboratories, as well as our own Wistar strain. Two strains are utilized, since they exhibit different patterns of adipocyte size increase (7). In the Sprague-Dawley rat, the epididymal fat pad adipocytes continue to increase in size throughout the life span, whereas in Gerontology Research Center Wistar rats, hypertrophy ceases after roughly 4-6 months of age; and one can compare the mature and senescent animals without having to worry about the effects of cell size superimposed on the effects of cell age.

Another reason we chose the epididymal fat pad adipocyte system is that it is a relatively static postmitotic cell system. Cell numbers remain relatively constant throughout the life, so one can be reasonably confident of dealing with the same population of cells in the senescent animals as in the young animals. We don't have to worry about complex shifts in cell populations, so we can be relatively confident that the change we are looking at is restricted to this particular cell type, rather than including the loss of a small population of hormone responsive cells. We have examined glucocorticoid receptor levels by the method of Scatchard (4) in cells of three age groups (Fig. 3). As with the dopamine receptors mentioned above, there is no change in the slope, therefore, no change in the binding affinity. However, there is a progressive reduction with increasing age in the apparent concentration of receptor sites.

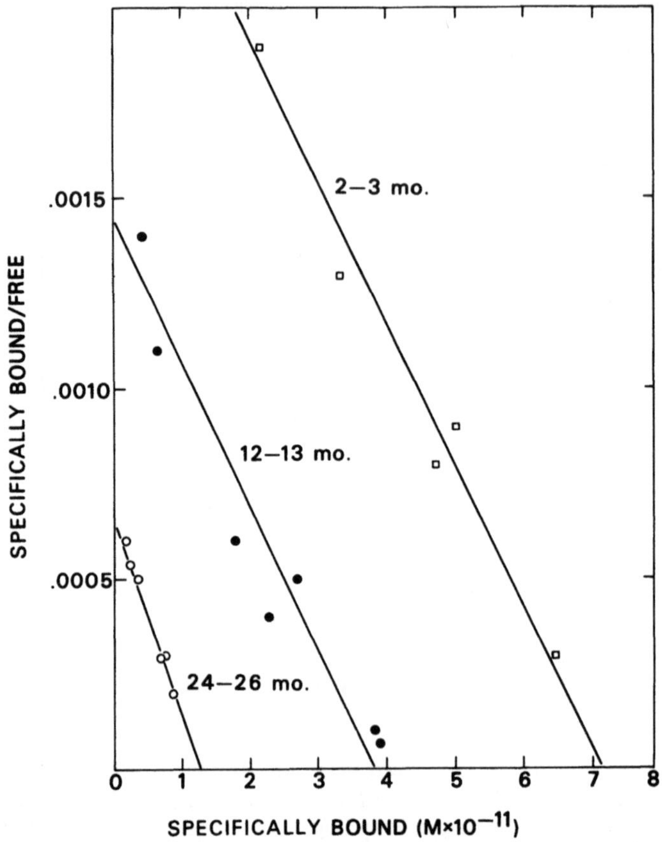

Fig. 3. Scatchard analyses of specific glucocorticoid binding in adipocyte cytosols. Cytosols of adipocytes from 2-3 mo. (□), 12-13 mo. (●), and 24-26 mo. (○). Wistar rats were prepared, and specific dexamethasone binding was assessed as described in ref. 7.

We are also interested--in fact, more interested--in the action of the hormone and how it changes with age. Thus, we have examined one particular response of adipocytes to glucocorticoid hormones, the ability of glucocorticoids to inhibit the rate of glucose utilization by these cells. Dexamethasone is the synthetic glucocorticoid that we used for this effect. We measured the ability of this synthetic corticoid to inhibit glucose oxidation in fat cells from the three age groups. Again, as with the dopamine-sensitive adenylate cyclase data shown above, progressive reduction with increasing age in glucocorticoid responsiveness is also observed (Fig. 4).

Figure 5 shows some statistics with respect to the reduction in binding sites for glucocorticoid hormone receptors in the three age

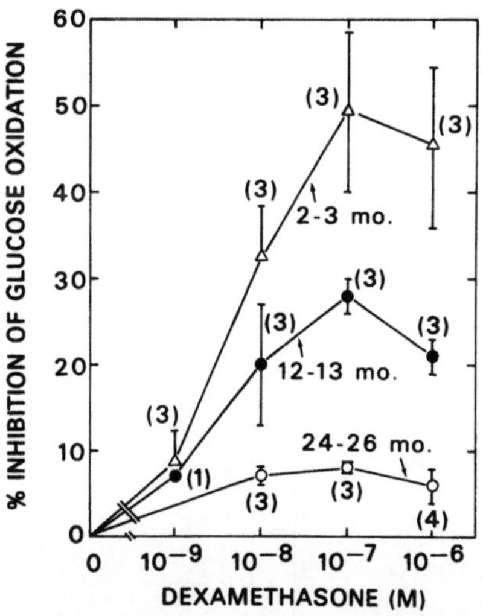

Fig. 4. Effect of dexamethasone concentration on inhibition of glucose oxidation in young, mature, and senescent rat adipocytes. Dexamethasone inbibition of glucose oxidation in Wistar rat adipocytes was determined as in ref. 7. Values are the mean ± standard errors for the number of experiments in parentheses.

groups and the reductions in the ability of the hormone to inhibit glucose utilization. There is a fairly close relationship between the two. In fact, it has been demonstrated that if the receptors are blocked with other types of steroids, they are inactive with respect to this particular response. No dexamethasone effect can be observed. So, there appears to be very close, if not causal, relationship between the receptor and the response loss.

DISCUSSION

Now, I would like to digress a bit, using the same system to discuss what we feel is the change in the cell membrane which may in part contribute to some of the change in responsiveness to glucocorticoid. For a number of reasons, we were enticed to look a little bit more closely at the changes that occur between young adulthood and maturity, although this is not the true senescence phase of the life span. In looking at the literature, we realized that many people felt that the effect of glucocorticoid hormones on glucose metabolism was secondary to inhibition of the glucose transport system within the cell membrane. In other words, people felt that any inhibition of glucose oxidation was simply the consequence of the reduced entry of glucose into the cell in the presence of dexamethasone. Indeed, if one looks at the effect of dexamethasone on both

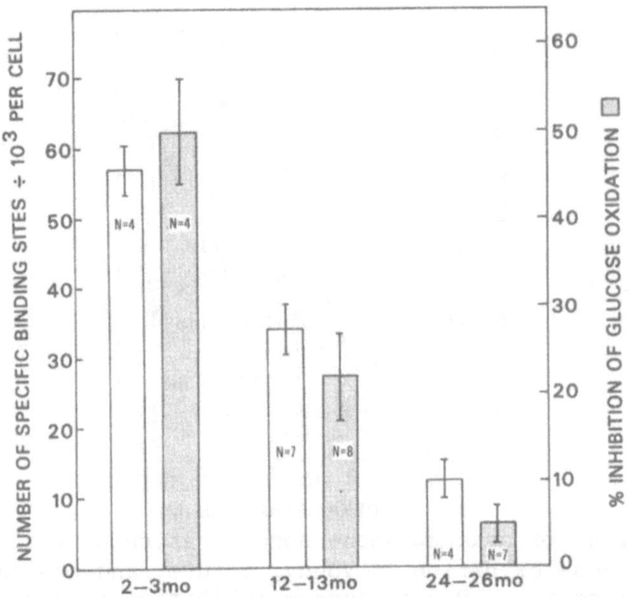

Fig. 5. Effect of age on glucocorticoid receptor concentration and inhibition of glucose oxidation in rat adipocytes. Data as for Figs. 3 and 4 were compiled for the number of experiments shown inside the bars. Values are the means ± standard errors.

glucose transport and metabolism in cells from the young 2-3 month old animals, there is essentially no difference in the response curves. However, if one looks at the mature animals, one still can get a pretty good effect on inhibition of glucose by dexamethasone, but there is no effect on glucose transport (Fig. 6). This suggests that the two processes may be dissociable, at least under conditions of increased age or increased cell size. In the senescent animals, there is a statistically significant dexamethasone effect on glucose oxidation, but again, no effect on the transport system (8).

The possibility exists that this apparent decrease in the ability of dexamethasone to effect transport has something to do with the metabolism of glucose. We therefore used two other glucose analogs, 2-deoxyglucose and 3-O methyl glucose, both of which are either minimally metabolized or not metabolized at all, and repeated our experiments. Again we found large inhibition of sugar transport in the young animals, but essentially no effect at all in the mature or senescent animals.

We can also express our data in terms of molecules of glucose which are either taken into the cell or metabolized. These basal

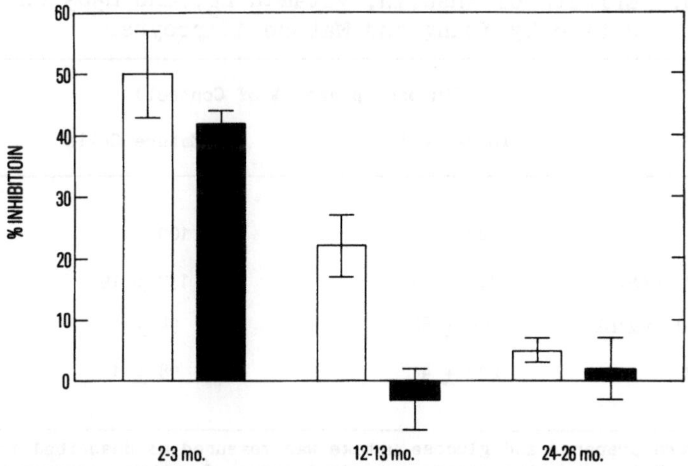

Fig. 6. Effect of age on the ability of dexamethasone to inhibit glucose transport and metabolism. Effects of dexamethasone on adipocyte glucose transport and metabolism were determined as described in ref. 8. Values are the means ± standard errors for 3-8 separate experiments for each group. Open bars, glucose oxidation; shaded bars, glucose transport.

levels of glucose uptake are essentially unchanged with age, so that when we express our values as percentages, we might equally well express them in terms of absolute molecules of sugar transported or metabolized. Thus, the effect that we observed is not due to some intrinsic change in the basal rate of transport of metabolism.

Since in the mature animals, there did not appear to be any effect of dexamethasone on glucose transport, we examined the glucose phosphorylation system. In the 2-3 month old animals, there is a very good correlation between the inhibition of glucose oxidation and the inhibition of glucose phosphorylation. This, of course, is due to the fact that transport is inhibited. However, in the mature 12 to 13 month old animals, where there is no effect at all of dexamethasone on glucose transport, we do observe that the effect on glucose phosphorylation is comparable to the amount of inhibition of glucose oxidation. Thus, there appears to be some sort of compensatory mechanism whereby the phosphorylation step is independently effected by dexamethasone. We don't know the mechanism here, but this does appear to account for the fact that one can still inhibit glucose oxidation without inhibiting transport in these older cells.

We think that the insensitivity to dexamethasone that we see is the consequence of the generalized refractoriness of the membrane with increasing age or increasing cell size. Other agents which can

Table 5. Effects of Insulin, Vitamin K_5, and H_2O_2 on Glucose Uptake by Young and Mature Adipocytes

Addition	Glucose Uptake (% of Control)	
	Young Cells	Mature Cells
None	100	100
Insulin, 500 μU/ml	467 ± 51	132 ± 19
Vitamin K_5, 10 μg/ml	559 ± 62	94 ± 1
H_2O_2, 0.3 mM	222 ± 4	98 ± 1

Adipocytes were prepared and glucose uptake was measured as described in reference 8. Values are the means ± standard errors for three experiments.

moderate glucose transport are also less effective in older animals (Table 5). Insulin, vitamin K-5, and hydrogen peroxide, all of which stimulate the glucose transport system, show this decreased sensitivity.

We are now interested in possible molecular mechanisms that might be involved in these changes, such as reduced rates of glucocorticoid receptor synthesis, increased rates of receptor degradation, malformation or blocking of aged receptors, and possible neuroendocrine-systemic mechanisms that may be involved.

SUMMARY

A variety of hormone receptor concentrations appear to decrease during aging. Such reductions seem to be closely, if not causally, related to reduced responsiveness. The receptors appear to be lost from target cells during aging. The simple loss of target cells from target tissues is not a sufficient explanation for decreased hormone concentrations, since we can observe these changes in static cell populations. Currently, we are attempting to elucidate the molecular and neuroendocrine mechanisms that are involved in these changes, and we would like to apply some of the mechanisms of hormone receptor control to these problems of altered responsiveness.

REFERENCES

1. G. S. Roth, Mech. Ageing Dev. 9:497 (1979).
2. G. S. Roth, Fed. Proc. (in press).

3. J. A. Joseph, R. E. Berger, B. T. Engel, and G. S. Roth, J. Gerontol. 33:643 (1978).
4. G. Scatchard, Ann. N.Y. Acad. Sci. 51:660 (1949).
5. C. E. Finch (personal communication).
6. M. H. Makman, H. S. Alin, L. J. Thal, N. Sharpless, B. Dvorkin, S. G. Horowitz, and M. Rosenfeld, Fed. Proc. (in press).
7. G. S. Roth and J. N. Livingston, Endocrinology 99:831 (1976).
8. G. S. Roth and J. N. Livingston, Endocrinology (in press).

CELLS, SIGNALS, AND RECEPTORS: THE ROLE OF PHYSIOLOGICAL AUTOANTIBODIES IN MAINTAINING HOMEOSTASIS

Marguerite M.B. Kay

Laboratory of Molecular and Clinical Immunology
Geriatric Research, Education and Clinical Center (691/11G)
V.A. Wadsworth Medical Center
Los Angeles, California 90073, USA

INTRODUCTION

Macrophages can distinguish mature "self" from senescent "self" cells. This is reflected by their ability to phagocytize cells which have reached the end of their functional lifespan, while sparing the mature cells. For example, mononuclear phagocytes of the liver and spleen remove syngeneic lymphocytes as well as antibody-coated red blood cells (RBC) (1,2,3). Erythrophagocytosis also occurs in lymph nodes (4). Studies on the fate of aged RBC indicate that they are eliminated intracellularly by mononuclear phagocytes rather than by osmotic lysis both in vitro and in situ (5 6,7,8,9). In this way, mononuclear phagocytes may perform an essential homeostatic role by permitting the more efficient mature cells to carry out their vital functions without hindrance from the less efficient senescent cells, or by preventing pathological reactions which could arise as a consequence of senescent cells dying and decaying within the organism.

The mechanism by which macrophages make such a fine distinction between mature and senescent cells has fascinated and eluded biologists for years. This paper summarizes my investigations into the mechanisms by which macrophages may make this distinction.

Initially, I hypothesized that Ig in normal human serum attaches to the surface of senescent RBC until a critical level is reached which results in phagocytosis (3,10). Human RBC were utilized as a model system because mononuclear phagocytes routinely phagocytize RBC at the end of their 120-day lifespan and because they are an ideal experimental system in many respects. Large numbers of RBC are readily available, and senescent cells can be easily separated from mature cells. RBC membranes have been extensively characterized biochemically and they have a smooth regular surface which does not "cap" or ingest labels.

MATERIALS AND METHODS

Isolation of Ig from old RBC. Blood was obtained from 41 healthy individuals. Young RBC were removed, and the remaining RBC were washed 3 times with 50 volumes of phosphate buffered saline (PBS), pH 7.4. Ig was eluted from 50-250 ml of packed RBC by the method of Kochwa and Rosenfield (11), as methods of elution which did not result in dissociation of antigen-antibody bonds (e.g., temperature and glycine-NaOH buffer, pH 8), did not result in Ig elution in our hands. Preliminary experiments indicated that Ig could be eluted from old, but not young, RBC. The RBC eluate from 31 individuals was assessed without further purification. Antibody from the RBC eluates of each of 10 individuals was isolated with an anti-Fab immunoabsorbent column. Fab was obtained from normal human IgG by papain digestion and column chromatography (12,13, An Chaun Wang, personal communication). Purity was determined by immunodiffusion (ID), immunoelectrophoresis (IEP), and polyacrylamide gel electrophoresis (PAGE). Antisera to Fab was obtained by immunizing a goat with eight weekly injections of 1 mg of pure Fab, as determined by ID and IEP. After 10 weeks, the goat was bled and the immune serum incubated with an immunoabsorbent that was made by binding Fab covalently to Sepharose 4B through a 13 atom spacer (aminohexyl derivative of Sepharose 4B; 14). After thorough washing, the beads were poured into a 7.5 ml glass column (Bio Rad) and the antibodies specific for Fab were eluted with 0.1 M glycine-HCl, pH 2.3. The eluted antibody, determined with a recording spectrophotometer, was neutralized with 1 N NaOH, concentrated, and dialysed against PBS, pH 7.4. The anti-Fab antibodies obtained by this procedure were specific for Fab and reacted with pure IgA and IgM as well as IgG, as determined by ID and IEP. Conversely, specific anti-IgA, IgG, and IgM reagents reacted only with the specific Ig class. Anti-Fab specific antibodies were coupled to aminohexyl Sepharose 4B and used to isolate Ig from RBC eluates. The Ig was eluted from the anti-Fab column in the same manner as described for anti-Fab antibodies, then concentrated with an Amicon Diaflow with PM 10 filter. The quantity of IgG eluted per ml of packed RBC was 270 $\pm$ 60 ng (mean $\pm$ std. error), as determined by radial immunodiffusion with Ultra Low Level Diffu-gen plates, lot #55822, Oxford Laboratories, Foster City, Calif.

Mononuclear phagocytes. Mononuclear cells from human peripheral blood were isolated on "Lymphoprep" and washed three times with Medium 199. The percentage of mononuclear phagocytes was determined by spreading an aliquot of mononuclear cells on a slide, or by making a cytocentrifuge preparation of mononuclear cells and staining with May-Gruenwald-Giemsa or with esterase (15), and performing differential cell counts with a 64X or 100X oil immersion objective (Zeiss). The number of mononuclear phagocytes was calculated by multiplying the total number of mononuclear cells times the percentage of mononuclear phagocytes. Polymorphonuclear leukocyte contamination was less than 1%. Mononuclear cells were diluted with bicarbonate buffered Medium 199 with Methicillin/Gentamycin (100 μg/ml) and glutamine so that the concentration of mononuclear phagocytes was 6-10 x 10^5/ml, and 1 ml was pipetted into each tube. After a 1 hr incubation at 37°C in an atmosphere of humidified air containing 5% CO^2, nonadherent cells were removed by vigorous washing.

<u>Phagocytosis assay</u>. The phagocytosis assay utilized for these studies measured phagocytosis rather than attachment, osmotic lysis, or adhesion of RBC to glass tubes. Light microscopy and transmission electron microscopy of cultures after 30 mins and 3 hrs demonstrated that RBC in various stages of degradation were present inside mononuclear phagocytes with some phagocytes having as many as 20 RBC inside them (16). Scanning electron microscopy of the cultures after 3 hrs demonstrated that only RBC which were partially engulfed were visible on the surface (16). When young RBC were added to 20 tubes containing mononuclear phagocytes, 100% of the RBC were recovered 3 hrs later. When RBC stored without Ig were added to 16 tubes containing mononuclear phagocytes, 98-100% of the RBC were recovered 3 hrs later. Negative controls were utilized throughout the study. These included young RBC, RBC aged *in vitro* and incubated in medium <u>without</u> serum or in Ig depleted serum, neuraminidase treated RBC incubated in culture medium, and young RBC incubated in allogeneic Ig eluted from senescent cells. These cells were not phagocytized, as indicated by the recovery rates noted above. Mononuclear phagocyte viability at the end of culture was 98-100% as determined by trypan blue dye exclusion.

<u>Young and senescent RBC</u>. RBC from freshly drawn blood were depleted of white cells and reticulocytes, then separated into young, middle-aged and old (senescent) populations by their differences in density (17). At the end of the density separation, young RBC are at the top of the gradient and the old RBC are at the bottom, as determined by the distribution of recently synthesized Fe-labeled RBC (18).

<u>Stored RBC</u>. Freshly isolated young RBC were washed 3 times with 50 volumes of Medium 199, resuspended at a concentration of 10% in Medium 199 without serum, to avoid IgG binding, or alpha minimum essential medium (AMEM) with 10% fetal calf serum (FCS), and transferred to tissue culture flasks. RBC were stored for 2-4 wks at 4°C.

Not all of the RBC populations were needed for the purpose of these experiments. Those in excess of the required numbers remained in storage for a total of five months. When these cells were subsequently examined, it was found that all old RBC and approximately half of the middle-aged RBC had lysed. The young RBC populations, however, were essentially free of lysed cells. This reaffirms that the method of cell separation employed in the present experiment is successful and that different cell populations have different membrane properties. It suggests that storage of RBC *in vitro* may be a reasonable parallel model for aging *in vivo*, because young RBC survive at least 150 days, and that old RBC have the potential for lysis if stored, without macrophages, for an extended period of time. It is possible that the mechanism by which membrane lesions are generated during storage *in vitro* may not be the same as that by which lesions are generated *in vivo* as cells age. However, the lesions themselves may be identical.

Incubation of RBC with Ig eluted from senescent cells. Stored RBC were washed and resuspended to a concentration of 1.5-2.0 x 10^9 RBC per ml. Twenty micrograms of Ig were added to 1 ml of the cell suspension, which was incubated at 37°C for 30-60 mins in a shaking water bath. The RBC were then washed three times with medium and incubated with mononuclear phagocytes. Approximately 10-15 RBC were added per phagocyte and the volume was adjusted to 0.24-0.40 ml per tube. Following incubation for three hours at 37°C, the percent of phagocytized RBC was calculated as described previously (3). This culture method supports a maximum of ≃ 50% phagocytosis.

The maximum percent phagocytosis obtainable appears to be limited by depletion of nutrients in the media. Addition of new medium at the end of 3 hrs results in additional phagocytosis of RBC: 46 ± 11% of the RBC were phagocytized during 6 hrs when new media was *not* added, whereas 61 ± 2% were phagocytized when new media was added after the first 3 hr incubation. If old RBC are added to cultures that have been incubated without RBC for the first 3 hrs, without changing media, there is no significant phagocytosis (only 8 ± 7% of the RBC were phagocytized). Finally, an additional 40 ± 3% of the old RBC, harvested from cultures after a 3 hr incubation, are phagocytized when added to new cultures with fresh media.

Neuraminidase treated RBC. Freshly isolated young RBC were washed 3 times with 50 volumes of Medium 199; incubated with 3.35 units of *Vibrio cholerae* neuraminidase (Behring Diagnostics, which was tested and found to be lipase and protease free) per 10^{10} RBC at 37°C in PBS, pH 6.8, for 30-60 min; and washed again. They were incubated in Medium 199 containing 20 μg of either autologous or allogeneic Ig eluted from senescent cells, washed 3 times, and incubated with autologous mononuclear phagocytes.

Scanning Immunoelectron Microscopy. Aliquots of the RBC used in

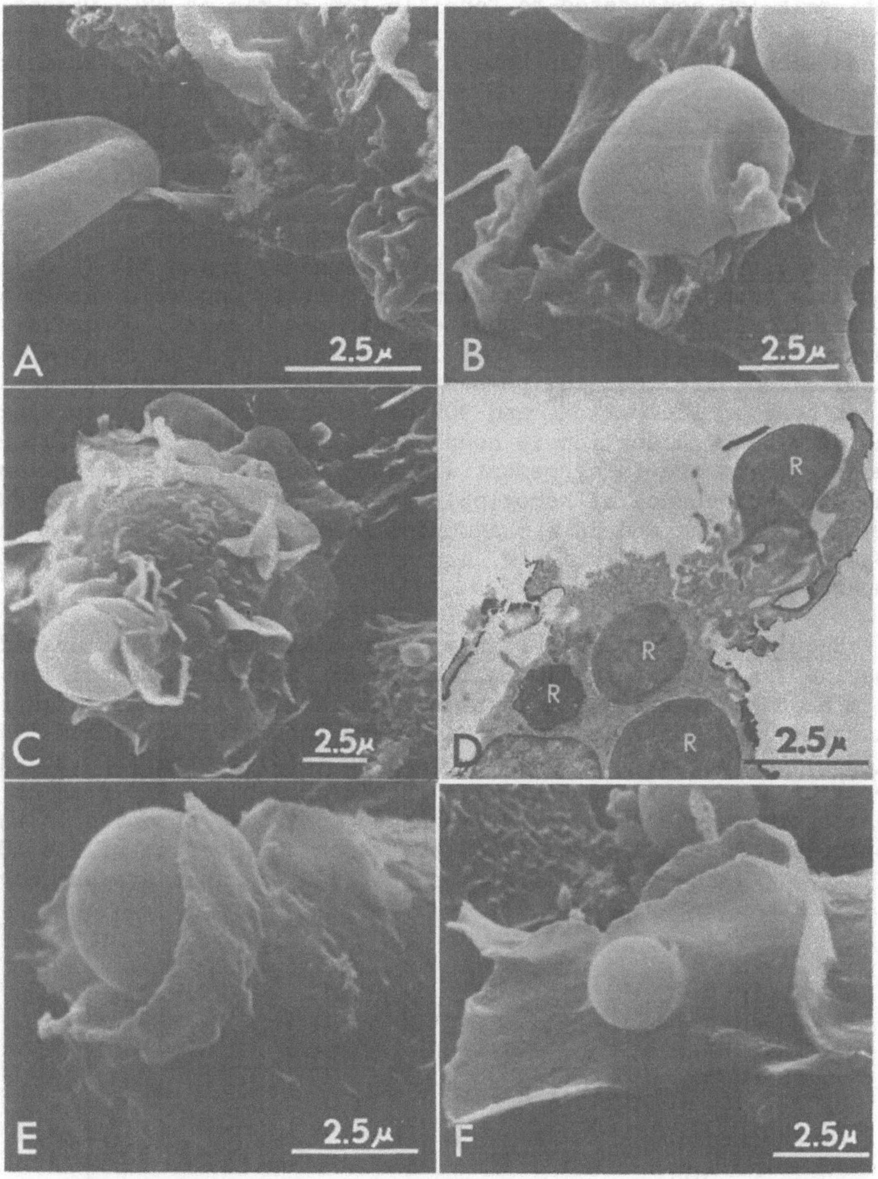

Fig. 1. Scanning electron micrographs of stages in the phagocytosis of senescent RBC by macrophages. D is a transmission electron micrograph showing RBC (indicated by "R") inside of a macrophage. From (63).

phagocytosis experiments were incubated in the IgG fraction of goat antihuman IgG for 30 min at 37°C, washed, incubated in rabbit anti-goat IgG conjugated to ferritin for 30 min at 4°C, washed, and prepared for scanning electron microscopy (3,10,19,20,21). Preparations were viewed with an Hitachi HFS-2 field emission, scanning electron microscope with 3 nm resolution. Between 200 and 300 cells were viewed in each preparation at magnifications from 20,000 to 100,000. Scanning time per preparation was 18-36 hrs.

RESULTS

Kinetics of Phagocytosis of RBC. Freshly drawn RBC were separated into young and old populations by density and were washed and stored *in vitro* and then incubated with macrophages. Samples were removed for analysis at various intervals up to 6 hr (Fig. 1). The results indicate that the percent phagocytosis is greatest during the first hour of incubation, and 90% of the phagocytosis occurring during a 6 hr incubation is complete by the end of 2 hr (Fig. 2). These results are in agreement with those of Morita and Perkins (6), who used absorbance of hemoglobin to determine the number of RBC remaining at the end of a phagocytosis experiment. Based on the results of these experiments, a 3 hr incubation time was selected for subsequent studies.

Requirement for Ig. Freshly drawn human RBC were incubated with the IgG fraction of rabbit anti-human RBC antibody (Cappel Lab.) for 30 min at 37°C, washed three times with Medium 199, and added to macrophages. Controls consisted of RBC incubated in Medium 199 or Ig-depleted serum. Sixty-three percent (63%) of the RBC (standard error of mean, 19%) treated with rabbit anti-human RBC reagent were phagocytized, whereas only 3-7% phagocytosis was observed in the controls. Rabbit IgG was demonstrated on the surface of the RBC with SIEM (3). These results indicate that IgG can initiate phagocytosis

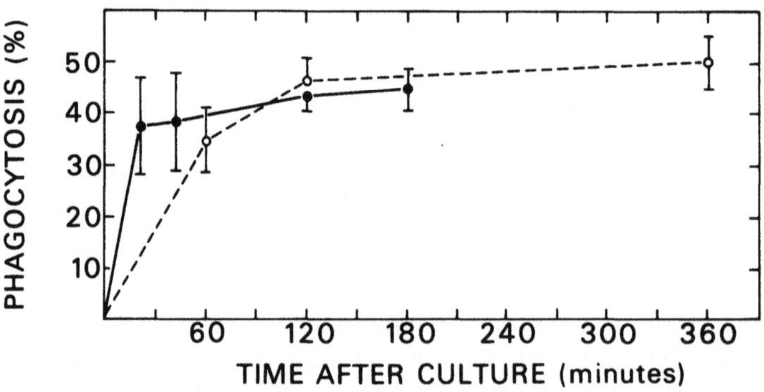

Fig. 2. Kinetics of phagocytosis of RBC aged *in situ* (o) and stored RBC (•). Zero time samples were not taken in the experiment since preliminary studies consistently showed no phagocytosis at this time. Sample size per culture, 4. Vertical bars indicate standard error. From (3).

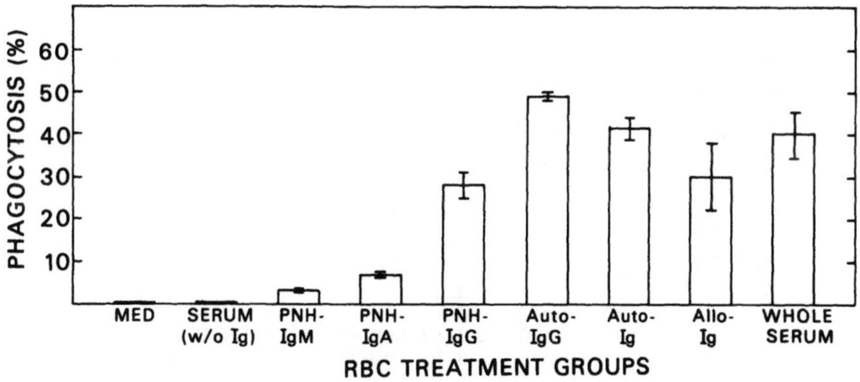

Fig. 3. Phagocytosis of stored RBC. Stored RBC were washed and incubated in Medium 199, autologous Ig-depleted or agamma serum (serum w/o Ig), pooled normal human IgM, IgA, or IgG (PNH-Ig), autologous IgG (Auto-IgG), autologous Ig (Auto-Ig), allogeneic Ig (Allo-Ig), or autologous, fresh, whole serum. RBC were then washed and incubated with macrophages. Vertical bars indicate one standard error of the mean. From (3).

and might be required. However, the RBC were deliberately coated with foreign IgG in the form of a specific antibody. Therefore, it could not be determined from this procedure whether normal circulating Ig would attach to RBC. In order to test this, human RBC were stored <u>in vitro</u> for 14 days at 4°C in Medium 199. They were then incubated for 1 hr in Medium 199, autologous Ig, autologous IgG, another individual's allogeneic Ig, or pooled, normal human (PNH) IgG, PNH-IgM, PNH-IgA, washed, and incubated with the individual's macrophages. The results of these experiments (Fig. 3) demonstrated that (a) the percent phagocytosis of stored RBC ("O"-RBC) incubated in IgM and IgA is only slightly more than that in medium alone ($\leq$ 10%); (b) the percent phagocytosis of stored RBC incubated in autologous IgG was essentially the same as that of stored RBC incubated in either autologous whole serum or the Ig fraction (42-49%); and (c) allogeneic Ig and PNH-IgG ($\geq$ 30% phagocytosis) were not as effective as autologous whole serum, Ig, or IgG in promoting phagocytosis, although they had not been tested for blood group compatibility. These results, which confirm the requirement for Ig, indicate that normal circulating Ig can attach to RBC, and suggest that the Ig that attaches is IgG. They further suggest that macrophages discriminate not only between classes of Ig, but also between their own and "foreign" Ig. These experiments support, but do not prove, the initial working hypothesis which states that immunoglobulins attach to the surface of aging RBC until a threshold level is reached, at which time macrophages no longer recognize the RBC as a "self" cell.

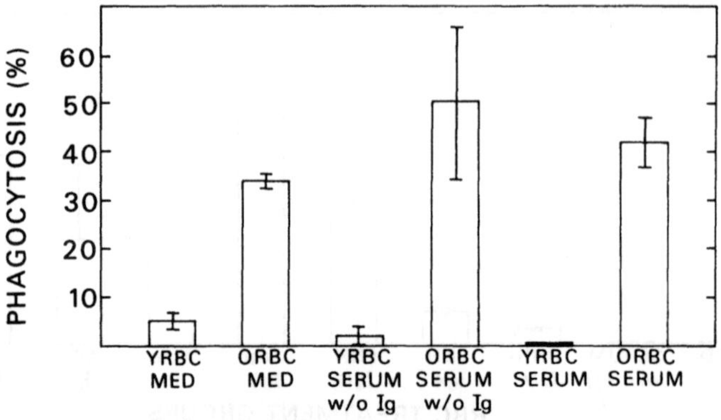

Fig. 4. Phagocytosis of RBC aged _in situ_. Freshly drawn RBC were separated by density into young and old RBC populations, washed, resuspended in Medium 199 (Med), autologus agamma serum (serum w/o Ig), or autologous fresh, whole serum (serum), and incubated with autologous macrophages. Vertical bars indicate one standard error of the mean. From (3).

Demonstration of Phagocytosis of Aged RBC Bearing Autologous IgG In Situ. In an attempt to test this hypothesis directly, and to determine whether the Ig which attached _in situ_ was IgG, the following experiments were performed.

Freshly drawn human RBC were separated into young and old populations according to their different densities and washed three times with Medium 199. Aliquots from each population were incubated with scanning immunoelectron microscopy marker conjugates and prepared for scanning electron microscopy. At the same time, each population was incubated with macrophages in Medium 199, Ig-depleted serum, or whole serum. A consistent difference in phagocytosis, greater than 30%, was observed between young and old populations of RBC whether the final incubations were performed in medium _without_ serum, in autologous Ig-_depleted_ serum, or whole serum containing Ig (Fig. 4). This indicated that the Ig was attached _in situ_ to the RBC, and that phagocytic recognition was not inhibited by other serum components. Scanning immunoelectron microscopy of the two populations revealed that young RBC were essentially unlabeled, whereas senescent RBC were heavily labeled with SV40 anti-human IgG, but not with T2 anti-human IgA or with KLH anti-human IgM. The fact that only 30-40% of the senescent RBC were ingested suggests that a threshold level of IgG may be required.

This tentative view is consistent with the observation, using scanning immunoelectron microscopy, that the number of IgG molecules

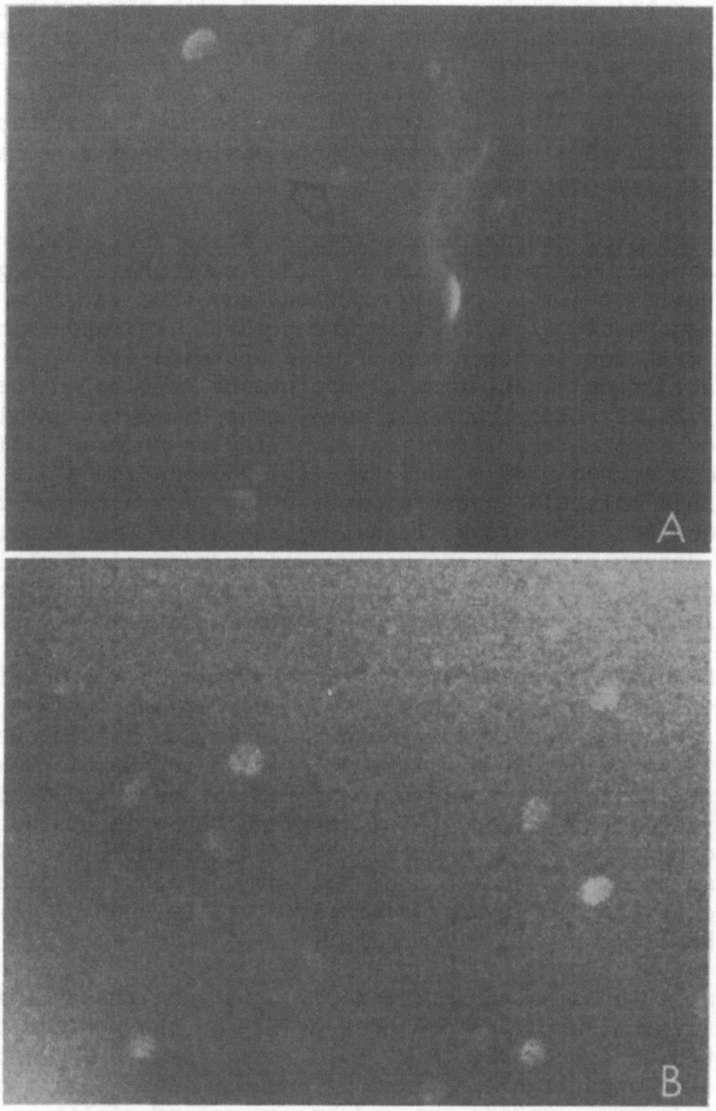

Fig. 5. A. Surface of a young RBC treated with neuraminidase, incubated in IgG, washed, and incubated with ferritin-conjugated antihuman IgG. From (16).

B. A higher magnification of ferritin-labeled RBC. From (16).

on senescent RBC varied between 20 to 50 per half cell. It is also possible that the macrophages were engorged with RBC and had, therefore, ceased ingesting. However, this seems unlikely as the macrophage:RBC ratio was 1:10.

On the basis of these findings, it can be concluded that IgG attaches in situ to senescent human RBC, making them vulnerable to phagocytosis by macrophages.

Phagocytosis of Neuraminidase-Treated Young RBC. The preceding experiments elucidate a mechanism by which macrophages recognize "senescent-self" cells. The next obvious question is, "How does IgG recognize senescent cells?" It is known that: (a) approximately 10% of the RBC membrane is comprised of glycoproteins (22); (b) removal of sialic acid from circulating glycoproteins results in their removal (23,24,25); (c) transient autoimmune hemolytic anemias sometimes follow respiratory infection with viruses such as influenza which contain neuraminidase, and that (d) "autoantibody" is generally formed against molecular precursors of blood groups rather than intact molecules. Therefore, it was hypothesized that autologous IgG recognizes determinants which are exposed by removal of sialic acid from membranes of RBC as they age. The following experiments were performed in order to test this hypothesis.

Young RBC were incubated with neuraminidase, a microbial enzyme which cleaves sialic acid groups from glycoproteins, washed, then incubated in either Medium 199, autologous Ig, or autologous IgG, washed again, and incubated with autologous macrophages. Results were that: (a) neuraminidase-treated young RBC incubated in medium were not phagocytized (0% phagocytosis), whereas those incubated with either autologous Ig or IgG were ($\geq$ 45% phagocytosis); (b) IgG is as effective as total Ig; and (c) the percent phagocytosis of neuraminidase-treated young RBC is approximately equal to that of in situ aged senescent RBC.

Scanning immunoelectron microscopy, utilizing the tri-labeling technique, demonstrated the presence of IgG on the surface of neuraminidase-treated young RBC (Fig. 5). These results suggest that young RBC can be artificially aged by neuraminidase treatment and that IgG binds to receptors exposed by removal of sialic acid (presumably carbohydrate moieties).

The results presented thus far suggest that macrophages can distinguish senescent from mature self RBC on the basis of selective attachment of autologous IgG to the membrane of senescent RBC. The presence of IgG on senescent cells is presumptive evidence that an immunological receptor-IgG binding has occurred. However, such evidence by itself does not establish that the Ig is a homeostatic autoantibody directed against normal constituents of the cell membrane. Definitive evidence for the role autoantibodies play in the selective removal of senescent cells can be obtained by first dissociating the antibodies from senescent cells and then by demonstrating their specific immunologic reattachment to homologous senescent, but not to mature cells, leading to destruction of only the senescent cells by mononuclear phagocytes.

Identification and Characterization of Old RBC Ig. Ig was eluted from RBC aged *in situ*. It was shown to be an IgG containing kappa and lambda light chains by immunodiffusion and immunoelectrophoresis. Other Igs were not detected by immunodiffusion, immunoelectrophoresis, or polyacrylamide gel electrophoresis. Thus, the antibody attached to senescent cells is an IgG which is polyclonal with respect to light chains.

IgG Binding and Specificity Experiments. In order to determine whether the IgG eluted from old RBC aged *in situ* would reattach to homologous cells, the IgG was incubated with autologous or allogeneic young stored RBC. These RBC were then washed and incubated with autologous mononuclear phagocytes. The percent phagocytosis, of stored RBC incubated with autologous IgG and then with autologous mononuclear phagocytes (46 ± 0%), was essentially the same as that of RBC aged *in situ* (50 ± 4%). Mononuclear phagocytes phagocytized autologous stored RBC incubated with autologous IgG (27 ± 0% phagocytosis), as well as allogeneic stored RBC incubated with autologous IgG (56 ± 4% phagocytosis). However, they did not phagocytize allogeneic cells which had not been incubated with IgG (0% phagocytosis), nor did they phagocytize young allogeneic cells which were incubated with allogeneic IgG (5 ± 3% phagocytosis). IgG was demonstrated on the surface of stored RBC incubated with IgG eluted from autologous or allogeneic cells with scanning immunoelectron microscopy. Absorption of the eluted IgG with stored RBC, but not with freshly isolated young RBC, abolished its phagocytosis-inducing ability (Table 1).

These binding and specificity experiments indicate that: (a) IgG is required for the phagocytosis of stored autologous and allogeneic RBC; (b) non-specific binding of IgG does not play a major role in these experiments because absorption of both pooled normal human IgG and IgG eluted from senescent cells with stored RBC abolishes its phagocytosis-inducing activity; (c) IgG eluted from senescent RBC is reactive against stored, but not young, cells; and, (d) IgG eluted from senescent RBC cannot discriminate between autologous and allogeneic cells. The last two findings suggest that the receptor site appearing on the surface of cells aged *in situ* and that appearing on stored cells is the same, or closely related, for all individuals. Likewise, absorption of pooled normal human IgG with stored RBC abolished its phagocytosis-inducing ability (Table 2).

To confirm these findings and to determine the nature of the membrane molecules that are altered during RBC aging *in situ*, young RBC were treated with neuraminidase, the microbial enzyme that cleaves

Table 1. Phagocytosis of Stored RBC ("O" RBC) Incubated with IgG Eluted from Senescent Cells Before and After Absorption with Stored RBC or Freshly Isolated Young RBC (YRBC)

EXPT	QUANTITY*	PHAGOCYTOSIS (%) ± SEM+		
		Before Absorption	After Absorption with YRBC	After Absorption with "O" RBC
1	3	49 ± 2	43 ± 9	0
2	3	35 ± 1	34 ± 7	0
3	3	43 ± 11	46 ± 16	0

*Quantity (μg) of IgG added to 1.5 x 10^8 RBC in 1 ml of Medium 199.

+SEM, standard error of the mean of triplicate or quadruplicate cultures.

sialic acid groups from glycoproteins. Neuraminidase treated RBC incubated in medium alone were not phagocytized (0% phagocytosis), whereas those incubated in autologous and allogeneic IgG eluted from old RBC aged in situ were phagocytized (% phagocytosis: 35 ± 2 and 46 ± 6, respectively). IgG was observed with scanning immunoelectron microscopy on the surface of neuraminidase-IgG treated RBC, but not on RBC treated with neuraminidase alone.

The observation that the IgG eluted from RBC aged in situ recognizes the receptor exposed by removal of sialic acid groups suggests that the receptor exposed as cells age naturally in situ may be the same as, or analogous to, that exposed by the removal of sialic acid in vitro. Membrane glycoproteins may be losing sialic acid as cells age, thus exposing the molecular determinants to which IgG binds. Another possibility is that the structural association between glycoproteins and integral membrane proteins may be disrupted during aging, leading to exposure of cryptic antigens. In such a case, one could speculate that neuraminidase acts, not by exposing new sugars, but by changing glycoprotein-protein interactions through removal of sialic acid.

To determine whether the Fab or Fc portion of IgG attaches to

Table 2. Phagocytosis of Stored RBC Incubated with Pooled Human IgG Before or After Absorption of the IgG with Stored RBC*

EXPT	QUANTITY of IgG (μg)+	PHAGOCYTOSIS (%) Before Absorption (Mean ± SEM)++	After Absorption
1	30	42 ± 17	0
2	30	32 ± 4	0
3	300	52 ± 2	0
4	300	28 ± 6	0

*IgG was absorbed over night at 4°C with RBC aged *in vitro*.

+The quantity of IgG (μg) was added to 2 x 10^8 RBC which were incubated for 30 min at 24°C and then 30 min at 4°C, washed, and incubated with autologous mononuclear phagocytes. The quantity of IgG (μg) was adjusted so that it was the same both for absorbed and unabsorbed IgG, as determined by radial immunodiffusion.

++Mean ± the standard error of the mean of quadruplicate cultures.

RBC, receptor blockade studies were performed. The results are summarized in Figure 6. Stored RBC were incubated for 30 minutes with either pooled normal human IgG, its Fab or its Fc fragment. The RBC were washed, and all three groups were incubated with IgG for another 30 mins. RBC were washed again and incubated with autologous mononuclear phagocytes (Fig. 6A). For the control cultures, stored RBC were treated with IgG, Fab, or Fc before they were exposed to mononuclear phagocytes (Fig. 6B). Control results show that phagocytosis was achieved by exposing the RBC to IgG. Treatment with Fab or Fc did not promote phagocytosis. Experimental results show that treatment of RBC with Fab prior to incubation with IgG reduced the

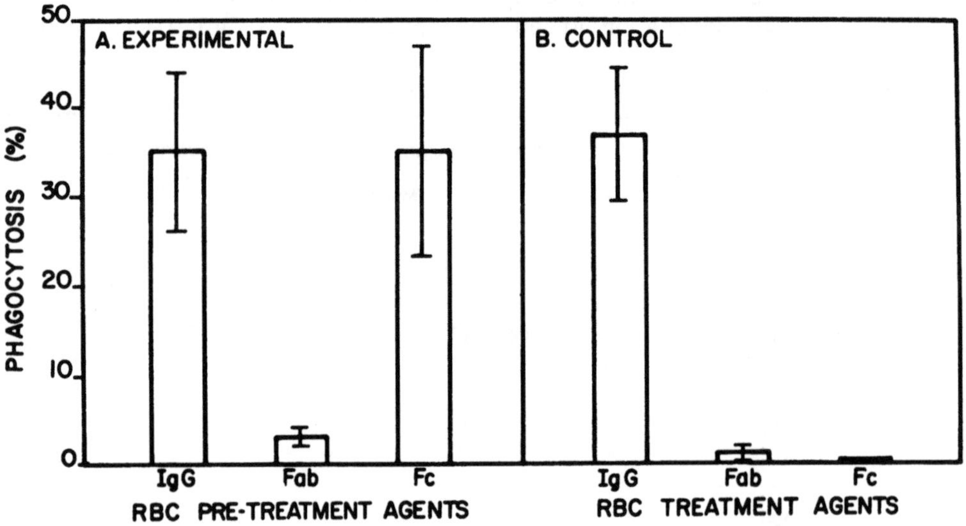

Fig. 6. A. Susceptibility to phagocytosis of aged RBC as influenced by their pretreatment with either IgG, Fab or Fc before exposure to IgG. Stored RBC were incubated with either IgG, Fab, or Fc for 30 min, washed, and incubated with IgG for 30 min. The RBC were washed and incubated with mononuclear phagocytes for 3 hr.

B. Susceptibility to phagocytosis of aged RBC as influenced by their exposure to either IgG, Fab, or Fc. Stored RBC were incubated with either IgG, Fab or Fc for 30 min, washed and then incubated with mononuclear phagocytes for 3 hr. Bars indicate standard error of the mean; sample size, 6.

phagocytosis to essentially 0, whereas pretreatment with Fc did not inhibit phagocytosis (Fig. 1A). Thus, these blockade studies demonstrate that IgG binds to old RBC via its Fab region. Binding of Fab but not Fc was also demonstrated with scanning electron microscopy. Binding of the IgG molecule to aged RBC via the Fab region is consistent with an immunological binding of IgG with a surface receptor. The Fc portion of IgG would then be available to the macrophage Fc receptor.

These experiments suggest that the IgG eluted from senescent RBC is an autoantibody, as it specifically reattaches to homologous RBC via its Fab region and initiates their selective destruction by mononuclear phagocytes.

Receptor Identification Studies. (The preliminary experiments directed toward identifying the IgG-binding receptor on old RBC were performed in collaboration with Dr. Hans Lutz, Department of Biochemistry, Swiss Federal Institute of Technology, Zurich, Switzerland. Details of these experiments will be published elsewhere.)

There are several possible explanations for the mechanisms by which appearance of a "new" receptor, such as the IgG-binding receptor, could occur with age. One possibility is the exposure of cryptic or hidden antigens that have existed as long as the cell has. These antigens could be blocked, for example, by steric hindrance of neighboring molecules. Alteration of the "shielding" molecules with age, possibly through loss of one of their subunits, could result in exposure of the receptor. Likewise, age-associated alterations in membrane fluidity or in the interactions of molecules within the membrane could result in exposure of cryptic antigens by allowing molecular drift.

Another possible explanation is that subunits of surface molecules are lost with aging, thus exposing "new" antigenic determinants. In this case, the altered molecule, itself, would be the receptor. Loss of a subunit could result in a change in the conformation of the protein. The receptor could be a sugar or amino acid sequence behind the lost subunit, or it could result from a conformational change in the molecule.

As an initial approach to this issue, we decided to isolate molecules that were potential receptor candidates. Based on data derived from previous studies (3,26), which indicated that neuraminidase treatment can increase IgG binding and phagocytosis of RBC, we suspected that the receptor was a sialoglycoprotein or sialopeptide. For this reason, we prepared glycophorin enriched vesicles (27). The vesicles contain the sialoglycoproteins (PAS_1-PAS_4), a sialoglycoprotein that appears in the tracking dye region on polyacrylamide gel electrophoresis, and trace contaminants of other minor proteins that are not sialoglycoproteins (27). We used vesicles rather than soluble antigen for four reasons. First, it was necessary to determine whether the receptor was indeed a sialoglycoprotein before proceeding to isolate and purify it. Second, we were concerned with the possibility that membrane glycoproteins would aggregate when isolated or when manipulated in an aqueous environment. Third, it is easier to work with vesicles than with soluble antigens. Finally, other membrane components, such as protein component 3 or lipids, can be added to the vesicles, enabling us to investigate the effect of these components on the receptor and IgG binding.

Isolation of potential receptors away from other membrane components allows differentiation between binding through exposure of cryptic antigens and binding through alteration of the receptor itself. If the appearance of an IgG-binding receptor on senescent cells were due to exposure of a cryptic antigen, then the receptor from young and old cells should bind IgG equally when isolated. On

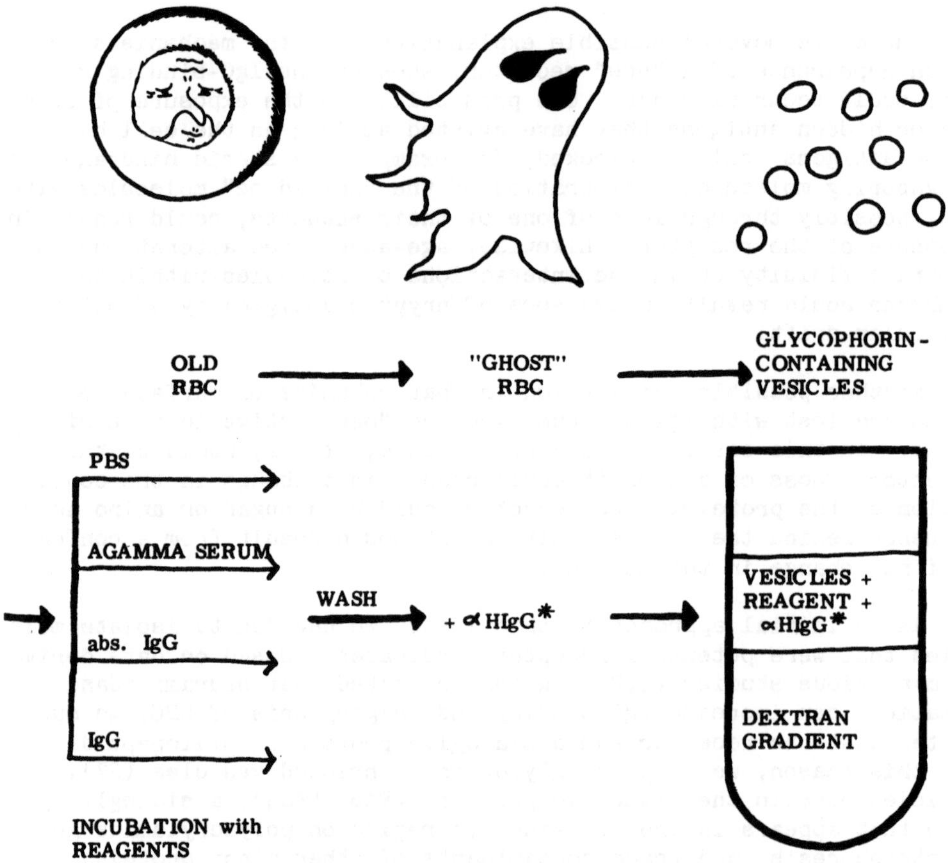

Fig. 7. Design of receptor identification experiments. Serum and buffy coat were removed from one unit of freshly obtained human blood. Cells were then resuspended in Medium 199 and placed in tissue culture flasks at 4°C if they were to be stored, or were separated into young and old populations and processed on the same day. For vesicle preparation, cells were washed 4 times with PBS and lysed with hypotonic PBS (27). RBC ghosts were incubated in 10mM sodium acetate, washed with 0.1 mM ETDA, then 0.5 M NaCl, followed by 5 mM phosphate buffer, pH 7.4. The RBC ghosts were extracted with Triton X-100 (0.15%). After centrifugation, extracted supernates were washed with Bio Beads SM 2 overnight at 4°C, resulting in vesicle formation (for details, see ref. 27). The vesicles were then incubated with PBS, agamma serum, autolgous IgG (10.5 mg), IgG or absorbed with stored RBC, for 1 hr at 4°C. After 2 washes with PBS, vesicles were incubated with ^{125}I labeled

the other hand, if the receptor were a membrane molecule that has been altered by a deletion or addition, then the receptor from senescent cells should bind more IgG than the receptor from young cells.

Binding of IgG to Glycophorin-Containing Vesicles Prepared from Stored RBC. The experiments were performed with vesicles prepared from stored RBC as described in Figure 7. After equilibrium centrifugation (Fig. 8), vesicles incubated with PBS or agamma serum remained in the upper half of the gradient and the ^{125}I labeled anti-human IgG remained in the upper third of the gradient. Vesicles incubated with autologous IgG pelleted on the bottom of the tube along with bound anti-human IgG.

The amount of anti-human IgG bound to the vesicles was estimated from the amount of free anti-IgG (786 cpm per μg) on the gradient, after correcting for recovery of anti-IgG as determined by cpm, because of technical difficulties. Approximately 284 ng of anti-IgG was bound per μg protein to vesicles incubated with human IgG, while approximately 28 ng was bound to vesicles incubated with Ig-depleted serum. The amount of IgG bound is probably the same as the amount of anti-human IgG bound (3). However, it could be twice as much, since IgG has two binding sites. These results suggest that the IgG binding receptor on stored RBC copurifies with sialoglycoproteins.

Binding of IgG to Glycoprotein Containing Vesicles Prepared from RBC Aged in Situ. Vesicles were prepared from young, middle-aged, and old RBC populations. They were incubated with Ig reagents as described in Fig. 4. The results, which are summarized in Table 3, show that more ^{125}I labeled anti-human IgG or Protein A binds to vesicles from the senescent cell fraction than to vesicles from the middle-aged RBC fraction. The least label is bound to vesicles from the young RBC population. Increasing the amount of protein component 3 by increasing the amount of Triton X-100 used for extractions enhanced total IgG binding to vesicles from both young and old fraction cells, but not the difference in the amount of IgG bound between the fractions.

---

specific antibodies of goat anti-human IgG (anti-H IgG) prepared by the affinity chromatography and labeled by the lactoperoxidase method for 1 hr at 4°C. The mixture was then layered on a dextran gradient (ρ 1.005, 1.008, 1.012, 1.016, 1.020, and 1.025). Gradients were centrifuged for 8 hours in a SW27 rotor in a Beckman LS-50 preparative centrifuge at 25,000 rpm. Fractions were monitored during collection with a recording spectrophotometer. Radioactivity of the fractions was measured with a Searle gamma counter, and protein was determined by the method of Lowry.

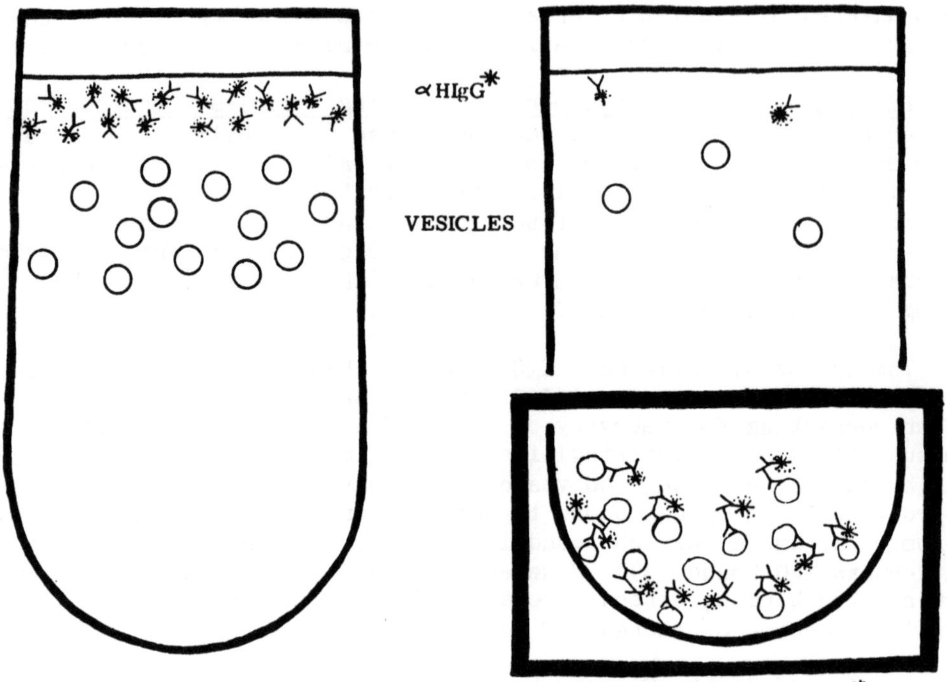

Fig. 8. Binding of IgG to glycoprotein-containing vesicles prepared from stored RBC. Vesicles were incubated with Ig reagents as described in Figure 4. After centrifugation on a dextran gradient, ^{125}I-labeled anti-human IgG that was not bound to vesicles was in the upper third of the gradient, and vesicles that were not labeled were in the upper half of the gradient. Labeled vesicles were on the bottom of the gradient. No radioactivity was detected in the bottom of the control gradient (incubated with PBS or agamma serum and then anti-human IgG). Fifty-nine percent of the radioactivity recovered from the gradient containing vesicles incubated with IgG was in the pellet.

Binding of ^{125}I labeled anti-human IgG or Protein A to vesicles from the young population could be due to technical problems, such as trapping of the label between vesicles during pelleting of the vesicles, influx of the label into the vesicles during incubation with subsequent resealing of the vesicles, sub-optimal separation of RBC populations, or damage to young RBC during the preparative

Table 3. Binding of ^{125}I Labeled Anti-Human IgG or Protein A to Glycophorin-Containing Vesicles Isolated from Young, Middle-Aged, or Senescent RBC Populations Pre-Incubated with Autologous or Allogeneic IgG[1]

Expt. No	IgG Source	IgG Binding[2] (ng Protein A or anti-human IgG bound per μg sialic acid) Cell Fraction: Young	Middle-aged	Old
1	autologous	50	70	90
		(0)	(20)	(40)
2	allogeneic	14	21	39
		(0)	(7)	(25)
3	allogeneic	9	21	26
		(0)	(12)	(17)

[1]Vesicles were incubated with autologous or allogeneic IgG, washed, and incubated with ^{125}I labeled anti-human IgG (Expt 1) or Protein A (Expt 2 and 3).
[2]Numbers in parentheses indicate relative anti-human IgG or Protein A binding when the amount bound to vesicles from the young cell fraction is subtracted from that bound to the middle-aged and old fraction. This calculation was performed because total binding of label to vesicles from young RBC incubated with IgG was not significantly different from that of old RBC that were incubated with IgG that had been absorbed before use with RBC ghosts.

procedure. On the other hand, such binding could indicate the presence of a small number of the IgG binding receptor molecules in the membranes of young cells.

As an independent method of assessing binding of IgG to vesicles,

Table 4. Phagocytosis-Inducing Ability of IgG Absorbed with Glycophorin-Containing Vesicles (GCV) from Young, Middle-Aged, or Senescent Cell Fractions

Expt No	Quantity (ug) of IgG per 50 μg GCV[1]	Vesicle Components[2]		Phagocytosis (%)[3] Mean ± SEM Source of Vesicles Used for Absorption		
		protein	lipids	YG	MA	OLD
1	250	+	-	36±3	ND	5±5
2a	125	+	-	55±6	38±9	0
2b	125	+	+	42±3	34±7	0
2c	125	-	+	32±3	38±5	ND

[1]IgG was absorbed with vesicles from young (YG), middle-aged (MA), or senescent (OLD) cell fractions for 24-48 hrs at 4°C. Vesicles were removed by centrifugation and the supernate was incubated with approximately 150 x 10^6 stored RBC for 1 hr at 4°C. RBC were washed and incubated with macrophages.

[2]Vesicle components: a plus (+) indicates that the component was present; a minus (-) indicates that it was not.

[3]SEM, one standard error of the mean. The percent phagocytosis of RBC incubated with IgG that was not also absorbed was 41±3% for Expt 1 and 32±2% for Expt 2.

the phagocytosis inducing ability of IgG absorbed with vesicles from young, middle-aged, and old cell fractions was examined. The results, which are summarized in Table 4, show that absorption of IgG with vesicles prepared from senescent cells abolished the phagocytosis inducing ability of IgG, whereas absorption with vesicles prepared from young cells did not. Addition of lipids to the vesicles did not significantly alter the results. Absorption of IgG with lipids alone did not alter its phagocytosis-inducing ability. The phagocytosis-inducing ability of IgG eluted from senescent cells could be absorbed with vesicles prepared from senescent cells.

The results of the preceding experiments indicate that the IgG binding receptor on senescent RBC copurifies with the sialoglycoproteins and is not a lipid. The receptor is not merely a cryptic antigen, but is a "new" antigen that appears on RBC membranes as they age because there is a significant difference in IgG binding between vesicles isolated from young and old cells, as determined by two independent assays. If the receptor were merely a cryptic antigen, then isolation of the receptor in vesicles, without the other "shielding" molecules, should result in equal binding of the IgG, regardless of the cell fraction from which it was prepared. This was not the case. Furthermore, addition of lipids to the vesicles does not alter IgG binding.

DISCUSSION

The results presented herein confirm the earlier studies from this laboratory (3,10,20) by demonstrating that macrophages distinguish between senescent and mature RBC on the basis of selective IgG attachment, and firmly establishing the existence of autoantibodies with intrinsic physiologic and homeostatic functions. The IgG that binds to senescent RBC _in situ_ and stored RBC _in vitro_ is an autoantibody, as it specifically attaches to old cells via the Fab region, thus initiating their selective destruction by macrophages. The IgG autoantibody is directed against an altered membrane protein or sialoglycoprotein, not a cryptic antigen. It is interesting to speculate that the IgG binding antigen may be a fragment of a higher molecule weight membrane molecule that is produced through the action of endogenous proteases or results from a change in activity of a membrane bound enzyme(s) which maintains membrane integrity.

The IgG autoantibody protects RBC from lysis for the first 10-15 days of storage _in vitro_ in serum (Kay, unpublished). It also induces phagocytosis of senescent RBC by macrophages. As a result, senescent cells are removed from the circulation instead of lysing (4,5,6,8). Thus, the membranes and hemoglobin of the approximately 1.93×10^{11} (Footnote *) senescent cells that are removed daily are enzymatically degraded by macrophages rather than being released into the circulation by lysis. Lysis of RBC could be detrimental to an individual's survival. For example, individuals with elevated plasma

*The number of senescent cells removed per day is calculated as follows: 5.1×10^9 RBC/ml blood divided by 120 days = 4×10^7 senescent RBC per ml at the end of their life span. This is multiplied by the blood volume (69 ml/Kg times 70 Kg = 4830 ml).

iron levels, as are seen with overt hemolytic anemia or destruction of ferritin-containing liver cells (e.g., viral hepatitis), are extremely susceptible to even a small innoculum of invading pathogens (29). Iron enhances the virulence of bacteria and can neutralize the microbiostatic action of serum (for review of the subject, see 28).

The IgG described herein is a physiologic autoantibody, as it contributes to the maintenance of homeostasis by permitting the more efficient mature cells to carry out their vital functions without hindrance from the less efficient senescent cells, or from pathological reactions which could arise as a consequence of senescent cells dying or decaying within the organism. Thus, the existence of homeostatic autoantibodies has been demonstrated experimentally probably for the first time. Since these autoantibodies are part of the normal immune mechanism for removing cells, the B cell clones producing these antibodies cannot be "forbidden" (29), nor need the presence of these autoantibodies be attributed to an age-related decrease in suppressor cell function (30,31).

Some authors have attributed macrophage removal of senescent cells to a reduction in net negative surface charge with aging of RBC (32,33). However, recent reports indicate that there are no differences between young and senescent RBC in net surface charge densities, as determined by several different methods (34,35).

Other investigators have attributed removal of senescent RBC to direct interaction between desialylated RBC and macrophages that is not mediated by IgG (36). This assumption is based on the observation that neuraminidase treated rat RBC bind to Kupffer cells and to unseparated spleen cells (36). There are several problems with this assumption. First, it has been shown that attachment of a cell or particle to a specific receptor on a macrophage is not sufficient to trigger phagocytosis (37,38). The following examples clearly demonstrate that attachment does not lead to phagocytosis.

Complement coated RBC are bound to the macrophage membrane but are not ingested. When IgG coated pneumococci are added to the macrophage preparations which have already bound complement coated RBC, the macrophages ingest an average of 15-20 pneumococci, but not the attached RBC (38). Thus, the response of the macrophage membrane to a phagocytic stimulus is highly selective.

In addition, the distribution of IgG molecules on the potential particle is of great importance to a macrophage. For example, macrophages will ingest B lymphocytes if they are diffusely coated with antibodies against lymphocyte surface antigens which do not cap. Capped lymphocytes treated with IgG anti-immunoglobulin are bound but not ingested. Surprisingly, macrophages will clean capped immunoglobulins from the surface of lymphocytes without apparently damaging them.

Evidence from many different laboratories has shown that IgG is required for phagocytosis of RBC. Jancik and Schauer (39) have shown that the phagocytosis of desialylated erythrocytes in vitro requires serum factors and that circulating erythrocytes are coated with IgG following desialylation. Durocher (40) has shown that immunoglobulins bind to desialylated rat RBC. In contrast to the studies on removal of desialylated serum glycoproteins (23,24,25), galactose oxidase treatment of desialylated RBC does not improve their survival nor does it reduce immunoglobulin binding (40). Cellular deformability does not seem to contribute to destruction of RBC (40).

Steer (41) has shown that infusion of desialylated chromium labeled lymphocytes into rabbits results in rapid uptake of these cells by the liver. However, incubation of desialylated lymphocytes with Fab fragments prior to infusion results in a marked decrease in hepatic uptake. This is consistent with the finding reported here and elsewhere (26) that the Fab portion of IgG binds to RBC, leaving the Fc portion free to interact with the Fc receptor on macrophages.

There is still some controversy regarding sialic acid content of aged RBC. Some authors report that senescent RBC have slightly lower levels of sialic acid (35), while others found identical levels of sialic acid in glycophorin of both young and senescent RBC (43). It is possible that sialic acid is lost from sialoglycoproteins besides glycophorin.

It has been suggested that the autoantibody described here and in previous studies from my laboratory may simply be the T-agglutinin which binds to an exposed β-galactose residue on desialylated RBC. However, the T-agglutinin belongs to the IgM class. The antibody which binds to senescent RBC is IgG, as determined by four different methods. Furthermore, IgM antibodies have not been observed on senescent RBC (3). A recent investigation using two mouse strains, one with and one without serum T agglutinin, demonstrated that T-agglutinin does not participate in the removal of desialylated RBC (44).

The concept of self-tolerance is a basic tenet of immunology. Ehrlich used the term, "horror autotoxicus" to describe autoimune disease which was felt to result from a breakdown in internal regulation that prevented reactions against "self." The demonstrated existence of physiologic autoantibodies requires a revision of this view. Besides the physiologic autoantibody described herein, for which a homeostatic function has been demonstrated and a mechanism of action has, in part, been elucidated (Fig. 9), autoantibodies are being found with increasing frequency in normal, healthy individuals (45-48). Essentially 100% of the young healthy individuals tested in this laboratory have low levels of antibodies to thyroglobulin (Kay, unpublished). Injection of the polyclonal activator, lipopolysaccharide (LPS), into mice results in production of IgM antibodies which are specific for mouse IgG (48). Immunogen injection has the same effect. Plaque-forming cells producing IgM anti-IgG autoantibody have been demonstrated (48). Autoantibodies against mouse RBC treated with bromelain have been described, and plaque forming cells producing autoantibody against bromelain treated mouse RBC have been demonstrated (49,50). The function or significance of cells capable of responding to bromelain treated RBC is unclear at this time because bromelain hydrolyzes proteins, peptides, amides and esters of amino acids and peptides, and because bromelain treatment represents a non-physiologic situation. The implication of such studies is that mice have a high proportion (≥ 50%) of cells that recognize endogenous antigens. The problem with these studies is that bromelain may generate many "new" antigens by altering many molecules. Further, alteration of a self recognition antigen, such as one of the H-2 antigens, could result in recognition of the molecule as "non-self" or "altered self" (51), just as addition of a single sugar (α-N-acetyl-galactosamine) to a glycosphingolipid produced by adenocarcinoma of the stomach and colon leads to a "non-self" antigen passing as a "self" antigen (52).

In 1964, Swartzendruber (53) described removal of plasma cells by macrophages in the spleen of mice between 3 and 6 days after primary immunization, as determined by electron microscopy. Phagocytosis of plasma cells was most extensive on day 6. Jerne et al. (54), utilizing a plaque assay, reported a 90% decrease in the number of antibody-producing cells in the mouse spleen between 4 and 7 days after primary immunization with the same antigen. Schooley (55), using autoradiography, estimated the mean-life of a plasma cell at 8-12 hr after the last division in a stimulated lymph node. In addition, the phagocytosis of plasma cells observed by Swartzendruber correlates with the log phase of antibody appearance in the circulation (56). In view of the preceding, it is tempting to speculate that a clone(s) of plasma cells, and thus, antibody production to a specific immunogen, is terminated at the log phase of antibody appearance <u>in situ</u> by phagocytic macrophages. It is possible that an autoantibody similar to the one described herein is responsible for initiating the phagocytosis of terminally differentiated plasma cells. Anti-idiotypic antibody directed toward the Fab or Fc region might be responsible for initiating phagocytosis.

One of the implications of such speculation is that multiple myeloma might result from a defect in macrophages or a regulatory autoantibody allowing plasma cells to function autonomously. Freed of their normal mechanism of destruction, plasma cells could then accumulate and the plasmacytosis of multiple myeloma would result.

It is possible that autoantibodies may also function as a regulatory mechanism for initiating and/or terminating metabolic processes. This is suggested by studies into the pathophysiology of certain disease processes. For example, thyroid-stimulating immunoglobulin

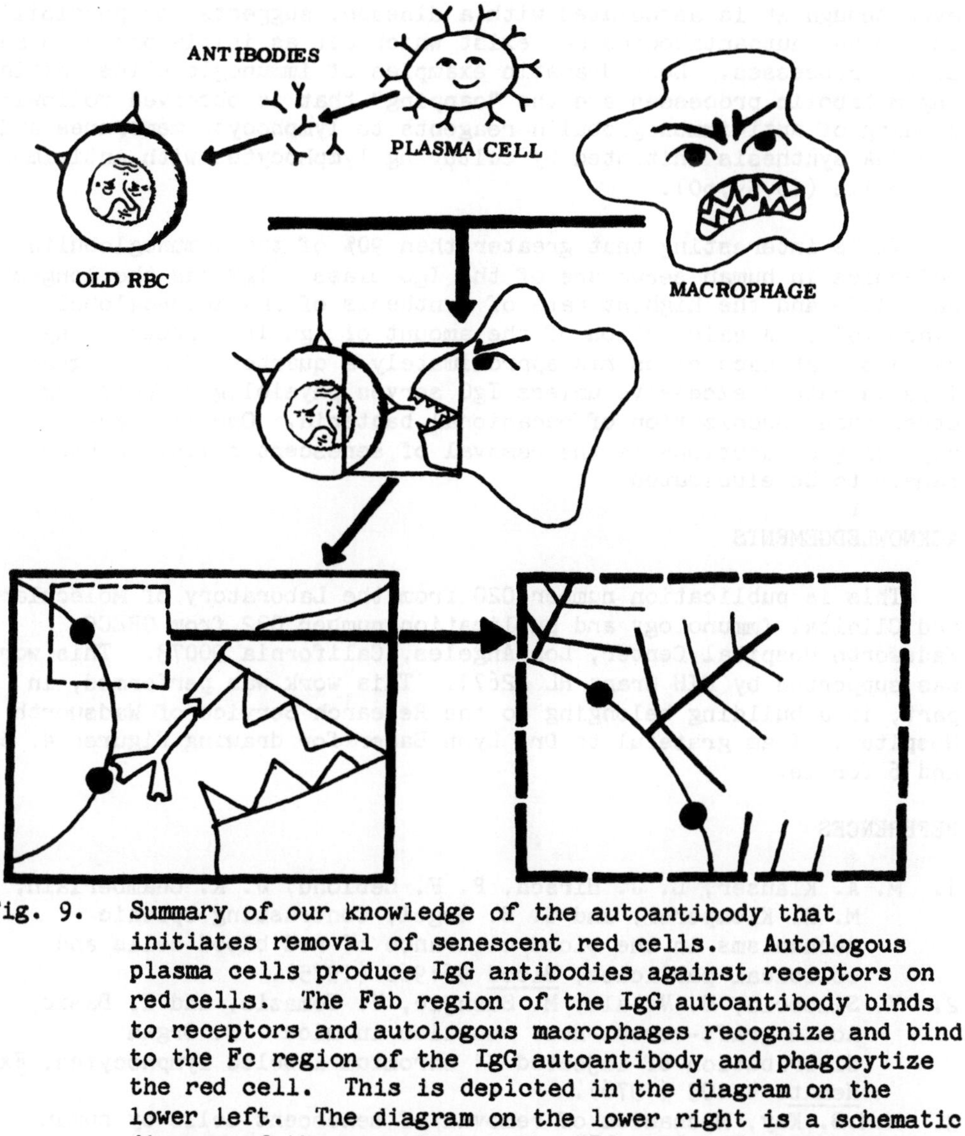

Fig. 9. Summary of our knowledge of the autoantibody that initiates removal of senescent red cells. Autologous plasma cells produce IgG antibodies against receptors on red cells. The Fab region of the IgG autoantibody binds to receptors and autologous macrophages recognize and bind to the Fc region of the IgG autoantibody and phagocytize the red cell. This is depicted in the diagram on the lower left. The diagram on the lower right is a schematic diagram of the receptor on the RBC, which is represented as a branched glycoprotein. The circles represent adjacent membrane proteins.

(TSI) is an IgG autoantibody that binds to the thyroid follicular cell's receptor or a component thereof. TSI stimulates cyclic adenosine monophosphate and endocytosis of colloid droplets, displaces thyroid stimulating hormone from membrane sites and results in excessive levels of circulating thyroid hormone (58). The existence of an autoantibody that can initiate the activities of an endocrine gland, even though it is associated with a disease, suggests the possibility that other autoantibodies may exist which act as initiators of homeostatic processes. Less dramatic examples of immunoglobulins initiating metabolic processes are the "capping" that is observed following binding of anti-immunoglobulin reagents to lymphocyte membranes and the DNA synthesis initiated by culturing lymphocytes with anti-immunoglobulin (19,59,60).

It is interesting that greater than 90% of the immunoglobulin molecules in human serum are of the IgG class. IgG has the longest half-life and the highest rate of synthesis of any immunoglobulin class (61). A calculation of the amount of IgG in a human being reveals that each of us has approximately a quarter of a kilogram. This is rather excessive unless IgG serves physiologic functions other than opsonization of occasional bacteria. One of these physiologic functions is the removal of senescent cells. Others remain to be elucidated.

ACKNOWLEDGEMENTS

This is publication number 020 from the Laboratory of Molecular and Clinical Immunology and publication number 032 from GRECC, Wadsworth Hospital Center, Los Angeles, California 90073. This work was supported by NIH Grant HL 22671. This work was performed, in part, in a building belonging to the Research Service of Wadsworth VA Hospital. I am grateful to Dr. Lynn Baker for drawing Figures 4, 5, and 6 for me.

REFERENCES

1. M. A. Klauser, L. J. Hirsch, P. F. Leblond, J. K. Chamberlain, M. R. Klemperer, and G. B. Segel, Contrasting splenic mechanisms in the blood clearance of red blood cells and colloidal particles, Blood 46:965 (1975).
2. V. Silobcic, B. Vitale, M. Susnjic, V. Tomazic, and I. Basic, Acute graft-versus-host reaction in mice. 3. Organ distribution of injected 51 chromium labeled lymphocytes, Exp. Hemat. 4:103 (1976).
3. M.M.B. Kay, Mechanism of removal of senescent cells by human macrophages in situ, Proc. Natl. Acad. Sci. USA 72:3521 (1975).
4. F. Smith, Erythrophagocytosis in human lymph-glands, J. Path. Bact. 78:383 (1958).
5. C. R. Jenkin and K. Karthigasu, Elimination hepatiques des erythrocytes age et alteres chez le rat, Compt. Rend. Soc. Biol. 161:1006 (1967).
6. T. Morita, and E. H. Perkins, A simple quantitative method to assess the in vitro engulfing and degradative potentials of mouse peritoneal phagocytic cells. J. Reticuloendothel. Soc. 2:406 (1965).

7. A. E. Stuart, and R. A. Cumming, A biological test for injury to the human red cell, Vox Sang. 13:270 (1967).
8. D. S. Nelson, Macrophages in auto-immunity, the disposal of effete cells and chronic inflammation, in:"Macrophages and Immunity," Amer. Elsevier Pub. Co., New York (1969).
9. D. Gemsa, C. H. Woo, H. H. Fudenberg, and R. Schmid, Erythrocyte catabolism by macrophages in vitro. The effect of hydrocortisone on erythrophagocytosis and on the indication of heme oxygenase, J. Clin. Lab. Invest. 52:812 (1973).
10. M. M. B. Kay, Mechanism of macrophage recognition of senescent red cells, Gerontologist 14(5):33 (1974).
11. S. Kochwa and R. Rosenfield, Immunochemical studies of the Rh system. I. Isolation and characterization of antibodies, J. Immunol. 92:682 (1964).
12. A. Nisonoff, F. C. Wissler, L. N. Lipman, and D. L. Woernley, Separation of univalent fragments from the bivalent rabbit antibody molecule by reduction of disufide bonds, Arch. Biochem. Biophys. 89:230 (1960).
13. J. J. Cebra, D. Guval, H. I. Silman, and E. Katchalski, A two-stage cleavage of rabbit y-globulin by a water-insoluble papain preparation followed by cysteine, J. Biol. Chem. 236:1720 (1961).
14. C. L. Cambiasco, A. Goffinet, J.-P. Vaerman, and J. F. Feremans, Glutaraldehyde-activated aminohexyl-derivative of Sepharose 4B as a new versatile immunoabsorbent, Immunochemistry 12:272 (1975).
15. J. Mueller, R. G. del Brun, H. Buerki, H.-U. Keller, M. W. Hess, and H. Cottier, Non-specific acid esterase activity: A criterion for differentiation in mouse lymph nodes, Eur. J. Immunol. 5:270 (1975).
16. M. M. B. Kay, Kupffer cells: Homeostatic functions during aging, in:"Liver and Ageing," D. Platt, ed., F.K. Schattauer Verlag, Stuttgart (1977).
17. J. R. Murphy, Influence of temperature and method of centrifugation on the separation of erythrocytes, J. Lab. Clin. Med. 82:334 (1973).
18. E. R. Borun, M. G. Figueroa, and I. M. Perry, The distribution of Fe^{59}-tagged human erythrocytes in centrifuged specimens as a function of cell age, J. Clin. Invest. 36:676 (1957).
19. M. M. B. Kay, Multiple labeling technique used for kinetic studies of activated human B lymphocytes, Nature 245:425 (1975).
20. M. M. B. Kay, Multiple labeling technique for scanning immunoelectron microscopy, in:"Principles and Techniques of Scanning Electron Microscopy," M.A. Hayat, ed., Van Nostrand and Reinhold Co., New York, (1978).
21. M. M. B. Kay, High resolution scanning electron microscopy and its application to research on immunity and aging, in:"Immunity and Aging," T. Makinodan and E. Yunis, eds., Plenum Press, New York (1978).

22. T. Steck, The organization of proteins in the human red blood cell membrane, J. Cell Biol. 62:1 (1974).
23. C. J. A. van den Hamer, G. Morell, I. H. Scheinberg, J. Hickman, and G. Ashwell, Physical and chemical studies on ceruloplasmin. IX. The role of glactosyl residues in the clearance of ceruloplasmin from the circulation. J. Biol. Chem. 245:4397 (1970).
24. A. G. Morell, G. Gregoriadis, I. H. Scheinberg, J. Hickman, and G. Ashwell, The role of sialic acid in determining the survival of glycoproteins in the circulation, J. Biol. Chem. 246:1461 (1971).
25. W. E. Pricer Jr. and G. Ashwell, The binding of desialylated glycoproteins by plasma membranes of rat liver, J. Biol. Chem. 246:4825 (1971).
26. M. M. B. Kay, Role of physiologic autoantibodies in the removal of senescent human red cells, J. Supra. Mol. Stuct. 9:555 (1978).
27. H. U. Lutz, A. von Daniken, G. Semenza, and T. H. Bachi, Glycophorin-enriched vesicles obtained by a selective extraction of human erythrocyte membranes with a non-ionic detergent, Biochim. Biophys. Acta., in press.
28. E. D. Weinberg, Iron and susceptibility to infectious disease, Science 148:952 (1974).
29. F. M. Burnet, "Immunological Surveillance," Pergammon Press, Oxford, England (1970).
30. H. H. Fudenberg, Genetically determined immune deficiency as the predisposing cause of "autoimmunity" and lyphoid neoplasia, Amer. J. Med. 51:295 (1971).
31. M. E. Gershwin and A. D. Steinberg, Suppression of autoimmune hemolytic anemia in New Zealand (NZB) mice by syngeneic young thymocytes, Clin. Immunol. Immunopath. 4:38 (1975).
32. Y. Marikovsky, D. Danon, and A. Katchalsky, Agglutination by polylysine of young and old red blood cells, Biochim. Biophys. Acta 124:154 (1966).
33. E. Skutelsky, Y. Marikovsky, and D. Danon, Immunoferritin analysis of membrane antigen density: A. Young and old human blood cells. B. Developing erythroid cells and extruded erythroid nuclei, Eur. J. Immunol. 4:512 (1974).
34. G. V. F. Seaman, R. J. Knox, F. J. Nordt, and D. H. Regan, Red cell aging. I. Surface charge density and sialic acid content of density-fractionated human erythrocytes, Blood 50:1001 (1977).
35. S. J. Luner, D. Szklarek, R. J. Knox, G. V. H. Seaman, J. Y. Josefowicz, and B. R. Ware, Red cell charge is not a function of cell age, Nature 269:719 (1977).
36. D. Aminoff, W. F. V. Bruegge, W. C. Bell, K. Sarpolis, and R. Williams, Role of sialic acid in survival of erythrocytes in the circulation: Interaction of neuraminidase-treated and untreated erythrocytes with spleen and liver and the cellular level, Proc. Natl. Acad. Sci. USA 74:1521 (1977).

37. A. F. LoBuglio, R. S. Cotran, and J. H. Jandl, Red cells coated with immmunoglobulin G: Binding and sphereing by mononuclear cells in man, Science 158:1582 (1967).
38. J. Michl and S. C. Silverstein, Role of macrophage receptors in the ingestion phase of phagocytosis, in:"Birth Defects: Original Article Series," 14 (2), R.A. Lerner and D. Bergsma, eds., The National Foundation--March of Dimes, White Plains, New York (1978).
39. J. M. Janicik, R. Schauer, K. H. Andres, and M. von During, Sequestration of neuraminidase-treated erythrocytes. Studies on its topographic, morphologic and immunologic aspects, Cell. Tiss. Res. 186:209 (1978).
40. J. R. Durocher, J. Supramol. Struct. Suppl. 2:199 (1978).
41. C. J. Steer, Kupffer cells and glycoproteins: Does a recognition phenomenon exist? Bull. Kupffer Cell Fdn. I:26 (1978).
42. A. Baxter and J. G. Beeley Surface carbohydrates of aged erythrocytes, Biochem. Biophys. Res. Commun. 83:466 (1978).
43. H. U. Lutz and J. Fehr, Total sialic acid content in glycophorin remains unchanged during senescence of human red cells, submitted.
44. G. Perret, D. Bladier, L. Gattegno, and P. Cornillot, The role of T-agglutinin in the disappearance of erythrocytes artificially aged by desialylation, Mech. Ageing Dev., in press.
45. W. J. Martin and S. E. Martin, Thymus reactive IgM autoantibodies in normal mouse sera, Nature 254:716 (1975).
46. J. C. Roder, D. A. Bell, and S. K. Singhal, Regulation of the autoimmune plaque-forming cell response to single-strand DNA (sDNA) in vitro, J. Immunol. 121:38 (1978).
47. D. W. Dresser and A. M. Popham, Induction of IgM anti-(bovine)-IgG response in mice by bacterial lipopolysaccharide, Nature 264:552 (1976).
48. D. W. Dresser, Most IgM-producing cells in the mouse secrete auto-antibodies (rheumatoid factor), Nature 274:480 (1978).
49. A. E. Bussard, M.-A. Vinit, and J. M. Pages, Immunochemical characterization of the autoantibodies produced by mouse peritoneal cells in culture, Immunochemistry 14:1 (1977).
50. E. J. Stelle and A. J. Cunningham, High proportion of IgG producing cells making autoantibody in normal mice, Nature 274:483 (1978).
51. G. M. Shearer, Cell-mediated cytotoxicity to trinitrophenyl-modified syngeneic lymphocytes, Eur. J. Immunol. 4:527 (1974).
52. P. Levine, Self-nonself concept for cancer and diseases previously known as "autoimmune" diseases, Proc. Natl. Acad. Sci. USA 75:5697 (1978).
53. D. C. Swartzenbruber, Phagocytized plasma cells in mouse spleen observed by light and electron microscopy, Blood 24:432 (1964).
54. N. K. Jerne, A. A. Nordin, and C. Henry, The agar plaque technique for recognizing antibody-producing cells, in:"Cell-Bound Antibodies," D.B. Amos and H. Koprowski, eds.,

Wistar Press, Philadelphia (1963).
55. J. C. Schooley, Autoradiographic observations of plasma cell formation, J. Immunol. 86:331 (1961).
56. C. G. Congdon and T. Makinodan, Splenic white pulp after antigen injection: Relation of time of serum antibody production, Am. J. Path. 39:697 (1961).
58. D. H. Solomon, The nature of Graves' hyperthyroidism, in:"Autoimmune thyroid diseases--Graves' and Hashimoto's," J. Brown, moderator, Ann. Intern. Med. 88:379 (1978).
59. M. C. Raff, Two distinct populations of peripheral lymphocytes in mice distinguishable by immunofluorescence, Immunology 19:637 (1970).
60. D. J. Scribner, H. L. Weiner, and J. W. Moorhead, Anti-immunoglobulin stimulation of murine lymphocytes. V. Age-related decline in Fc receptor-mediated immunoregulation, J. Immunol. 121:377 (1978).
61. H. N. Eisen, "Immunology," Harper and Row Publishers, Inc., Hagerstown, Md (1974).
62. M. M. B. Kay, Hodgkin's Disease: A war between T lymphocytes and transformed macrophages? in:"Lymphocytes and Macrophages in Cancer Patients, Vol. 1, Recent Results in Cancer Research," G. Mathe, I. Florentn, and M.-C. Simmler, eds., Springer-Verlag, New York (1976).

CHANGES IN SYNAPTIC STRUCTURE AFFECTING NEURAL TRANSMISSION IN THE SENESCENT BRAIN

William Bondareff

Department of Anatomy and
Institute of Psychiatry
Northwestern University Medical School
Chicago, Illinois, USA

INTRODUCTION

Neural transmission involves electrochemical interactions between two neurons along a region of interneuronal contact known as a synapse. In vertebrate nervous systems these interactions are mediated by transmitter substances, which react with receptor sites on synaptic membranes affecting their permeability to various ions. Synaptic membranes are modified segments of neuronal plasma membranes, and their properties vary in different types of synapses.

Among synapses found in mammalian brains, axodendritic synapses are probably most numerous. They involve the axonal plasma membrane of one neuron and the dendritic plasma membrane of another. They consist of three parts: an axonal terminal or presynaptic component; a dendritic or postsynaptic component; and a modified segment of the extracellular space, the synaptic cleft. The interaction between presynaptic and postsynaptic components, which facilitates both initial contact in early embryogenesis and functional interactions later, appears to depend in part upon the presence of complex macromolecules. These include glycoproteins and glycolipids, which are structural components of the pre- and post-synaptic membranes. It is believed that the side chains and terminal groups of these plasma membrane-associated macromolecules extend into the synaptic cleft, where they may interact with one another and with other macromolecules, perhaps proteoglycans.

A relationship between synaptic structure and function is indicated by the fact that interneuronal transmission in the fetus is heralded by the appearance of synapses with adult-like structure.

The return of function after deafferentation in young and adult animals is similarly associated with the appearance of synapses, and the character of the returning function appears to depend upon the accuracy with which synaptic connections are remade with previously deafferentated neurons (1). As a relationship between synaptic structure and function exists in immature and mature animals, it seems reasonable to anticipate that a similar relationship exists in senescence and that senescent changes in neuronal function can be associated with changes in synaptic structure and distribution. Age-related changes in the structure/function relationship of synapses are, however, not well known. They have been the subject of recent studies (2,3), and their discussion here is predicated upon the observation that synaptic loss typically occurs in the brain of the senescent rat, and is not necessarily dependent upon an antecedent loss of neurons (4), although neuronal loss in senescence is well known (5).

MATERIALS AND METHODS

Axo-dendritic synapses of the dentate gyrus molecular layer were compared in hippocampi of young adult and senescent male Fischer-344 rats. The hippocampus was chosen for study because of its presumed relationship to memory and learning functions, and the dentate gyrus because its anatomy is well known. The animals, bred under pathogen-free conditions, were commercially available from the Charles River Breeding Laboratories (Wilmington, Massachusetts). Their natural history and pathology has been characterized (6). The 50% mean survival age is 29 months; the maximal survival age appears to be about 36 months; and the incidence of pathological changes in the brain is small. Rats of the Fischer-344 strain of 24 and 3 months of age, therefore, seemed well suited for studies of aging.

RESULTS

Attention was focused on the axo-dendritic synapses of a specific part of the dentate gyrus portion of the hippocampus (see refs. 14,19). The postsynaptic component of these synapses appears to consist primarily of dendrites of dentate gyrus granule cells, but the presynaptic component is less well-defined. Synapses were first counted in an electron microscope study of the middle third of the molecular layer (4). When compared with synaptic counts of the same region of 3-month-old rats, a 27% decrease in the number of synapses per unit of square area of neuropil was found in the 24-month-old animals (Fig. 1). Unfortunately, it was difficult to determine whether this loss of synapses reflected an antecedent age-related insult to the pre- or post-synaptic neurons involved in the synapses. There was, however, no age-related change in the number of postsynaptic granule cell bodies (nor in synaptic size, nor in tissue volume), and it appeared, therefore, to depend upon changes to the presynaptic component (7). This conclusion was supported by a later

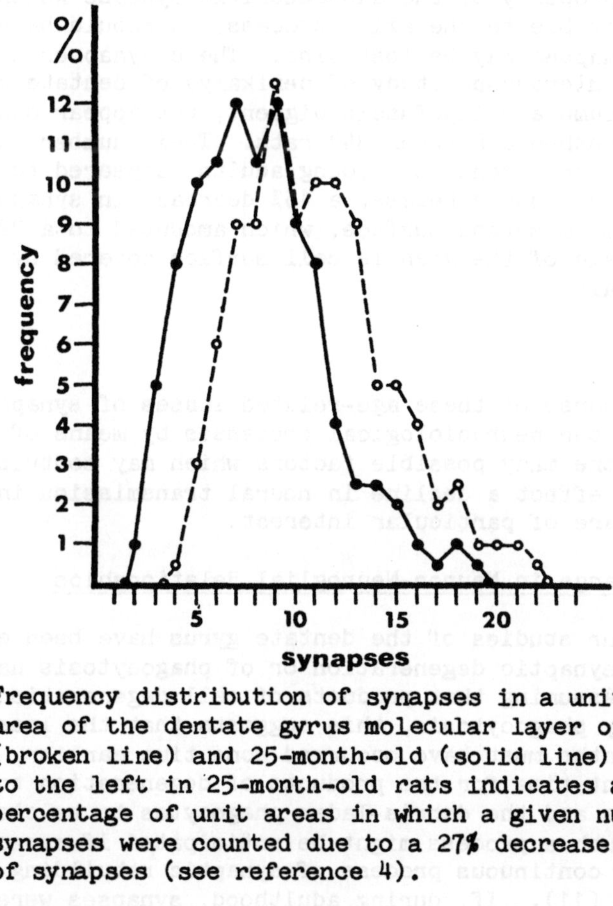

Fig. 1. Frequency distribution of synapses in a unit of square area of the dentate gyrus molecular layer of 3-month-old (broken line) and 25-month-old (solid line) rats. A shift to the left in 25-month-old rats indicates a smaller percentage of unit areas in which a given number of synapses were counted due to a 27% decrease in the number of synapses (see reference 4).

electron microscope study (8) in which an almost identical loss of synapses was found in the supragranular portion of the molecular layer, where presynaptic elements have been shown to be different from those found in the middle third portion. Again, no decrease in the number of postsynaptic granule cell bodies could be demonstrated.

A loss of axo-dendritic synapses has also been found in the visual area of the cerebral cortex of the senescent Fischer-344 rat (9) and the cerebellar cortex (10). In the latter, a 33% decrement in the axo-dendritic synapses of 25-month-old Fischer-344 rats was found to involve axo-spinous synapses selectively. The number of these synapses, between parallel fibers (axons) and Purkinje cell dendritic spines, seemed to decline in senescence, while those between climbing fibers and dendritic shafts were spared.

Lest the misinterpretation be given that synaptic loss in the senescent hippocampus involves only axo-dendritic synapses and that there is some property of the axo-dendritic synapse which makes it uniquely susceptible to the aging process, it should be noted that axo-somatic synapses may be lost also. These synapses were counted in an electron microscope study of perikarya of dentate gyrus granule cells which accumulate lipofuscin pigment, but appear otherwise normal in 25-month-old Fischer-344 rats. Their number, as compared with that of 3- to 4-month-old young adults, appeared to be constant. There was, nevertheless, a 15% decrease in synapses per length of plasma membrane surface, which amounted to a 22% decrease in the percentage of the granule cell surface covered by synapses in senescent animals.

DISCUSSION

The time course of these age-related losses of synapses is not known; nor are the neurobiological processes by means of which they occur. Among the many possible factors which may contribute to synaptic loss and effect a decline in neural transmission in senescence, the following are of particular interest.

Age-Related Change in Neuron-Neuroglial Relationships

Although our studies of the dentate gyrus have been extensive, no indication of synaptic degeneration or of phagocytosis has ever been encountered. Assuming that products of cell degeneration are generally removed by phagocytosis, this suggests that the loss of synapses found at 24 months must have occurred some time earlier, so as to allow sufficient time for the products of degeneration to be removed by phagocytosis and the debris-laden phagocytes to be cleared from the tissue. Such a process might be anticipated if synaptic loss were part of a continuous process of synaptic rebuilding, as was suggested earlier (11). If, during adulthood, synapses were being formed and deformed, the rate of deformation would increase with age such that, as senescence were approached, more synapses would be lost than formed. The number of microglial cells, which are the principal phagocytes of the central nervous system, might increase with age, as has been found in cerebral cortex (12). There is no evidence that the number of microcytes increases in the senescent dentate gyrus, and no evidence that microcytes laden with phagocytized remains of synapses are cleared from the dentate gyrus prior to the 24th month. There is, however, evidence that a process of remodelling occurs in the dentate gyrus as a function of age.

Although there appears to be no change in the number of microglial cells in the hippocampus of the senescent rat, there is evidence of an increase in the number of astrocytes (13). An electron microscope study of the supragranular region selected for morphometric analysis of synapses (14) did not demonstrate any change in the number of astrocytic cell bodies, but did show a 45% increase in the volume fraction of astrocytic processes (Table 1). As no change in

Table 1. Number and Volume Fraction of Astroglial Process Profiles in the Supragranular Zone of the Dentate Gyri of Young Adult (3 months of age) and Senescent (25 months of age) Rats (14)

	Volume Fraction	
	3 Months	25 Months
Mean ± S.E.M. per animal	0.114 ± 0.006 0.083 ± 0.006 0.098 ± 0.007 0.094 ± 0.007 0.082 ± 0.007	0.184 ± 0.008 0.141 ± 0.008 0.120 ± 0.007 0.136 ± 0.007 0.097 ± 0.007
Mean ± S.E.M. per group	0.094 ± 0.006	0.136 ± 0.014
Percent of 3-month-old group		144.7
Significance level		$P < 0.01$

the dimensions of the whole dentate gyrus could be demonstrated, there would appear to be a redistribution of its parts in the senescent rat.

Injury of Postsynaptic Neurons

Although a voluminous literature might lead to the assumption that synaptic loss is associated with an antecedent loss of neurons in the dentate gyrus, available data indicate no such loss. The data, however, are conflicting. On the one hand, counts of granule cells in senescent Fischer-344 rats have failed to demonstrate any significant age-related decrease (7,8). On the other hand, a whittling away of the dendritic trees of neurons appears to be a fairly generalized characteristic of aging, and has been described in several areas of the brain (9,15-18).

Decreases in both the volume fraction and surface area of dendrites, coincident with the age-related changes in synapses and astrocytes described above, have been demonstrated by morphometric analysis of the supragranular portion of the dentate gyrus and shown to reflect an absolute loss of dendrites (19). That these decreases are disproportionate (Table 2) probably indicates the selective loss

Table 2. Volume Fraction and Surface Area of Dendritic Shafts in 3-Month-Old and 25-Month-Old Rats (19)

	Volume Fraction		Surface Area	
	3 Months	25 Months	3 Months	25 Months
Mean ± S.E.M. per Animal	0.407 ± 0.016	0.346 ± 0.012	2.13 ± 0.07	1.31 ± 0.08
	0.421 ± 0.011	0.406 ± 0.015	1.90 ± 0.06	1.63 ± 0.06
	0.422 ± 0.015	0.395 ± 0.012	1.77 ± 0.07	1.46 ± 0.06
	0.365 ± 0.013	0.329 ± 0.011	1.78 ± 0.08	1.21 ± 0.04
	0.451 ± 0.015	0.333 ± 0.015	1.91 ± 0.07	1.29 ± 0.06
Mean ± S.E.M. per group	0.413 ± 0.014	0.362 ± 0.016	1.90 ± 0.06	1.38 ± 0.07
% of 3-month-old group		87.6		72.6
Significance		P < 0.05		P < 0.001

of smaller diameter, distal dendritic branches in the dentate gyrus, as might have been predicted from the findings of others (see above) in other parts of the brain. The mechanism of this loss is unknown and its relationship to synaptic loss in the dentate gyrus is unknown. However, it does not appear to be prerequisite for synaptic loss, because the loss of synapses is the same whether it is determined relative to the square area of neuropil or to a unit length of dendrites found in the senescent dentate gyrus (8) (Table 3).

Injury of Presynaptic Neurons

There has been no systematic enumeration of neurons presynaptic to synapses found in the dentate gyrus. There is evidence, however, that neurons of the septal nucleus, which contribute presynaptic cholinergic afferents to synapses in the supragranular region of the dentate gyrus, take up and incorporate ^{3}H-fucose into glycoproteins similarly in animals 24 and 3 months of age (20). Yet, the intraneuronal transport of fucose-labeled glycoproteins through axons of the septohippocampal pathway was shown to be slowed in 25-month-old Fischer-344 rats. This was shown by labeling the medial septal nucleus of young adult and senescent rats with ^{3}H-fucose and comparing the times of arrival of ^{3}H-fucose labeled glycoproteins in the hippocampus as a function of age (20). The arrival times differed significantly, reflecting a 30% reduction in the rate of axonal transport of glycoproteins to synapses remaining in the dentate gyrus of senescent rats (Fig. 2). Since glycoproteins are components of presynaptic membranes, such an age-related decrement in the amount

Table 3. Number of Synapses Involving Dendritic Shafts and Spines in the Supragranular Zone of the Dentate Gyrus of Young Adult (3-month-old) and Senescent (25-month-old) Rats (19)

	Per Tissue Square Area (66 sq. μm)				Per Dendrite Unit Length (10 μm)			
	Shafts		Spines		Shafts		Spines	
	3 Months	25 Months	3 Months	25 Months	3 Months	25 Months	3 Months	25 Months
Mean ± S.E.M. per Animal	2.6 ± 0.2	1.6 ± 0.1	17.0 ± 0.5	13.1 ± 0.4	6.3 ± 0.9 (n = 248)	4.7 ± 0.9 (n = 195)	4.2 ± 0.6	3.5 ± 0.6
	3.5 ± 0.2	1.0 ± 0.1	14.2 ± 0.6	13.6 ± 0.4	8.4 ± 1.3 (n = 253)	3.1 ± 0.6 (n = 239)	3.7 ± 0.8	3.6 ± 0.6
	2.4 ± 0.2	2.0 ± 0.2	14.6 ± 0.5	11.2 ± 0.4	7.2 ± 1.1 (n = 265)	3.2 ± 0.6 (n = 230)	7.7 ± 1.4	3.7 ± 0.6
	2.1 ± 0.2	2.3 ± 0.2	14.7 ± 0.4	9.7 ± 0.5	6.2 ± 0.8 (n = 300)	5.4 ± 1.0 (n = 225)	7.4 ± 0.9	3.5 ± 0.7
	2.5 ± 0.2	1.7 ± 0.1	13.6 ± 0.6	8.2 ± 0.4	7.0 ± 1.0 (n = 320)	4.2 ± 0.9 (n = 211)	6.0 ± 1.1	3.3 ± 0.7
Mean ± S.E.M. per Group	2.6 ± 0.2	1.7 ± 0.2	14.8 ± 0.6	11.2 ± 1.0	6.8 ± 0.2	4.1 ± 0.4	5.8 ± 0.8	3.5 ± 0.1
Per Cent of 3-month-old group		65.4		75.7		60.4		60.3
Significance Level	$P < 0.02$		$P < 0.02$		$P < 0.001$		$P < 0.05$	

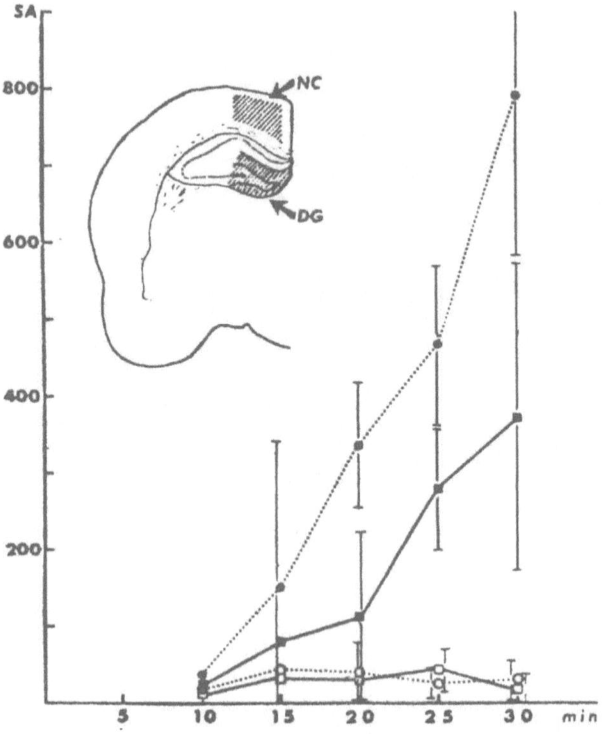

Fig. 2. Specific activities of the TCA-PTA-insoluble fractions of the dentate gyrus (closed symbols) and neocortex (open symbols) at various time intervals after ^{3}H-fucose injection into the medial septal nucleus of young adult (dotted line) and senescent (solid line) rats. The dentate gyrus (DG) with its hilus and the neocortex (NC) overlying the hippocampal formation were excised from a 1 mm thick coronal brain section through the most rostral part of the dentate gyrus (left upper corner). Each point on the graphs represents the mean specific activity obtained for a group of 5 rats, and 95% confidence intervals of the means are indicated by bars. Time after the end of ^{3}H-fucose injection is plotted on the abscissa against specific activities of the corresponding fraction on the ordinate (see reference 20).

and/or rate of glycoproteins transported to axonal terminals can be expected to indicate a failure of presynaptic neurons to maintain the integrity of their synaptic membranes in senescence.

Change in the Extraneuronal Microenvironment

The formation and maintenance of synaptic structure depends upon adequate neuronal metabolism. Neuronal metabolism, in turn, depends upon a physiological relationship between neurons, blood vessels supplying them, and the extracellular space through which neuronal-vascular exchanges occur. Although little is known about the vascular compartment of aging Fischer-344 rats, it has been shown that the blood-brain barrier, at least that to ^{14}C-sucrose, is intact at 28 months (21). It has been shown that the depth of penetration of ruthenium red from the free ventricular surface into the substance of the dentate gyrus decreases in the 25-month-old Fischer-344 rat (22), indicating a change in charge density of intercellular polyanions in the extracellular spaces of senescent brain. The nature of this change is unknown, but it correlates directly with the 50% reduction in volume of the extracellular space which was described in the rat cerebral cortex by Bondareff and Narotzky (23).

This description of structure/function relationships in the senescent brain has focused on the rearrangement of structural components and the presumed relationship between this rearrangement and faulty intraneuronal transport of glycoproteins. That the latter might be more than merely temporarily related to structural alterations of synaptic membranes is suggested by two peculiarities of neurons in senescent rats. First, a change in Concanavalin A binding patterns of neurons isolated from the lateral vestibular nuclei of 24-month-old rats was demonstrated by fluorescence microscopy (24). Second, a decrease in the sensitivity of cationized ferritin binding capacity of synaptosomes isolated from the brains of senescent rats was demonstrated to neuraminidase (25). Both suggest age-related changes in glycoprotein composition and are compatible with structural changes in presynaptic membranes. It is unknown how such changes might be related to functional impairment or to the rearrangement of structural components in the dentate gyrus of senescent rats.

REFERENCES

1. A. Globus, Brain morphology as a function of presynaptic morphology and activity, in:"The Developmental Neuropsychology of Sensory Deprivation," H. Reisen, ed., Academic Press, New York (1975).
2. W. T. Greenough, R. W. West and T. J. DeVoogd, Subsynaptic plate perforations: Changes with age and experience in the rat, Science 202:1096 (1979).
3. P. W. Landfield and G. Lynch, Impaired monosynaptic potentiation in in vitro hippocampal slices from aged, memory-deficient rats, J. Gerontol. 32:523 (1977).
4. W. Bondareff and Y. Geinisman, Loss of synapses in the dentate gyrus of the senescent rat, Am. J. Anat. 145:129 (1976).
5. W. Bondareff, The neural basis of aging, in:"Handbook of the Psychology of Aging," J. E. Birren and K. W. Schaie, eds., Van Nostrand Reinhold, New York (1976).

6. G. L. Coleman, S. W. Barthold, G. W. Osbaldiston, S. J. Foster, and A. M. Jones, Pathological changes during aging in barrier-reared Fischer-344 male rats, J. Gerontol. 32:258 (1977).
7. Y. Geinisman and W. Bondareff, Decrease in the number of synapses in the senescent brain: A quantitative electron microscopic analysis of the dentate gyrus molecular layer in the rat, Mech. Ageing Dev. 5:11 (1976).
8. Y. Geinisman, W. Bondareff, and J. T. Dodge, Partial deafferentation of neurons in the dentate gyrus of the senesent rat, Br. Res. 134:541 (1977).
9. M. L. Feldman, Aging changes in the morphology of cortical dendrites, in:"Neurobiology of Aging," R. D. Terry and S. Gershon, eds., Raven Press, New York (1976).
10. R. Glick, and W. Bondareff, Synapses in the cerebellar cortex of the senescent rat, J. Gerontol. (in press).
11. C. Sotelo and S. L. Palay, Altered axons and axon terminals in the lateral vestibular nucleus of the rat, Lab. Invest. 25:653 (1971).
12. D. W. Vaughan and A. Peters, Neuroglia cells in the cerebral cortex of rats from young adulthood to old age, J. Neurocyt. 3:405 (1974).
13. P. W. Landfield, G. Rose, L. Sandles, T. C. Wohlstadtes, and G. Lynch, Patterns of astroglial hypertrophy and neuronal degeneration in the hippocampus of aged, memory-deficient rats, J. Gerontol. 32:3 (1977).
14. Y. Geinisman, W. Bondareff, and J. T. Dodge, Hypertrophy of astroglial processes in the dentate gyrus of the senescent rat, Am. J. Anat. 153:3 (1978).
15. D. W. Vaughan, Age-related deterioration of pyramidal cell basal dendrites in the rat auditory cortex, J. Comp. Neur. 171:501 (1977).
16. J. W. Hinds and N.A. NcNelly, Aging of the rat olfactory bulb: Growth and atrophy of constituent layers and changes in size and number of mitral cells, J. Comp. Neur. 171:345 (1977).
17. M. E. Scheibel, R. D. Lindsay, U. Tomiyasu and A. B. Scheibel, Progressive dendritic changes in aging human cortex, Expt. Neurol. 47:392 (1975).
18. M. E. Scheibel, R. D. Lindsay, U. Tomiyasu and A. B. Scheibel, Progressive dendritic changes in aging human limbic system, Ep. Neurol. 53:420 (1976).
19. Y. Geinisman, W. Bondareff, and J. T. Dodge, Dendritic atrophy in the dentate gyrus of the senescent rat, Am. J. Anat. 152:321 (1978).
20. Y. Geinisman, Y. Bondareff, and A. Telser, Transport of ^{3}H-fucose labeled glycoproteins in the septo-hippocampal pathway of young adult and senescent rats, Br. Res. 125:182 (1977).
21. S. I. Rapoport, K. Ohno, and K. D. Pettigrew, Society for Neuroscience Abstracts (1978).

22. W. Bondareff and S. Lin-Liu, Age-related change in the neuronal microenvironment: Penetration of ruthenium red into extracellular space of brain in young adult and senescent rats, Am. J. Anat. 148:57 (1977).
23. W. Bondareff and R. Narotzky, Age changes in the neuronal microenvironment, Science 176:1135 (1972).
24. K. D. Bennett and W. Bondareff, Age-related differences in binding of Concanavalin A to plasma membranes of isolated neurons, Am. J. Anat. 150:175 (1977).
25. S. Lin-Liu and W. Bondareff (unpublished).

ROLE OF THE IMMUNE SYSTEM IN AGING*

Takashi Makinodan

Geriatric Research, Education and Clinical Center (GRECC)
Wadsworth Medical Center
Los Angeles, CA 90073
and the Department of Medicine, UCLA
Los Angeles, CA 90024

INTRODUCTION

Since the turn of the century, there has been a continuum of medical breakthroughs controlling life-shortening diseases. As a consequence, more people are now living longer than they were at the turn of the century. Unfortunately, life extension means chronic disorders to many of the elderly. This has created a trememdous socio-economic burden throughout the world. Thus, during the past decade, there has been a growing emphasis in biomedical research towards control of age-related chronic disorders, in order to enable the elderly to extend their healthy years of life.

To this end, various physiologic systems are being investigated, with the major emphasis on those with systemic homeostatic functions. Among them is the immune system. It is an attractive model system for the following reasons: (a) loss of immunologic vigor is one of the characteristics of perhaps all aging mammals; (b) the decline in normal functions of the immune system seems to trigger infectious, neoplastic, autoimmune and immune complex diseases; (c) the pattern of rise and fall in activity of the immune system with age is inversely related to the death rate; (d) our understanding of the immune system's differentiation process at the cellular, molecular and genetic levels is more comprehensive than that of perhaps

*This is publication no. 026 from GRECC, VA Wadsworth Medical Center, which has been supported in part by The Medical Research Service of VA and the Department of Energy (Grant no. ET 76-S-03-0034 P.A. 264).

any other system, and therefore it appears to be amenable to successful manipulation; and (e) circumvention of the declining function of the immune system may minimize the severity of diseases of the elderly.

My task is to present an overview of the two major issues confronting us on aging and immunity or immunologic aging. One is at the cellular level and the other at the organismic level. At the cellular level, it concerns the nature of decline in normal immunologic vigor with age. At the organismic level, it concerns the causal nature of the inverse relationship between immunologic aging and increase in susceptibility to various diseases. These discussions will be preceded by a brief discussion of age-related changes in immune functions.

LOSS OF IMMUNOLOGIC VIGOR WITH AGE--IMMUNOLOGIC AGING

The immune system protects the body in a highly specific manner against foreign invasion by viruses, bacteria, fungi and protozoans, and against one's own somatic cells which have been damaged or undergone transformation into cancer cells. Obviously, any factor or event that can decrease the normal surveillance activity of the immune system will permit growth of invasive antigens (e.g., bacteria and cancer cells) which can, in turn, disrupt various physiological functions of the body. Hence, it should be apparent that the immune system plays a major role in the preservation of life.

The bone marrow, thymus, spleen and lymph nodes comprise the major organs of the mammalian immune system. The bone marrow and thymus are generally referred to as the primary or central organs of the immune system because they become lymphocytic first in embryogenesis, and thereafter serve as the source of precursor cells. The spleen and lymph nodes, on the other hand, are referred to as secondary or peripheral organs. It is in these peripheral organs that immunity is initiated. The cells of the immune system can be subdivided into (a) stem cells, (b) thymus-derived T lymphocytes, (c) bone marrow-derived B lymphocytes, which upon antigen stimulation give rise to plasma cells, and (d) macrophages. In a typical immune response, the latter three cell types communicate with each other in a highly specific manner, and undergo proliferation and maturation (i.e., clonal differentiation).

In general, immunologic activity increases rapidly after birth to a peak level at sexual maturity followed by a gradual decline. The onset and rate of decline, however, will vary with the type of immune response and the species. The decline with age appears to be characteristic of aging mammals, as it has been observed not only in humans (1), but also in all experimental mammals examined (2-7). Therefore, it has been commonly referred to as "immunologic aging."

Moreover, as with immunodeficient children (8) and immunosuppressed adults (9), the decline is associated with an increase in the incidence of infectious, autoimmune, immune complex, and cancerous diseases (1,10). Thus, there are two major issues in Immunogerontology. At the cellular level, it concerns the nature of cellular and humoral changes responsible for immunologic aging. At the organismic level, it concerns the causal nature of the inverse relationship between immunologic aging and the increase in susceptibility to immunologically involved diseases of aging (infections, autoimmune and immune complex diseases, cancer, amyloidosis, etc.).

FACTORS RESPONSIBLE FOR IMMUNOLOGIC AGING

The immunologic network is highly complex and multifaceted, so the multifactorial etiology of immunologic aging should not be a surprise (1,10-14). At the tissue level, changes in both the environment and the immune cells have been shown to be responsible.

Very little is known of the nature of the responsible factor(s) in the cellular environment, but the findings indicate that two types of factors are involved: deleterious substances of molecular and viral natures, and essential substances of nutritional and hormonal natures. Support for the first possibility came initially from the cell-impermeable diffusion chamber studies by Price and Makinodan (15), who showed that young mouse cells can be inhibited in their immunologic performance when exposed to in vivo plasma fluid factors of old mice. More recently, Rivnay et al. (16) found that the lipid microviscosity is 20% higher in the plasma membrane of lymphocytes of old than that of young mice, due mainly to the age-related elevation of the cholesterol/phospholipid ratio. Elevation in lipid microviscosity could be a major contributory factor in the kinetic sluggishness of old cells, as it can decrease the rate of protein diffusion. Support for the second possibility comes from the observation of Bach et al. (17), who found that secretion of thymic factors essential for T cell maturation decreases with age in parallel with thymic involution, and of Bilder and Denkla (18), who found that hypophysectomy plus hormonal replacement therapy had a pronounced immunorestorative effect on old but not young rats.

There are 3 possible types of cellular changes which can cause immunologic aging: (a) an absolute decrease in the number of antigen-responsive cells through cell death caused possibly by autoimmune cells or by the Hayflick phenomenon (19), (b) functional alteration of immune cells caused by genetic and epigenetic events, and (c) a relative decrease in the number of antigen-responsive cells as a result of interference by specific and nonspecific factors. Studies over the past decade show that all 3 types of change do indeed occur with age. Perhaps the least dramatic and consistent is the decrease in number of antigen-responsive cells, which varies with population sampling, ranging from no change with age to only a modest decrease (10). Changes intrinsic to immune cells include findings such as:

a) Decrease with age in the number of surface theta receptor antigens of mouse splenic T cells (20), which differentiate into stem cells, T cells, B cells and macrophages.
b) Increase with age in the frequency of aneuploidy in circulating human T cells (21).
c) Decrease with age in the number of nuclear actinomycin binding sites in circulating human lymphocytes (22).
d) Decrease with age in nuclear histone acetylation of circulating human lymphocytes (23).
e) Decrease with age in the ability of mouse bone marrow stem cells to repair ionizing radiation-induced DNA damage (24).
f) Decrease with age in the Fc receptor-mediated immunoregulation of mouse splenic B cells (25).
g) Decrease with age in the ratio of cyclic AMP/cyclic GMP levels of unstimulated and stimulated mouse spleen cells (26).

Changes caused by alteration in the regulatory factors with age include such findings as:

a) The inability of precursor cells of old mice to interact with each other as efficiently as those of young mice in response to antigenic stimulation (15,27,28).
b) An increase with age in the number of suppressor T and B cells (28-30).
c) A decrease with age in the number of suppressor T cells in short-lived autoimmune-susceptible mice and in humans (31-33).
d) An increase with age in the number of helper T cells in humans (33).
e) A decrease with age in the ability of carrier-primed mouse T cells to enhance B cells in their antibody response (34).
f) A parabolic pattern of change with age in the avidity of antibody (35).

RELATIONSHIP BETWEEN IMMUNOLOGIC AGING AND DISEASES OF AGING

An issue that has not been resolved satisfactorily is whether the decline to a threshold level predisposes an individual to disease, or whether disease compromises normal immunologic activities. Circumstantial evidence tends to favor the former possibility.

One appproach toward resolving this issue is to perturb the immune system of adult individuals before their normal activities decline, and then to assess the immunologic, pathologic, and actuarial changes kinetically. The system can be perturbed by altering either the onset of the decline and/or the rate of decline. Another approach is to perturb the immune system of old individuals whose normal immune functions are already reduced, and then assess the immunologic, pathologic and actuarial changes kinetically. The system can be perturbed by further reductive, by preventive, or by restorative means. Although all three approaches should be attempted to resolve this complex triangular relationship of aging, decreased immune function and increased incidence of disease, the latter two approaches are preferred. They would lend themselves more effectively to the study of both cellular and molecular mechanisms responsible for the decline in normal immunologic activities with age. For these reasons the discussion will be limited to these latter approaches.

Intervention by Preventive Methods

Internal Body Temperature Control. Liu and Walford demonstrated that the life span of an annual fish can be extended by subjecting it to mild hypothermia during the last half of its life (36). The immunologic implication of this observation is intriguing. However, further studies are required to understand the significance of the life extending effect of hypothermia on the relationship between immunity and disease.

Tissue Ablation. In controlling a disease that can disrupt normal immune functions and shorten the life span, one approach is to remove the tissue from which a disease originates or that promotes it (provided the tissue is not essential). This approach was first employed successfully by Furth over 30 years ago (37). He thymectomized a short-lived, thymoma-susceptible AKR strain of mice at young adulthood. The incidence of leukemia decreased drastically; as a consequence, the mice lived significantly longer. This approach was also used successfully by us in long-lived hybrid mice (38). We found that the survival time of mice splenectomized at about 100 weeks of age can be nearly doubled over that of sham-splenectomized mice. Splenectomy was performed at about 100 weeks because previous studies had shown that many old mice were dying at about 2 years of age of reticulum cell sarcoma originating in the spleen (39).

Although this method is not practical in humans, it could be used in experimental animals to resolve the types of diseases emerging late in life that can compromise general and specific immune functions.

Genetic Manipulation. Genetic manipulation has been performed in both long-lived and short-lived strains of mice In studies with long-lived mice, it was reasoned that aging is influenced genetically by only a limited number of regulatory genes, that the immune system plays a major role in aging (40), and that a "super-regulatory gene complex system" of the immune system (41), i.e., the H-2 region of chromosome 17 in the mouse and the HLA region of chromosome 6 in the human, is the major histocompatibility complex (MHC) system. Inbred congenic strains of mice differing only at the H-2 region were therefore assessed for their age-related immune functions, age-specific diseases and life spans (42,43). Variation in these parameters between congenic mice within a given inbred strain was as great as that observed between different inbred strains of mice. One would have expected a greater uniformity in life span, immunologically associated disease pattern, and immunologic activities between congenic sets of mice within an inbred strain than between inbred strains, if the MHC system in the mouse did not exert a significant influence upon aging, age-related immunologic abnormalities and life span. It can be argued, therefore, that the MHC system plays a major role in age-associated immunologic abnormalities and life span in mice.

The focus with short-lived mice has been on susceptibility to autoimmune and immune complex manifestations (44). These studies showed that more than one gene is involved in susceptibility to autoimmune and immune complex diseases. An example is reflected in a comparison of life spans of different inbred mouse strains and their hybrids; e.g., the mean life span of autoimmune-susceptible NZB, NZW, $(NZB \times NZW)F_1$, $(NZB \times CBA)F_1$ and nonautoimmune-susceptible CBA mice were 12, 21, 12, 29, and 28 months, respectively.

Genetic manipulation is not practical in humans, but it can be used to dissociate the relative roles that genetic and environmental factors play in aging. To this end, Greenberg and Yunis have been studying the influence of HLA haplotype on immune responsiveness and life span in aging humans (45).

Dietary Manipulation. About 45 years ago, McCay et al. (46) first discovered that the life span of rats can be extended significantly by restricting their caloric intake during growth. Recently a more exhaustive study was carried out, also in rats, by Ross and Bras (47,48) that confirmed and extended the classical work. They found that early caloric restriction decelerates the aging rate, as judged by age-related biochemical and pathological changes. Walford et al. (49) subsequently demonstrated that the immune systems of long-lived mice subjected to a calorically restricted but nutritionally supplemented diet, mature slowly and manifest age-associated changes belatedly. Fernandes et al. (50,51) showed that a diet high in fat and relatively low in protein, which favors reproduction in experimental rodents, significantly increased cell-mediated autoimmune manifestations and shortened the life expectancy of short-lived, autoimmune-susceptible mice. In contrast, a diet low in fat, which is less favorable for reproduction, decreased autoimmune manifestations and prolonged the life expectancy of these mice. Further, they showed that the life span of these short-lived autoimmune-susceptible mice can be dramatically extended by restricting their caloric intake (52).

Intervention by Restorative Methods

Tissue Ablation. As mentioned earlier, the tissue ablation approach, has been used as a preventive method. It has also been recently used very effectively by Bilder and Denckla in an attempt to restore normal immune functions (18). Denckla hypothesized that hypothyroidism in old individuals could be caused by a substance(s) secreted by the pituitary that competes with thyroid hormones for the same target cell receptors, including those of the immune system, and that secretion of the substance begins shortly after sexual maturity (53). He reasoned that if this were correct, hypophysectomy of aging individuals supplemented with standard hormone replacement therapy should have a beneficial effect. Accordingly, old and young rats were hypophysectomized and subjected to hormone replacement therapy. The results showed that hypophysectomy had a pronounced immunorestorative effect on old rats, but had no effect on young rats.

This method is not practical in humans. However, hypophysectomized old rats could be used to resolve the problem of the relationship between the immune system's "aging clock" and its extrinsic "pacemaker." Moreover, if the pituitary substance can be purified, a specific antiserum reagent could be prepared and used clinically. It appears, then, that this type of tissue ablation study has both basic and clinical importance.

Cell Grafting. Grafting of thymus, spleen, lymph nodes and bone marrow has been attempted individually or in combinations in genetically compatible old recipients with varying success in terms of immunologic restoration and extension of life span.

Fabris et al. demonstratrated most impressively that the life span of short-lived, growth-hormone deficient, hypopituitary dwarf mice can be extended as much as 3- to 4-fold by injecting large doses of lymph node cells (54). A comparable life-prolonging effect was obtained by injecting growth hormone and thyroxin into dwarf mice with intact thymi, but not into dwarf mice whose thymi had been removed beforehand. These results indicate that the pituitary "turns on" the immune system through the thymus, and the T cells "turn on" the endocrine system through the pituitary. Injection of young spleen or thymus cells into old, autoimmune-susceptible, short-lived mice has had less spectacular results. The appearance of certain types of auto-antibodies (55) was delayed, but not prevented permanently, and the life-prolonging effect was minimal (56). Similarly, multiple thymus grafts did extend their life expectancy, but only by 1 month (57). Furthermore, the age-associated pathological changes were unaltered by these treatments (58).

The first attempts to graft young thymus or bone marrow cells into old nonautoimmune-susceptible, long-lived mice were also not too encouraging, as the life span was not extended appreciably, nor was the immune response elevated (59,60). Subsequent studies on the mechanism of decline with age in normal immune functions suggested to us the reason that these earlier cell grafting attempts were not successful. These studies revealed that the loss of immunologic vigor is due in part to changes in the T cell population (61), in part to the reduced rate at which stem cells can self-generate and generate progeny cells (62), and in part to the inability of involuted thymus to transform precursor cells to T cells efficiently (63). Therefore, we exposed long lived old mice to low dose radiation to destroy most of their immune cells and grafted into them both newborn thymus and young adult bone marrow stem cells. This treatment restored their immune functions to levels approaching those of adult mice (64) for at least six months after graft treatment in mice with a normal mean life span of 27 months (an equivalent to 0.22 of a mean mouse life span, or about 15 human years). Current immunorestorative studies by cell grafting should resolve what influence, if any, grafting will have on the frequency and severity of diseases of the aged and whether cell grafting can alter the life expectancy of short-lived and long-lived mice.

Studies by Perkins et al. (65) on susceptibility to infection have also generated encouraging data. These showed that old mice can be made to resist lethal doses of virulent *Salmonella typhimurium* by injecting them before exposure with spleen cells from young genetically compatible mice which had been immunized with the vaccine. Their findings also indicated that sensitized spleen cells can persist in the recipients for a long time after injection, and that spleen cells can be stored cryogenically for an extended period of time without loss of immunologic activity. This means that the method of Perkins et al. (65) may have a practical application in random bred species.

Chemical Therapy. Only a few chemical agents have been shown to possess immunorestorative activity. These include thymic hormones, certain free radical inhibitors (antioxidants), double-stranded polynucleotide, and mercaptoethanol.

It seems obvious that thymic hormones will be used to prevent immunologic aging or restore immunologic vigor, since the loss of the latter has been clearly shown to be associated with the failure of thymus to continue synthesizing T cell maturation hormones (17,63). Surprisingly, however, there has been no systematic study on their effectiveness in preventing immunologic aging, and studies on their use as immunorestorative agents have been few--but nevertheless encouraging. Friedman et al. (66) found that thymus humoral factor (THF), prepared by N. Trainin, can enhance the T cell dependent graft-vs-host activity *in vitro* of spleen cells from old but not young mice. This would indicate that THF is not acting as a nonspecific adjuvant agent. Otherwise, THF also would have enhanced the activity of young spleen cells. Less encouraging are the preliminary findings of Bach (67). Using T cell-dependent lymphocyte-mediated cytotoxicity (LMC) as the assay, she found that circulating thymic factor (TF) treatment in vivo is effective in preventing the accelerated decline in LMC activity of adult thymectomized mice, but ineffective in normal young and middle-aged (75-86 weeks old) mice. It would appear that TF may be promoting the emergence of suppressor cells in these normal mice. Whether or not it would be effective in old mice, as demonstrated by Friedman et al. (66), remains to be proven.

Weksler et al. (68) were able to partially restore the antibody-forming capacity of old spleen cells by exposing them to another preparation of thymic hormones, thymopoietin. In contrast, Martinez et al. (69) failed to demonstrate the effectiveness of thymopoietin, ubiquitin and synthetic serum thymic factor, prepared by G. Goldstein, in restoring T cell mitogenic response and resistance to tumor cells. The test mice were thymectomized either neonatally or at 1 month of age, and then subjected to treatment with one of the hormones. Unfortunately, no attempt was made to assess the effectiveness of a mixture of these hormones. According to A. Goldstein (70), T cell maturation requires many steps, and several different types of thymic hormones are necessary for the generation of mature functional T cells.

A. Goldstein et al. (70) using still another preparation of thymic hormone, thymosin, have found that repeated injections of the hormone can alleviate many of the symptoms in mice and humans manifesting immunodeficiency diseases. In addition, repeated injection of thymosin may also have immunorestorative effect on elderly humans manifesting reduced T cell-dependent immune functions according to a recent preliminary report showing that the number of T cells of old individuals can be increased by exposing their white blood cells to thymosin in vitro (71). However, before assessing the effect of thymosin on elderly individuals, it would seem prudent to carry out animal studies; i.e., assess the effects of repeated injection into aging short-lived and long-lived mice on their normal immune functions, disease patterns and life spans.

The use of free radical inhibitors stems from the hypothesis that aging is caused by somatic mutation (72), and, consequently, excess formation of free radicals should enhance aging, and the use of inhibitors delay aging (73). It was further reasoned that since the immune system plays a major role in aging (12), these agents should enhance immune functions of aging individuals. This notion was tested by Harman et al. (74) who incorporated these chemical agents into the diet of aging mice. Their preliminary results indicate that vitamin E and other free radical inhibitors can enhance the antibody response of adult and middle-aged (88 weeks) mice. These studies are being extended to assess the effectiveness of these agents on immune functions, disease pattern and life span of older mice. In a related study, Bliznakov (75) found that coenzyme Q_{10}, a nonspecific stimulant of mitochondrial electron transport, can enhance the level of antibody response of 2-year-old mice to that approaching adult mice. Both of these studies will require further investigation to identify the target cell(s) and the mechanism of action of these agents.

Braun et al. (76) were the first to demonstrate that double-stranded polynucleotides (e.g., polyadenlic-polyuridylic acid complexes) can restore the T cell-dependent antibody response of middle aged long-lived mice to that of young adult mice. Han and Johnson (77) not only confirmed this observation, but proceeded to demonstrate that the supernatant of cultures of thymocytes treated with double-stranded polynucleotides is equally effective as a immunorestorative agent. This suggests that the double-stranded polynucleotide restores immunologic vigor to aging mice by acting on T cells. Further studies are required to determine its mechanism of action on T cells and other immune cells, on both disease pattern and life span. One insight into a possible mechanism of action at the membrane level comes from an observation by Schmidt and Douglas (78), who found that double- and triple-stranded, but not single-stranded, polynucleotides increase the IgG binding activity of human monocytes *in vitro*. This would indicate that multi-stranded polynucleotides stimulate either by unmasking or by stimulating more synthesis of surface IgG binding receptors.

About a decade ago, when we became interested in intervention, we decided on the restorative method. We felt that a successful immunorestorative method would lend itself more effectively to the study of both cellular and molecular mechanisms responsible for the decline in normal immunologic activities with age. In our initial effort, immunorestoration of old mice was attempted by replacing their immune cells with those from syngeneic young mice (65). This was done by injecting spleen cells from young donors which had been previously immunized with *Salmonella typhimurium* vaccine into old mice that had received no prior treatment. Following this procedure, the old mice were able to resist lethal doses of virulent *Salmonella typhimurium* for an extended period of time. We then found that the combined treatment of old mice with 400 R of X-rays to destroy most of their radiosensitive immune cells, followed by injection of bone marrow cells and implantation of thymic tissues from young syngeneic donors can elevate the T cell dependent antibody response and T cell proliferative activity of the old mice to levels approaching those of young adult mice for an extended period (64). These results suggest that a cell replacement method could be used as a probe to identify the cell(s) responsible for the decline in immunologic vigor with age. However, its effectiveness as a molecular probe appears to be limited.

We therefore decided to focus our effort on chemically defined agents that are effective at the cellular level. We chose 2-mercaptoethanol (2-ME) because sulfhydryl compounds have been employed effectively in enhancing various nonimmunologic and immunologic cel lular activities in vitro (79-85), and because 2-ME is a simple 2-carbon compound effective at very low concentrations. We found that the reduced in vitro T cell-dependent antibody forming activities of spleen cells from four out of four genetically-defined old long-lived mice strains can be restored to levels approaching those of young adult mice by exposing the cells to 2-ME at very low concentration (4 µg/ml) (86-88). We demonstrated that the enhancing effect of 2-ME on old spleen cells is greater than that on young spleen cells, as judged by 2 different criteria. That is, the effect of 2-ME on old spleen cells was an order of magnitude greater than that on young spleen cells, in terms of its magnitude of enhancement of the antibody forming capacity of an optimum number of spleen cells, (i.e., 500 versus 30% enhancement). In terms of its ability to transform antigen-stimulated, nonantibody-responding cultures containing limiting numbers of spleen cells into antibody-responding cultures, the effect of 2-ME on old spleen cells was 6.5 times greater than that on young spleen cells.

We demonstrated that 2-ME is an effective immunorestorative agent in intact old mice by restoring the T cell-dependent antibody responding capacity of long-lived old mice to the level of young mice with appropriate doses (87-89). These results suggest that 2-ME and related chemicals may have practical applications.

The mode of action of 2-ME is not known. This is not surprising in view of the multitude of possible biochemical effects sulfhydryl compounds can have on cell structure and functions, ranging from SH/SS exchange reactions at the membrane level to the antioxidant and metal chelating effects (79,80,84). Moreover, various types of immunologic processes have been shown to benefit from the presence of 2-ME, including antibody response (81), mitogentic response of T and B cells to plant lectins (80,82,90), B cell colony formation (91), mixed lymphocyte reaction (83,92) and cytolytic killer T cell formation (93,94).

All three major cell types have been implicated as the target of 2-ME (80-83,90-95), as well as serum factor(s) in the tissue culture medium (90,95). Finally, it should be emphasized that in previous immunoenhancing studies of 2-ME, the source of immune cells has been limited to young adult donors whose magnitude of response in the presence of 2-ME, as demonstrated here, is not enhanced by more than two-fold (100%). Logistically, this could make it difficult to resolve the molecular mechanism of the enhancing action of 2-ME. The use of immune cells of old donors is therefore of obvious advantage, for, at a concentration as low as 4 µg/ml, 2-ME can enhance the primary antibody response of old spleen cells by as much as 11-fold

(1100%) (86-88). For these reasons, we are using 2-ME as a molecular probe to study the nature and mechanism of age-associated decline in normal immunologic activities.

CONCLUSION

The field of immunogerontology is still in its scientific infancy, but the immune system has already shown tremendous promise both as an experimental model for cellular and molecular aging and as a clinical model for diseases of the elderly.

What emerges from studies on the etiology of immunologic aging is that as individuals become old they lose their immunologic vigor primarily as a result of changes affecting the normal differentiation pathway of T cells. Consequently, aging individuals become susceptible to attack by microbial and other naturally occurring intrinsic and extrinsic agents (e.g., mutated cancer cells) that are routinely destroyed by T cells in healthy adults.

Six model intervention approaches have been used in attempts to prevent immunologic aging and to restore normal immunologic vigor. These studies are preliminary, but overall, the findings are most encouraging. Of the six approaches, genetic manipulation and chemical therapy appear to be most promising to use as probes in understanding the biochemical nature and mechanism(s) of the immune decline. The genetic approach should enable us to determine which gene(s) is primarily responsible for the decline in normal immune functions with age and the diseases associated with it. The chemical approach should enable us to determine the cell type(s) that is most severely affected functionally as well as the nature of associated changes at the subcellular level. However, dietary manipulation and chemical therapy appear to be the most promising in controlling immunologic aging, in terms of practical application. Cell grafting also appears to be promising. Perhaps the most effective approach in controlling immunologic aging is a combination of dietary manipulation, chemical therapy and cell grafting.

We still do not know what triggers the loss of immunologic vigor as individuals age. We may know in the near future, however, judging by the recent advances in areas such as genetic and chemical manipulations of immune functions. While the former approach is not appropriate in humans, no doubt clinical applications will arise from a better understanding of the specific genetic determinants of immunologic aging and its many consequences. The latter approach not only offers an understanding of age-related changes in cellular and subcellular function, but direct clinical applications as well. As we are now in the process of unravelling these puzzles, it is not unreasonable to predict that either retardation of immune decline or restoration of immune vigor in humans will be clinically feasible in the not too distant future.

REFERENCES

1. I. R. Mackay, Ageing and immunological function in man, Gerontologia 18:285 (1972).
2. H. Baer and R. T. owser, Antibody production and development of contact skin sensitivity in guinea pigs of various ages, Science 140:1211 (1963).
3. G. E. Bilder, Studies on immune competence in the rat: Changes with age, sex, and strain, J. Gerontol. 30:641 (1975).
4. B. N. Jaroslow, K. M. Suhrbier, and T. E. Fritz, Decline and restoration of antibody forming capacity in aging beagle dogs, J. Immunol. 112:1467 (1974).
5. T. Makinodan, and W. J. Peterson, Relative antibody-forming capacity of spleen cells as a function of age, Proc. Nat. Acad. Sci. U.S. 48:234 (1962).
6. M. Mathies, L. Lipps, G. S. Smith, and R. L. Walford, Age related decline in response to phytohemagglutinin and pokeweed mitogen by spleen cells from hamster and a long-lived mouse strain, J. Gerontol. 28:425 (1973).
7. T. A. Nomaguchi, Y. Okuma-Sakurai, I. and Kimura, Changes in immunological potential between juvenile and presenile rabbits, Mech. Ageing Dev. 5:409 (1976).
8. H. H. Fudenberg, R. A. Good, H. C. Goodman, W. Hitzig, H. G. Kunkel, I. M. Roitt, F. S. Rosen, D. S. Rowe, M. Seligmann, and J. R. Soothill, Primary immunodeficiencies, Bull. WHO 45:125 (1975).
9. I. Penn, and T. E. Starzl, Malignant tumors arising de novo in immunosuppressed organ transplant recipients, Transplantation 14:407 (1972).
10. M. M. B. Kay, and T. Makinodan, Immunobiology of aging: Evaluation of current status, Clin. Immunol. Immunopathol. 6:394 (1976).
11. "Tolerance, Autoimmunity and Aging," M. M. Seigel, and R. A. Good, eds., Charles C. Thomas, Springfield, Ill. (1972).
12. R. L. Walford, The immunologic theory of aging, current status. Fed. Proc. 33:2020 (1974).
13. "Immunology and Aging," T. Makinodan, and E. J. Yunis, eds., Plenum Medical Book Company, New York (1977).
14. D. Segre, and M. Segre, Age-related changes in B and T lymphocytes and decline of humoral immune responsiveness in aged mice, Mech. Ageing Dev. 6:115-129 (1977).
15. G. B. Price, and T. Makinodan, Immunologic deficiencies in senescence. II. Characterization of extrinsic deficiencies. J. Immunol. 108:413 (1972).
16. B. Rivnay, A. Globerson, and M. Shinitzky, Viscosity of lymphocyte plasma membrane in aging mice and its possible relation to serum cholesterol, Mech. Ageing Dev. 10:71 (1979).

17. F. J. Bach, M. Dardenne, and J. C. Solomon, Studies on thymus products. IV. Absence of serum thymic activity in adult NZB and (NZB x NZW)F1 mice, Clin. Exp. Immunol. 14:247 (1973).
18. G. E. Bilder, and W. D. Denckla, Restoration of ability to reject xenografts and clear carbon after hypophysectomy of adult rats, Mech. Ageing Dev. 6:153 (1977).
19. L. Hayflick, and P. S. Moorhead, The serial cultivation of human diploid cell strains, Exp. Cell Res. 25:585 (1961).
20. P. C. Brennan, and B. N. Jaroslow, Age-associated decline in theta antigen on spleen thymus-derived lymphocytes of $B6CF_1$ mice, Cell. Immunol. 15:51 (1975).
21. P. A. Jacobs, and W. M. Court Brown, Distribution of human chromosome counts in relation to age, Nature 191:1178 (1961).
22. A. M. Preumont, P. Van Gansen, and J. Brachet, Cytochemical study of human lymphocytes stimulated by PHA in function of donor age, Mech. Ageing Dev. 7:25 (1978).
23. Y. H. Oh, and R. A. Conrad, Effect of aging on acetate incorporation in nuclei of lymphocytes stimulated with phytohemagglutinin. Life Sciences 11:677 (1972).
24. M. G. Chen, Impaired Elkind recovery in hematopoeitic colony-forming cells of aged mice. Proc. Soc. Exp. Biol. Med. 145:1181 (1974)
25. D. J. Scribner, H. L. Weiner, and J. W. Moorhead, Anti-immunoglobulin stimulation of murine lymphocytes. V. Age-related decline in Fc receptor-mediated immunoregulation. J. Immunol. 121:377 (1978).
26. C. F. Tam, and R. L. Walford, Cyclic nucleotide levels in resting and mitogen-stimulated spleen cell suspensions from young and old mice, Mech. Ageing Dev. 7:309 (1978).
27. G. B. Price, and T. Makinodan, Immunologic deficiencies in senescence. I. Characterization of intrinsic deficiencies. J. Immunol. 108:403 (1972).
28. R. E. Callard, and A. Basten, Immune function in aged mice. IV. Loss of T cell and B cell function in thymus-dependent antibody response, Eur. J. Immunol. 8:552 (1978).
29. T. Makinodan, J. W. Albright, P. I. Good, C. P. Peter, and M. L. Heidrick, Reduced humoral immune activity in long-lived old mice: An approach to elucidating its mechanisms, Immunology 31:903 (1976).
30. D. Segre, and M. Segre, Humoral immunity in aged mice. II. Increased suppressor T cell activity in immunologically deficient old mice, J. Immunol. 116:735 (1976).
31. N. L. Gerber, J. A. Hardin, T. M. Chused, and A. D. Steinberg, Loss with age in NZB/W mice of thymic suppressor cells in the graft-versus-host reaction, J. Immunol. 113:1618 (1974).
32. H. M. Hallgren, and E. J. Yunis, Suppressor lymphocytes in young and aged humans, J. Immunol. 118:2004 (1977).

33. S. Gupta, and R. A. Good, Subpopulations of human T lymphocytes. X. Alterations in T, B, third population cells, and T cells with receptors for immunoglobulin M(tγ) or G(Tμ) in aging humans, J. Immunol. 122:1214 (1979).
34. R. L. Krogsrud, and E. H. Perkins, Age-related changes in T cell function, J. Immunol. 118:1607 (1977).
35. G. Doria, G. D'Agostaro, and A. Poretti, Age-dependent variation of antibody avidity, Immunology 38:601 (1978).
36. R. K. Liu, and R. L. Walford, Mid-life temperature-transfer effects on life span of annual fish, J. Gerontol. 30:129 (1975).
37. J. Furth, Prolongation of life with prevention of leukemia by thymectomy in mice, J. Gerontol. 1:46 (1946).
38. J. W. Albright, T. Makinodan, and J. W. Deitchman, Presence of life-shortening factors in spleens of aged mice of long life span and extension of life expectancy by splenectomy, Exp. Gerontol. 4:267 (1969).
39. F. Chino, T. Makinodan, W. E. Lever, and W. J. Peterson, The immune systems of mice reared in clean and in dirty conventional laboratory farms. I. Life expectancy and pathology of mice with long life spans, J. Gerontol. 26:497 (1971).
40. R. L. Walford, The immunologic theory of aging, current status, Fed. Proc. 33:2020 (1974).
41. "Immunogenetics and Immunodeficiency," B. Benacerraf, ed., University Park Press, Baltimore (1975).
42. G. S. Smith, and R. L. Walford, Influence of the main histocompatibility complex on aging in mice, Nature 270:727 (1977).
43. P. J. Meredith, and R. L. Walford, Effect of age on response to T and B cell mitogens in mice congenic at the H-2 locus, Immunogenetics 5:109 (1978).
44. G. Fernandes, R. A. Good, and E. J. Yunis, Attempts to correct age-related immunodeficiency and autoimmunity by cellular and dietary manipulation in inbred mice, in:"Immunology and Aging," T. Makinodan and E. J. Yunis, eds., Plenum Medical Book Company, New York (1977).
45. L. J. Greenberg, and E. J. Yunis, Histocompatibility determinants, immune responsiveness and aging in mice, Fed. Proc. 37:1258 (1978).
46. C. M. McCay, M. F. Crowell, and L. A. Maynard, The effect of retarded growth upon the length of life span and upon the ultimate body size, J. Nutrition 10:63 (1935).
47. M. H. Ross, Aging, nutrition, and hepatic enzyme activity patterns in the rat, J. Nutrition Suppl 1, part 2, 97:565 (1969).
48. M. H. Ross, and G. Bras, Lasting influence of early caloric restriction on prevalence of neoplasia in the rat, J. Nat. Cancer Inst. 47:1095 (1971).

49. R. L. Walford, R. K. Liu, M. Mathies, M. Gerbase-DeLima, and G. S. Smith, Response to sheep red blood cells and to mitogenic agents, Mech. Ageing Dev. 2:447 (1974).
50. G. Fernandes, E. J. Yunis, D. G. Jose, R. A. and Good, Dietary influence on antinuclear antibodies and cell-mediated immunity in NZB mice, Int. Arch. Allergy Appl. Immunol. 44:770 (1973).
51. B. Fernandes, E. J. Yunis, J. Smith, and R. A. Good, Dietary influence on breeding behavior, hemolytic anemia, and longevity in NZB mice, Proc. Soc. Exp. Biol. Med. 139:1189 (1972).
52. G. Fernandes, E. J. Yunis, and R. A. Good, Influence of diet on survival of mice, Proc. Nat. Acad. Sci. USA 73:1279 (1976).
53. W. D. Denckla, Role of pituitary and thyroid glands in the decline of minimal O_2 consumption with age, J. Clin. Invest. 53:572 (1974).
54. N. Fabris, W. Pierpaoli, and E. Sorkin, Lymphocytes, hormones and aging, Nature 240:557 (1972).
55. P. O. Teague, and G. J. Friou, Antinuclear antibodies in mice. II. Transformation with spleen cells, inhibition or prevention with thymus or spleen cells, Immunology 17:665 (1969).
56. E. J. Yunis, and L. J. Greenberg, Immunopathology of aging, Fed. Proc. 33:2017 (1974).
57. S. Kysela, and A. D. Steinberg, Increased survival of NZB/W mice given multiple syngeneic young thymus grafts, Clin. Immunol. Immunopath. 2:133 (1973).
58. E. J. Yunis, G. Fernandes, and O. Stutman, Susceptibility to involution of the thymus-dependent lymphoid system and autoimmunity, Am. J. Clin. Path. 56:280 (1971).
59. J. F. Albright, and T. Makinodan, Growth and senescence of antibody-forming cells, J. Cell Comp. Physiol. 67(Suppl. 1): 185 (1966).
60. D. Metcalf, R. Moulds, and B. Pike, Influence of the spleen and thymus on immune responses in aging mice, Clin. Exp. Immunol. 2:109 (1966).
61. T. Makinodan, and W. H. Adler, The effects of aging on the differentiation and proliferation potentials of cells of the immune system, Fed. Proc. 34:153 (1975).
62. J. W. Albright, and T. Makinodan, Decline in the growth potential of spleen-colonizing bone marrow stem cells of long lived aging mice, J. Exp. Med. 144:1204 (1976).
63. K. Hirokawa, and T. Makinodan, Thymic involution: Effect on T cell differentiation, J. Immunol. 114:1659 (1975).
64. K. Hirokawa, J. W. Albright, and T. Makinodan, Restoration of impaired immune functions in aging animals. I. Effect of syngeneic thymus and bone marrow cells, Clin. Immunol. Immunopathol. 5:371-376 (1976).

65. E. H. Perkins, T. Makinodan, and C. Seibert, Model approach to immunological rejuvenation of the aged, Infect. Immunity 6:518 (1972).
66. D. Friedman, V. Keiser, and A. Globerson, Reactivation of immunocompetence in spleen cells of aged mice, Nature 251:545 (1974).
67. M.-A. Bach, Lymphocyte-mediated cytotoxicity: Effects of ageing, adult thymectomy and thymic factor, J. Immunol. 119:641 (1977).
68. M. E. Weksler, J. B. Innes, and G. Goldstein, G. Immunological studies of aging. IV. The contribution of thymic involution to the immune deficiencies of aging mice and reversal with thymopoietin, J. Exp. Med. 148:996 (1978).
69. D. Martinez, A. K. Field, H. Schwam, A. A. Tytell, and M. R. Hilleman, Failure of thymopoietin, ubiquitin and synthetic serum thymic factor to restore immunocompetence in T cell deficient mice, Proc. Soc. Exp. Biol. Med. 159:195 (1978).
70. A. L. Goldstein, G. B. Thurman, T. L. Low, G. E. Trivers, and J. L. Rossie, Thymosin: The endocrine thymus and its role in the aging process, in:"Physiology and Cell Biology of Aging," A. Cherkin, C. E. Finch, N. Kharasch, T. Makinodan, F. L. Scott, and B. L. Strehler, eds., Raven Press, New York (1979).
71. J. Rovensky, A. L. Goldstein, P. J. L. Holt, J. Pwkarek, and T. Mistina, Obnova funkcie T lymfocytor tymosinom u klinicky zdravych asob vyssieho veku, Cas. Lek. Ces. 116:1063 (1977).
72. B. Strehler, "Time, Cells and Aging," Academic Press, New York (1977).
73. D. Harman, Prolongation of life: Role of free radical reactions in aging, J. Am. Geriatrics Soc. 17:721 (1969).
74. D. Harman, M. L. Heidrick, and D. E. Eddy, Free radical theory of aging: Effect of free-radical-reaction inhibitors on the immune response, J. Am. Geriatrics Soc. 25:400 (1977).
75. E. G. Bliznakov, Immunological senescence in mice and its reversal by coenzyme Q_{10}, Mech. Ageing Dev. 7:189 (1978).
76. W. Braun, Y. Yajima, and M. Ishizuka, Synthetic polynucleotides as restorers of normal antibody formation capacities in aged mice, J. Reticuloendothel. Soc. 7:418 (1970).
77. I. H. Han, and A. G. Johnson, Regulation of the immune system by synthetic polynucleotides. VII. Amplification of the immune response in young and aged mice, J. Immunol. 117:423 (1976).
78. M. E. Schmidt, and S. D. Douglas, Effects of synthetic single and multistranded polynucleotides on human monocyte IgG receptor activity in vitro, Proc. Soc. Exp. Biol. Med. 151:376 (1979).
79. W. Braun, W. M. Lichtenstein, and C. Parker, eds., "Cyclic AMP, Cell Growth and the Immune Response," Springer-Verlag, New York (1974).

80. J. D. Broome, and M. W. Jeng, Promotion of replication in lymphoid cells by specific thiols and disulfides in vitro, J. Exp. Med. 138:574 (1973).
81. C. Chen, and J. G. Hirsch, The effects of mercaptoethanol and of peritoneal macrophages on the antibody forming capacity of nonadherent mouse spleen cells in vitro, J. Exp. Med. 136:604 (1972).
82 M. W. Fanger, D. A. Hart, J. V. Wells, and A. Nisonoff, Enhancement by reducing agents of the transformation of human and rabbit peripheral lymphocytes, J. Immunol. 105:1043 (1970).
83. E. Heber-Katz, and R. E. Click, Immune responses in vitro. V. Role of mercaptoethanol in the mixed-leukocyte reaction, Cell. Immunol. 5:410 (1972).
84. N. Johnson, R. Jessup, and P. W. Ramwell, The significance of protein disulfide and sulphonyl groups in prostaglandin action, Prostaglandins 5:125 (1974).
85. W. Lands, R. Lee, and W. Smith, Factors regulating the biosynthesis of various prostaglandins, Ann. N.Y. Acad. Sci. 180:107 (1971).
86. T. Makinodan, J. W. Deitchman, G. H. Stoltzner, M. M. Kay, and K. Hirokawa, Restoration of the declining normal immune functions of aging mice, Proc. 10th Internat. Cong. Gerontol. 2:23 (1975).
87. T. Makinodan, Control of immunologic abnormalities associated with aging, Mech. Ageing Dev. 9:7 (1979).
88. T. Makinodan, and J. F. Albright, Restoration of impaired immune functions in aging animals. II. Effect of mercaptoethanol in enhancing the reduced primary antibody responsiveness in vitro, Mech. Ageing Dev. 10:325 (1979).
89. T. Makinodan, and J. F. Albright, Restoration of impaired immune functions in aging animals. III. Effect of mercaptoethanol in enhancing the reduced primary antibody responsiveness in vivo, Mech. Ageing Dev., in press.
90. M. G. Goodman, and W. O. Weigle, Nonspecific activation of murine lymphocytes. I. Proliferation and polyclonal activation induced by 2-mercaptoethanol and a-thioglycerol, J. Exp. Med. 145:473 (1977).
91. D. Metcalf, Role of mercaptoethanol and endotoxin in stimulation of B lymphocyte colony formation in vitro, J. Immunol. 116:635 (1976).
92 M. J. Bevan, R. Epstein, and M. Cohn, The effect of 2-mercapto-ethanol on murine mixed lymphocyte cultures, J. Exp. Med. 139:1025 (1974).
93. H. D. Engers, H. R. MacDonald, J. C. Cerottini, and K. T. Brunner, Effect of delayed addition of 2-mercaptoethanol on the generation of mouse cytotoxic T-lymphocytes in mixed leukocyte cultures, Eur. J. Immunol. 5:223 (1975).

94. T. Igarashi, M. Okada, T. Kishimoto, and Y. Yamamura, In vitro induction of polyclonal killer T cells with 2-mercapto-ethanol and the essential role of macrophages in this process, J. Immunol. 118:1697 (1977).
95. H. G. Opitz, U. Opitz, H. Lemke, H. D. Flad, G. Hewlett, and H. D. Schlumberger, Humoral primary immune response in vitro in a homologous mouse system: Replacement of fetal calf serum by a 2-mercaptoethanol or macrophage-activated fraction of mouse serum, J. Immunol. 119:2089 (1977).

NEUROENDOCRINE FUNCTION AND AGING

Arthur V. Everitt

Department of Physiology
University of Sydney
Sydney, Australia

The life program from conception through growth, development, physiological aging, and the onset of terminal diseases leading to death is determined by both genetic and environmental factors. The course of aging and duration of life are affected by environmental factors such as temperature (1), food supply (2), and stress (3). These factors affect body functions by mediations of the neuroendocrine and autonomic nervous systems. For example, a rat or mouse living in a cold environment secretes more thyroxine (4) and catecholamines (5), which increase heat production and enable the animal to survive under these conditions (6). Survival in a hostile or rapidly changing environment is dependent upon adequate functioning of both the autonomic nervous and endocrine systems. The secretions of these two systems, neurotransmitters and hormones, regulate the vast majority of physiological activities throughout the body. Obviously, a deficiency of a specific neurotransmitter or hormone will have far-reaching effects on body function. This forms the basis of the neuroendocrine regulatory failure hypothesis of aging.

THE NEUROENDOCRINE REGULATORY FAILURE HYPOTHESIS

This hypothesis states that peripheral aging phenomena are due to failure of neuroendocrine regulatory mechanisms. There is little doubt that impairments occur in old age in many functions. For example, the ability to maintain constant body temperature is greatly reduced in old age, both in man and in laboratory animals. When young adult mice (aged 10 months) are kept in a cool room at 9-10°C, body temperature decreased slightly (about 1°C) over a 3 hour period; whereas, in old mice (30 months) body temperature falls markedly (about 8°C) (7). The cause of this impairment of temperature regulation in old mice may be due to single or multiple defects in the thermoregulatory system. Impairments may develop in the temperature receptors (in skin, abdomen, spinal cord, or brain), the afferent nerves which relay information from the receptors to the hypothalamus, the thermoregulatory centers in the hypothalamus, the efferent autonomic nerves, and the neuroendocrine system which transmit instructions from the hypothalamus to the effector organs that control heat production (the liver and muscles) and the organs that control heat loss from the skin. At present, it is not possible to estimate the contribution of these different nervous and endocrine components to the age decrement in thermoregulation.

In a similar manner, age decrements are found in most endocrine functions in old age, and there is an increasing volume of evidence suggesting that central regulatory deficiencies in the rat contribute to the peripheral aging in the ovary (8,9,10), the testis (11), and the adrenal cortex (12). Aging of the regulatory mechanisms has been studied most extensively in relation to the aging ovary.

AGING OF THE HYPOTHALAMIC-PITUITARY-OVARIAN AXIS

This is a very complex system with environmental inputs, hypothalamic surge and tonic centers, hypothalamic release and release inhibitory factors, pituitary gonadotropic hormones (FSH and LH) and prolactin, and the negative and positive feedback of both ovarian hormones (estrogen and progesterone) producing 4 or 5 day cycle of changes in the ovary and accessory reproductive organs.

With increasing age (starting at 10 months) estrous cycle irregularities appear, the cycles cease, pseudopregnancies (estrus every 12-14 days) develop, permanent estrus (anovulatory state) occurs, and then, finally, anestrus, which indicates cessation of ovarian function (8,10).

ROLE OF THE HYPOTHALAMUS

Most evidence indicates that, in the rat, the primary age lesion is in the hypothalamus. The elegant transplant study of Peng and Huang (13) clearly showed that in old non-cycling rats, neither the pituitary nor the ovaries are responsible for the loss of cycles. They found that a young rat with old ovaries and an old pituitary is able to cycle normally. The site of the primary age defect is probably the preoptic area of the hypothalamus, which is the surge or cyclic area controlling the large preovulatory rise in luteinizing hormone (LH) secretion. This is supported by the work of Clemens and Bennett (9), who found that lesions in the preoptic area of young rats reproduced the pseudopregnancy state seen in old rats. These workers were able to restore normal estrous cycles in these lesioned rats by injecting lergotrile mesylate, which is a dopamine agonist. It is also possible to achieve partial restoration of estrous cycles in old rats by electric stimulation of the preoptic area (14) or by injections of epinephrine, L-dopa, or iproniazide (15). Both L-dopa and iproniazide increase catecholamine levels in the brain (16). These pharmacological studies implicate catecholamines in the age-related loss of estrous cycles, as suggested by other workers (17,18). In the basal medial hypothalamus of the old rat, there is a fall in the content of dopamine and norepinephrine, and the metabolism of these catecholamines is depressed, while the metabolism of serotonin is increased (17). These authors suggest that these changes in biogenic amine metabolism may in part account for the age-related increase in serum prolactin (secretion stimulated by serotonin) and decrease in serum LH and FSH (most data indicate that NE stimulates LH secretion).

The responsiveness of the hypothalamus to the negative feedback of ovarian steroid hormones is also impaired in old age. Dilman (19) has presented evidence suggesting that elevation of the hypothalamic threshold to feedback control is a signficant factor in aging. In the rat, an age-related elevation of the hypothalamic threshold to negative feedback has been demonstrated for corticosteroids (12) and gonadal steroids (20). The hypothalamus becomes less responsive to changes in ovarian hormones with increasing age. For example, a deficiency of ovarian hormones created by ovariectomy produces a much smaller rise in plasma LH in old rats than in young (21).

These studies generally emphasize the importance of the hypothalamus rather than the pituitary as the primary determinant of ovarian aging.

ROLE OF THE PITUITARY

Age changes in pituitary gonadotropic function may also contribute to the loss of estrous cycles. Pituitary responsiveness to LRH (luteinizing hormone releasing hormone) is reduced in old female rats, as shown by a smaller increase in serum LH in aged rats compared with young animals (22). This means that for the same amount of LRH secreted by the hypothalamus, less pituitary LH is secreted. Hence, there is less likelihood of the LH surge being large enough to initiate ovulation in the aged rat. LH is the pituitary hormone most concerned with cyclic behavior in the ovary. Of course, it can be argued that the loss of pituitary responsiveness to LRH is secondary to age changes in the hypothalamus.

There have been relatively few long-term studies which attempt to manipulate the course of ovarian aging. At least three different studies suggest that pituitary gonadotropins regulate the rate of ovarian aging.

Hemiovariectomy in the young rat produces a compensatory increase in both FSH and LH secretion, which stimulates the remaining ovary to enlarge (23). In the mouse the reproductive performance is halved; the total number of offspring is halved; and the duration of reproduction is halved (24). That is, the life span of the ovary is halved. In women, there is also evidence that after hemiovariectomy the remaining ovary becomes exhausted before the normal age of menopause (25). In the hemiovariectomized rat, the duration of breeding is normal (26), but the onset of senile deviations of the estrous cycle occurs prematurely (27). It is tempting to suggest that the high secretion of gonadotropins is responsible for aging of the remaining ovary.

Complete removal of gonadotropins by hypophysectomy in CBA mice is found to retard the age-related loss of oocytes from the ovary (28), but does not abolish the loss. Although such animals are sterile due to lack of pituitary gonadotropins, ovaries from old hypophysectomized mice well beyond the normal age of reproduction are quite fertile when transplanted into young ovariectomized mice. Thus, a lack of pituitary hormones has delayed the onset of sterility.

Caloric restriction acts in a similar manner to hypophysectomy because it reduces the plasma levels of pituitary gonadotropins (29). Starvation reduces hypothalamic LRH stimulation of the pituitary and so decreases LH secretion (30). The reproductive life of the underfed female rat is prolonged. Berg (31) obtained litters from 16 out of 24 food-restricted rats aged 730 to 790 days, an age when fully-fed rats are sterile.

THE PITUITARY HYPOTHESIS

According to this hypothesis, pituitary hormones accelerate aging processes and lead to an early onset of age-related pathology (32). This hypothesis is supported by the observation that hypophysectomy in the rat retards the rate of aging in tail tendon collagen, kidney, heart muscle, aorta, skeletal muscle, bone, and ovary (32,33).

The effects of hypophysectomy on aging are profound when operations are performed on young rats at age 70 days. Tail tendon collagen in a senescent 1000-day-old (33 months) hypophysectomized rat has the physical properties (breaking time in 7M urea) of a 500-day middle-aged control rat. Similarly, the kidney of the 1000-day-old hypophysectomized rat corresponds to that of a 200-day young adult control, in terms of the excretion of protein in urine. There are no histological signs of renal disease in old hypophysectomized rats. The wall thickness of the thoracic aorta of the 1000-day-old hypophysectomized rat is similar to that of a 100-day young adult control. The 1000-day-old senescent hypophysectomized rat is able to walk normally, whereas 70% of controls of that age have hind leg paralysis causing them to drag their hind legs; and in the remainder, walking is impaired. The incidence of tumors at autopsy in old hypophysectomized rats (800-1300 days) averages 5%, whereas in age-matched controls it is 64%. The tissues of the old hypophysectomized rat are almost free of obvious pathological changes, such as renal and cardiac hypertrophy, tumors, and hind leg paralysis. This suggests that hypophysectomy has delayed the immunologic decline, usually seen in old age, which is associated with the emergence of disease (34).

These studies clearly show that hypophysectomy in the rat at an early age (70 days) produces a general slowing of aging phenomena in many tissues. The effects of hypophysectomy performed in middle age (at 400 days) are not quite so dramatic, but still lead to significant retardation of both collagen and renal aging. This study indicates that pituitary hormones are accelerating aging phenomena at all ages, and not merely turning on an aging program in early life.

One serious problem with hypophysectomy studies is that food intake is markedly reduced. The anti-aging effects could be due to either the loss of pituitary hormones or to the lowered food intake. Food restriction is known to prolong life (35), to delay the onset of the diseases of old age (36,37), and to retard the aging of collagen fibers in tail tendon (38,39). Since the anti-aging effects of hypophysectomy and food restriction are almost identical, a common mechanism is suggested. The only real difference is in life duration. The untreated hypophysectomized rat has a significantly reduced life duration (40,41). However, hypophysectomized rats receiving corticosteroid replacement (1 mg cortisone acetate per week subcutaneously) have mean life duration equal to that of food-restricted rats eating the same amount of food. Their life duration is significantly greater than that of controls consuming almost three times the quantity of food. These obvservations have been confirmed by Denckla (personal communication), who found 20/95 survival at 34 months (1000 days) in hypophysectomized rats receiving cortisone succinate, desoxycorticosterone acetate and thyroxine in their drinking water, compared with only 2/125 for controls.

These studies indicate that there are several pituitary factors concerned in aging phenomena: 1) factors which prolong life (such as ACTH and TSH, which respectively stimulate corticosteroid and thyroxine secretion) probably acting by an immunological mechanism, and 2) factors which increase aging (such as excessive secretion of TSH, ACTH, and growth hormone), probably acting by some metabolic mechanism such as crosslinking. Since the secretion of these hormones is controlled principally by hypothalamic centers, it is tempting to postulate that the hypothalamus is the ultimate regulator of these aging phenomena and the duration of life. A number of workers have discussed the possibility that the aging program is timed or regulated by a clock or center in the hypothalamus. For example, Denckla (42) has proposed that the life span is regulated by a biological clock which acts on endocrine glands to produce failure of the immune and circulatory systems.

THE HYPOTHALAMIC CLOCK HYPOTHESIS

This hypothesis states that there is a clock or center in the hypothalamus which regulates the rate of peripheral aging by mediation of the nervous and endocrine systems (32,43,44). The proposed center would be analogous to the thermoregulatory, feeding, satiety, thirst, sleep, and vasomotor centers in the hypothalamus, which specifically regulate temperature, feeding, etc. It is largely because of the multiplicity of functions performed by the hypothalamus that this organ has been proposed as a central regulator of aging (32). Possibly even more important is its unique anatomophysiological position, which enables the hypothalamus to mediate many of the effects of environmental factors, and so adjust the rate of aging according to the demands of the environment.

Biological clocks have been postulated to regulate endocrine cyclic phenomena, such as the circadian rhythm of ACTH and corticosteroid secretion, where the highest plasma level occurs just before waking, and decreases throughout the day to the lowest level when going to bed late at night (45). The suprachiasmatic nucleus in the anterior hypothalamus has been implicated in the diurnal rhythm of corticosteroid secretion (45,46). This nucleus appears to be implicated in many biological rhythms, such as periodicity in locomotor behavior, periodicity of feeding and drinking activity, periodicity of body temperature, and estrous cycle periodicity. Since the suprachiasmic nucleus area appears to control a great number of biological cycles, perhaps it also controls life's major cycle--that from birth to death. This is probably unlikely, because the role of this area is apparently to initiate the cycle. The clock or regulator which we are searching for is that which controls the duration of the cycle. The duration of most biological cycles is relatively resistant to change by altering environmental conditions. This is certainly not true of the life cycle when one considers the enormous effect of temperature on life duration in poikilothermic animals like Drosophila (47) and the large increases possible in rat life duration by manipulating the diet (48). Again, in the case of the estrous cycle, exposure to continuous light (49) leads to failure of ovulation and the development of the constant estrous pattern as seen in old age. Furthermore, rats exposed to low temperatures (2°C) have longer estrous cycles due to increased duration of estrus or proestrus (50). These experiments show how the environment can influence an intrinsic biological process. In a clock or biological rhythm mechanism, there are three components: 1) a receptor to detect light, heat, etc.; 2) a clock to measure time and integrate the information received; 3) an effector system to modify body functions. In the hypothalamic-pituitary thyroid axis, Ooka-Souda et al. (51) have shown how light deprivation from birth delays the maturation of the pituitary-thyroid axis. Ooka-Souda (personal communication) has also shown that when the day length is reduced to 18 hours, the pituitary-thyroid axis develops more rapidly, the rats grow faster and have shorter estrous cycles. Is the whole program of aging accelerated?

It is clear that environmental factors can modify the rate of development and aging. Quite a number of these factors appear to be acting by mediation of the hypothalamus. It is tempting to suggest that the state of the environment is detected by the appropriate receptors, which delay this information to an aging center or clock. most probably located in the hypothalamus. After integration of all information received, the clock adjusts the level of body functions and the rate of aging by altering the quantities of hormones and neurotransmitters delivered to the tissues concerned. The rate of aging in a given tissue is presumed to be regulated by the hormones and neurotransmitters stimulating or depressing that tissue.

ACKNOWLEDGEMENTS

I am especially grateful to Mr. Frank Jones, who performed most of the hypophysectomies, and to Roussel Pharmaceuticals, Sydney, who generously supplied the cortisone acetate used in these studies. The hypophysectomy studies reported here were supported, in part, by grants from the Consolidated Medical Research Fund of the University of Sydney and the University Research Grant.

REFERENCES

1. R. K. Liu and R. L. Walford, The effect of lowered body temperature on life span and immune and non-immune processes, Gerontologia 18:363 (1972).
2. C. H. Barrows and L. M. Roeder, Nutrition, in:"Handbook of the Biology of Aging," C. E. Finch and L. Hayflick, eds., Van Nostrand Reinhold, New York (1977).
3. H. Selye and B. Tuchweber, Stress in relation to aging and disease, in:"Hypothalamus, Pituitary and Aging," A. V. Everitt and J. A. Burgess, eds., Charles C. Thomas, Springfield, Illinois (1976).
4. H. D. Johnson, H. H. Kibler, and H. Silsby, The influence of ambient temperature of 9°C and 28°C on thyroid function of rats during growth and aging, Gerontologia 9:18 (1964).
5. J. Ledvic, Catecholamine production and release in exposure and acclimation to cold, Acta Physiol. Scand. 53(Suppl. 183):1 (1961).
6. T. R. Bauman and C. W. Turner, The effect of varying temperatures on thyroid activity and the survival of rats exposed to cold and treated with L-thyroxine or corticosterone, J. Endocrinol. 37:355 (1967).

7. C. E. Finch, J. R. Foster, and A. E. Mirsky, Ageing and the regulation of cell activities during exposure to cold, J. Gen. Physiol. 54:690 (1969).
8. P. Aschheim, Resultats fournis par la greffe heterochrone des ovaires dans l'etude de la regulation hypothalamo-hypophyso-ovarienne de la ratte senile, Geontologia 10:65 (1964/5).
9. J. A. Clemens and D. R. Bennett, Do aging changes in the preoptic area contribute to loss of cyclic endocrine function? J. Gerontol. 32:19 (1977).
10. H. H. Huang and J. Meites, Reproductive capacity of aging female rats, Neuroendocrinology 17:289 (1975).
11. C. D. Riegle, J. Meites, A. Miller, and S. M. Wood, Effect of aging on hypothalamic LH-releasing and prolactin inhibiting activities and pituitary responsiveness to LHRH in the male laboratory rat, J. Gerontol. 32:19 (1977).
12. C. D. Riegle, Chronic stress effects on adrenocortical responsiveness in young and aged rats, Neuroendocrinology 11:1 (1973).
13. M. T. Peng and H. H. Huang, Aging of hypothalamic pituitary-ovarian function in the rat, Fert. Ster. 23:535 (1972).
14. J. A. Clemens, Y. Amenomorri, T. Jenkins, and J. Meites, Effects of hypothalamic stimulation, hormones, and drugs on ovarian function in old female rats, Proc. Soc. Exp. Biol. Med. 132:561 (1969).
15. S. Quadri, G. Kledzik, and J. Meites, Reinitiation of estrous cycles in old constant estrous rats by central acting drugs, Neuroendocrinology 11:248 (1973).
16. J. H. Dowson and I. Laszlo, Quantitative histochemical studies of formaldehyde-induced parenchymal fluorescence following L-DOPA administration, J. Neurochem. 18:2501 (1971).
17. J. W. Simpkins, G. P. Mueller, H. H. Huang, and J. Meites, Evidence for depressed catecholamine and enhanced serotonin metabolism in aging rats: Possible relation to gonadotropin secretion, Endocrinology 100:1672 (1977).
18. C. E. Finch, Monamine metabolism in the aging male mouse, in: "Development and Aging in the Nervous System," M. Rockstein and M. L. Sussman, eds., Academic Press, New York (1973).
19. V. M. Dilman, Age-associated elevation of hypothalamic threshold to feedback control and its role in development, ageing and disease, Lancet 1:1211 (1971).
20. C. J. Shaar, J. S. Enker, G. D. Riegle, and J. Meites, Effects of castration and gonadal steroids on serum LH and prolactin in old and young rats, J. Endocrinol. 66:45 (1975).
21. R. G. Gosden and L. Bancroft, Pituitary function in reproductively senescent female rats, Exp. Gerontol. 11:157 (1976).
22. B. E. Watkins, J. Meites, and C. D. Riegle, Age related changes in pituitary responsiveness to LHRH in the female rat, Endocrinology 97:543 (1975).

23. B. E. Howland and C. Preiss, Effects of aging on basal levels of serum gonadotropins, ovarian compensatory hypertrophy and hypersecretion of gonadotropins after ovariectomy in female rats, Fert. Ster. 26:271 (1975).
24. E. C. Jones and P. L. Krohn, The effect of unilateral ovariectomy on the reproductive lifespan of mice, J. Endocrinol. 20:129 (1960).
25. M. Magendie, I. Bernard, M. Kolenc, and Partimbene, Le comportment hormonal de l'ovaire restant! C.R. Soc. Franc. Gynec. 23:201 (1953).
26. C. E. Adams, Ageing and reproduction in the female mammal with particular reference to the rabbit, J. Reprod. Fert., Suppl. 12:1 (1970).
27. P. Aschheim, Aging in the hypothalamic-hypophyseal ovarian axis in the rat, in:"Hypothalamus, Pituitary and Aging," A. V. Everitt and J. A. Burgess, eds., Charles C. Thomas, Springfield, Illinois (1976).
28. E. C. Jones and P. L. Krohn, The effect of hypophysectomy on the number of oocytes in the adult albino rat, J. Endocrinol. 21, 497 (1961).
29. B. E. Howland, Effect of restricted feed intake on LH levels in female rats, J. Anim. Sci. 34:445 (1972).
30. G. A. Campbell, M. Kurcz, S. Marshall, and J. Meites, Effects of starvation in rats on serum levels of FSH, LH, thyrotropin, growth hormone and prolactin; response to LH-releasing hormone and thyrotropin releasing hormone, Endocrinology 100:580 (1977).
31. B. N. Berg, Nutrition and longevity in the rat. I. Food intake in relation to size, health and longevity, J. Nutrition 71:242 (1960).
32. A. V. Everitt, The hypothalamic-pituitary control of aging and age-related pathology, Expl. Gerontol. 8:265 (1973).
33. A. V. Everitt, Hypophysectomy and aging in the rat, in: "Hypothalamus, Pituitary and Aging," A. V. Everitt and J. A. Burgess, eds., Charles C. Thomas, Springfield, Illinois (1976).
34. T. Makinodan, Immunity and aging, in:"Handbook of the Biology of Aging," C. E. Finch and L. Hayflick, eds., Van Nostrand Reinhold Co., New York (1977).
35. C. M. McCay, M. F. Crowell, and L. A. Maynard, The effect of retarded growth upon the length of life span and upon the ultimate body size, J. Nutrition 10:63 (1935).
36. J. A. Saxon, Jr., Nutrition and growth and their influence on longevity in rats, Biological Symposia 11:177 (1945).
37. B. N. Berg and H. S. Sims, Nutrition, onset of disease and longevity in the rat, Can. Med. Assoc. J. 93:911 (1965).
38. M. Chvapil and Z. Hruza, The influence of aging and undernutrition on chemical contractility and relaxation of collagen fibres in rats, Gerontologia 3:241 (1959).

39. A. V. Everitt, Food intake, growth and the ageing of collagen in rat tail tendon, Gerontologia 17:98 (1971).
40. F. Verzar and H. Spichtin, The role of the pituitary in the aging of collagen, Gerontologia 12:48 (1966).
41. A. V. Everitt and L. M. Cavanagh, The ageing process in the hypophysectomized rat, Gerontologia 11:198 (1965).
42. W. D. Denckla, A time to die, Life Sciences 16:31 (1975).
43. M. Hasan, P. Glees, and E. El-Ghazzawi, Age-associated changes in the hypothalamus of the guinea pig: Effect of dimethylaminoethyl p-chlorophenoxyacetate. An electron microscopic and histochemical study, Exp. Gerontol. 9:153 (1974).
44. T. Samorajski, Central neurotransmitter substances and aging: A review, J. Amer. Geriatrics Soc. 25:337 (1977).
45. D. T. Krieger, Factors influencing the circadian periodicity of ACTH and corticosteroids, Medi. Clin. North Am. 62:251 (1978).
46. M. A. Slusher, Effects of chronic hypothalamic lesions on diurnal and stress corticosteroid levels, Amer. J. Physiol. 206:1161 (1964).
47. J. V. Burcombe and M. J. Hollingsworth, The relationship between environmental temperature and longevity in Drosophilia, Gerontologia 16:172 (1970).
48. M. H. Ross, Length of life and caloric intake, Amer. J. Clin. Nutr. 25:834 (1972).
49. I. E. Lawton and N. B. Schwartz, Pituitary-ovarian function in rats exposed to constant light: A chronological study, Endocrinology 81:497 (1967).
50. M. E. Denison and M. X. Zarrow, Changes in the estrous cycle of rat during prolonged exposure to cold, Proc. Soc. Exp. Biol. Med. 89:632 (1955).
51. S. Ooka-Souda, D. J. Draves, and P. S. Timiras, Developmental patterns of plasma TSH, T_4 and T_3 in rats deprived of light from birth, Mech. Ageing Dev. 6:287 (1977).

EFFECT OF ADULT THYMECTOMY ON IMMUNE POTENTIALS, ENDOCRINE ORGANS AND TUMOR INCIDENCE IN LONG-LIVED MICE

Katsuiku Hirokawa and Yoshio Hayashi

Department of Pathology
Medical Research Institute
Tokyo Medical and Dental University
Yushima, Bunkyo-ku, Tokyo-113
Japan

INTRODUCTION

The thymus is known to be a central lymphoid tissue playing an important role in the ontogenic development of the immune system. Neonatal thymectomy causes severe immunodeficiency in mice, which usually die from wasting disease in the conventional environment (1). In contrast, thymectomy performed at the adult state results in no immediate effect on the immune potentials of the mice (2). However, since the thymic functions to promote T cell-differentiation are known to be maintained in the thymus of mice of any age, although these functions decline progressively with age (3), it would be expected that removal of the adult thymus would result in a delayed impairment of T cell-dependent immune potentials (4,5). The T cell-dependent component of the immune system is also said to play an important role in immune surveillance (6). If so, the incidence of naturally occurring tumors would increase in adult thymectomized mice. Moreover, growth and involution of the thymus is said to be closely interrelated with normal function of the other endocrine organs (7). If so, adult thymectomy would also influence the function of the other endocrine organs.

METHODS

To test these questions, $B6C3F_1$ female mice were thymectomized at 6 weeks of age and then studied at 6, 12, and 24 months of age. Non-thymectomized $B6CF_1$ female mice were used as controls. Immunological assessment of the spleens of both groups was performed as described previously (3), and the organs were examined pathohistologically.

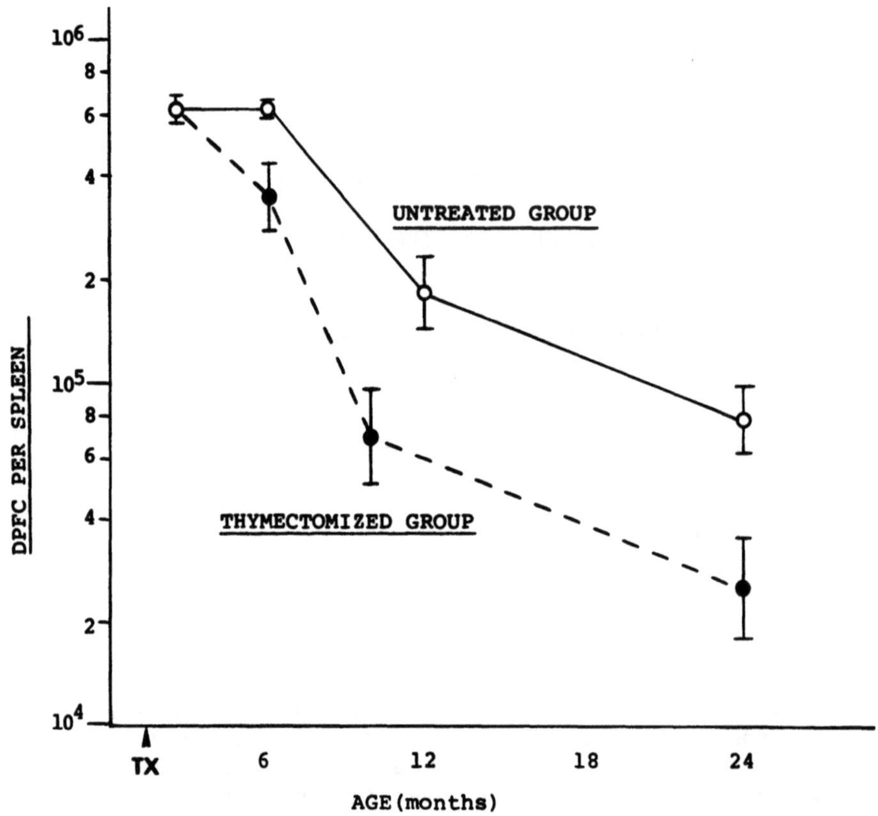

Fig. 1. Anti-SRBC antibody response measured by number of direct plaque forming cells (DPFC) per spleen in untreated control (open circles and solid lines) and thymectomized group (solid circles and broken lines). DPFC was assessed 5 days after i.p. injection of 3×10^8 SRBC. Each point, average of 3 to 6 samples. Vertical bars, one standard error of the mean. TX, thymectomy, performed at 6 weeks of age.

RESULTS AND DISCUSSION

Antibody response to sheep red blood cells (SRBC)

The level of anti-SRBC antibody response in untreated group declined gradually after 6 months of age, reaching the level of about 10% of the peak response at 24 months of age, as shown in Figure 1. In the thymectomized group, a significantly accelerated decline of this response was observed, showing 10% of the peak response at 12 months of age and 4% level at 24 months of age.

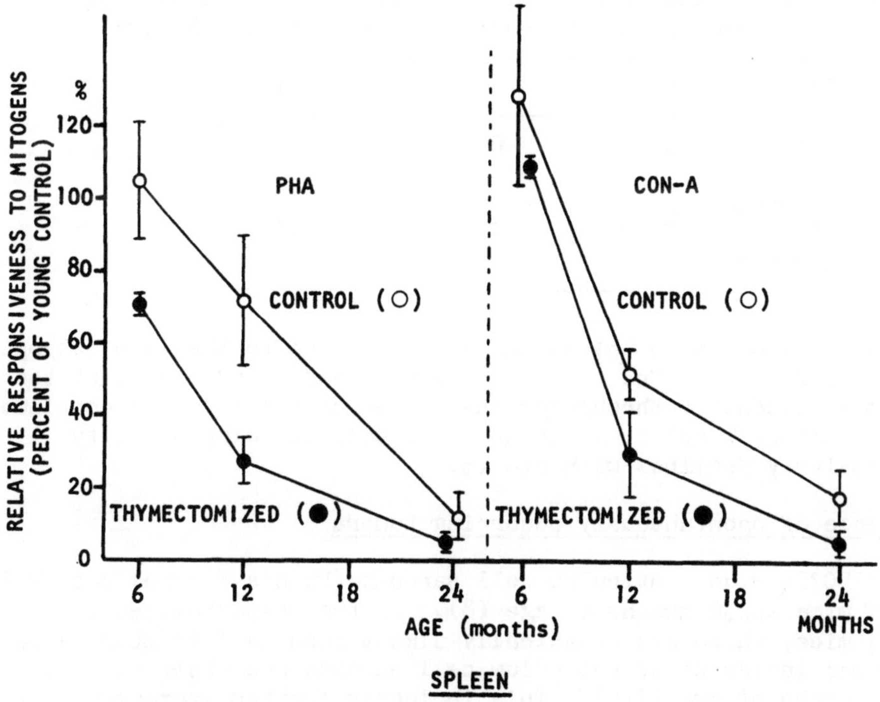

Fig. 2. Responsiveness of spleen cells to phytohemagglutinin (PHA) and concanavalin A (Con A), expressed by percent of the responsiveness of 3-month-old young control. Spleen cells, 5 x 10^5, in 0.2 ml of RPMI 1640 were cultured with 1.0 µg of either PHA or Con A in a microplate, pulsed 66 hr later with 0.25 µCi of ^{3}H-thymidine (sp. act. 8 Ci/mM) for 6 hr and processed. The responsiveness was expressed by cpm/culture. Open circles, untreated age-matched control. Solid circles, thymectomized group. Vertical bars, one standard error of the mean. TX, thymectomy performed at 6 weeks of age.

Mitogenic responsiveness of the spleen cells

Responsiveness of spleen cells to phytohemagglutinin (PHA) also progressively declined with age in controls (Fig. 2). An accelerated decline of this responsiveness in the thymectomized group was thought to be observed at 6 and 12 months of age, but the difference became marginal at 24 months of age. Responsiveness of the spleen cells to concananvalin A (Con A) also showed a similar pattern of age-associated decline, as observed in PHA-responsiveness in both treated and non-treated animals, but the acceleration of the declining responsiveness to Con A in the thymectomized group was not apparent until 12 and 24 months of age. These results suggest that PHA- and Con A-

Table I. Effect of Adult Thymectomy on the Incidence of Spontaneously Occurring Tumors in $B6C3F_1$ (♀)

Age.	6m	12m	24m
Control	0/3	0/6	2/7
Thymectomized at 6 wks old	0/3	1/6	4/6

responsive T cells in the spleen do not belong to the same subpopulation of T cells. The data in Figures 1 and 2 indicate that the thymus is necessary throughout the course of the life for continuous recruitment of T cells, although the T cell-inducing capacity progressively declines with age (3).

Incidence of spontaneously occurring tumors

In $BC3F_1$ mice, reticulum cell sarcoma (Dunn's A type) occurs in 50% of mice at 30 months of age (8). In the thymectomized group of $B5C3F_1$ mice, which are genetically almost identical to $BC3F_1$ mice, an increased incidence of reticulum cell sarcoma was observed as early as 12 months of age (1/6). This incidence further increased to 4/6 at 24 months of age. This incidence is significantly higher than that of the control group, which is 2/7 at 24 months of age (Table I). These results appeared to be compatible with the concept that the thymus-dependent component of the immune system does indeed perform the task of immune surveillance (6).

Weight of endocrine organs

The weight of adrenal and pituitary glands in the thymectomized group appeared to be less than that of the same endocrine organs in the age-matched control (Fig. 3). A significant difference was observed in the weight of the adrenal glands at 6 and 24 months of age. This difference might be ascribed to higher susceptibility of the thymectomized group to infection and tumor as compared with the control. However, at 6 months of age, both thymectomized and control mice were revealed to be healthy by pathological examination. Therefore, presence of the weight difference suggested that function of the adrenal and pituitiary glands is closely interrelated with the normal function of the thymus.

SUMMARY

The data presented here indicate that the thymus plays an important role not only in the early ontogenic development of the immune system, but also in the maintenance of the immune potentials

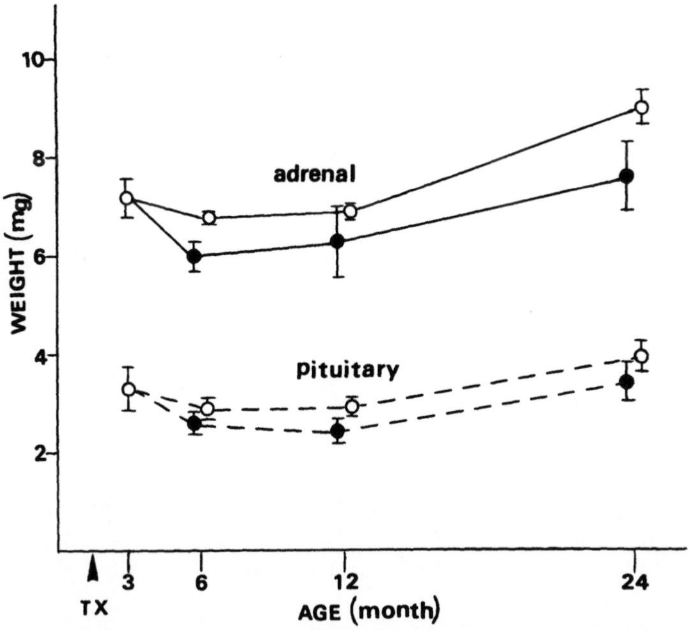

Fig. 3. Net weight of adrenal (solid lines) and pituitary glands (broken lines) in untreated, age-matched control (open circles) and thymectomized group (solid circles). TX, thymectomy, performed at 6 weeks of age. Vertical bars, one standard error of the mean.

throughout the course of life. Moreover, thymic function is closely interrelated with functions of the other endocrine organs.

REFERENCES

1. J. F. A. P. Miller, Lancet ii:748 (1961).
2. J. F. A. P. Miller and D. Osoba, Physiol. Rev. 47:437 (1967).
3. K. Hirokawa and T. Makinodan, J. Immunol. 114:1659 (1975).
4. D. Metcalf, Nature 208:1336 (1965).
5 L. C. Robson and M. R. Schwarz, Transplantation 11:465 (1971).
6. M. Burnet, "Immunological Surveillance," Pergamon Press, Oxford (1970).
7. N. Fabris, W. Pierpaoli, and E. Sorkin, Nature 240:557 (1972).
8. F. Chino, T. Makinodan, W. E. Lever, and W. J. Peterson, J. Gerontol. 26:497 (1971).

ENVIRONMENT AND AGING: AN APPROACH TO THE ANALYSIS OF AGING MECHANISMS USING POIKILOTHERMIC VERTEBRATES

Nobuo Egami

Zoological Institute, Faculty of Science
University of Tokyo
Hongo, Tokyo 113, Japan

INTRODUCTION

Epidemiological data and various circumstantial evidence suggest that the rate of aging in humans is influenced by many environmental conditions, such as nutrition, climate, or more complicated factors, including social conditions. Research designed to analyze the relationship between each environmental factor and the aging of organisms has been carried out using laboratory animals, particularly mice and rats. However, it is difficult to draw either specific or general conclusions regarding these relationships, since, in mammals, homeostatic mechanisms are well developed, and cells within the individuals are not always directly exposed to environmental conditions. One possible approach toward solving this problem would be to reevaluate the use of simple animal models, together with that of using cultured cells of animals and poikilothermic vertebrates. These animals reflect environmental conditions more directly than mammals do (Fig. 1). Data or comments on environmental effects, such as temperature, nutrition, photoperiod, radiation and chemical trace elements on the life span of small laboratory fish will be presented.

TEMPERATURE

It is difficult to analyze the effect of temperature on the life span of mammals directly, since body temperature is regulated by complicated mechanisms. However, animal longevity at various temperatures has been examined, and many zoologists have recorded long life spans in hibernators. In the case of poikilothermic animals, the situation is simpler. The life span of fish is, in general, longer at low temperatures, within a limited range. Under natural conditions, some fish species which live in cooler

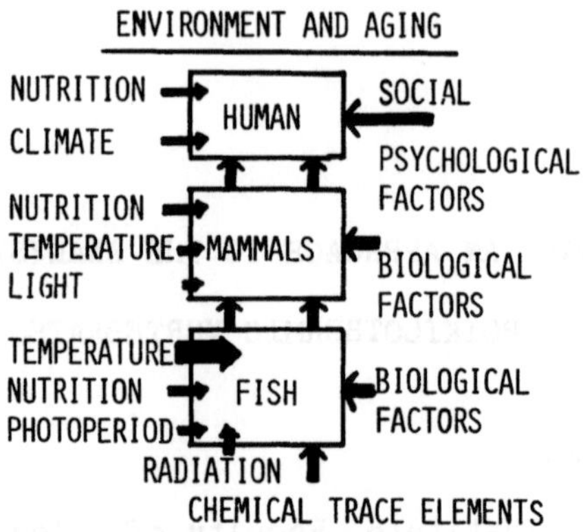

Fig. 1. Diagram showing relationsip between environment and aging in different classes of animals.

environments live longer than other members of the same species living in warmer localities. In 1970, Liu and Walford (1) used several species of Cynolebias as model animals in the laboratory. They concluded that the longer survival at low temperatures is due to a decrease in the rate of aging, since the slope of the survivorship curve at low temperatures decreased at about the same ratio as the increase in the mean survival time. Further studies using this model were performed by them in 1972, from an immunological perspective (2).

The small teleost fish Oryzias latipes, native to Japan, is a temperature-tolerant species. The fish is known to live in hot springs at 40°C, but the same species can survive under ice at 1°C. We have previously reported that if the fish are irradiated with 8 kR of X-rays, the proliferation of cells in the intestine is completely inhibited. Following this, the cell population of the intestinal epithelium decreases day by day, since the intestinal epithelium is a typical cell renewal system, and the life span of the epithelial cells is limited. Finally, so-called "intestinal death induced by radiation" occurred (3,4). The rate of development of this syndrome is temperature-dependent because the cell cycle time and life span of the cells are determined by the water temperature (Fig. 2). In other words, the survival time after irradiation with 8 kR is clearly dependent upon the water temperature (Fig. 3). We believe from autoradiographic examination that dependency of survival time of fish on the temperature is a reflection of the temperature dependency of the rate of the aging process in the differentiated intestinal epithelial cells.

Moreover, during the period between 1970 and 1974, I observed that the life span of non-irradiated fish is longer if the fish are kept in cool thermal surroundings in summer, and shorter if the fish are heated in winter (5) (Fig. 4). Furthermore, it was demonstrated

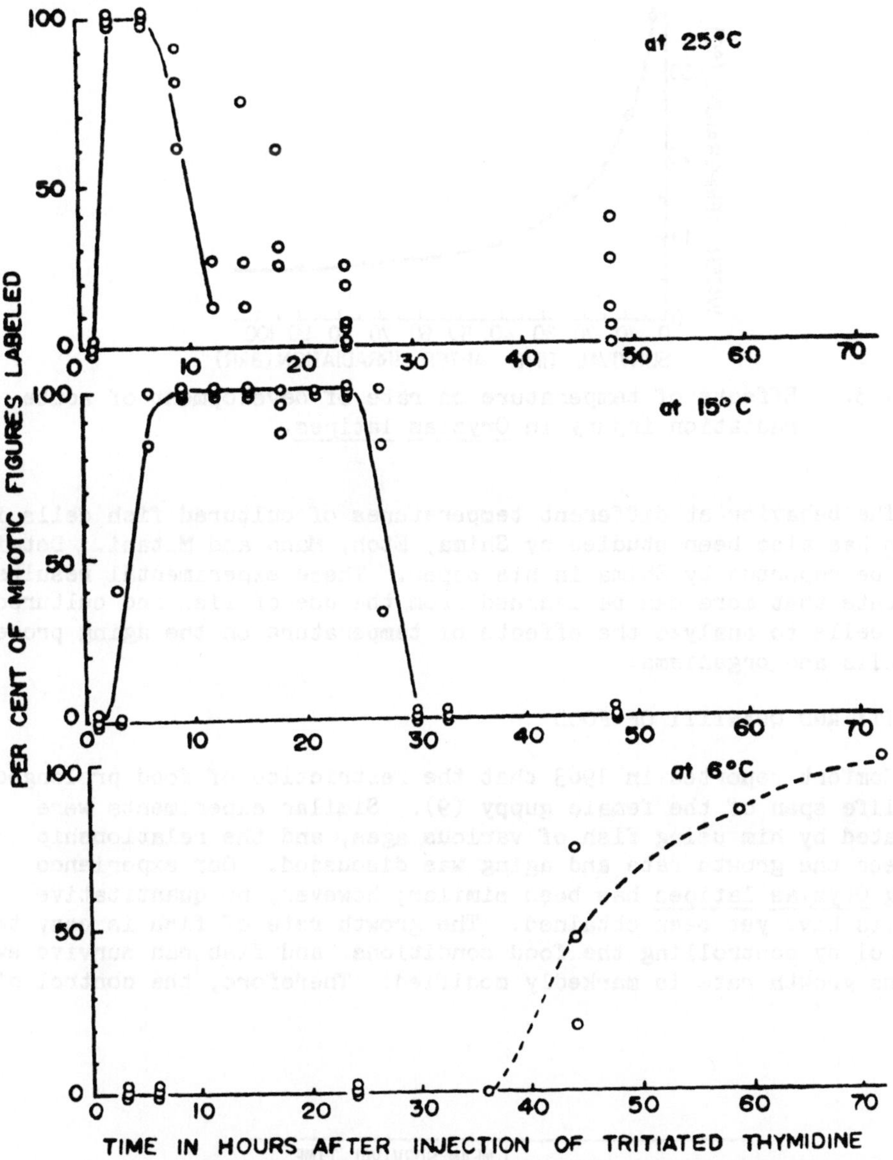

Fig. 2. Percent of labeled mitotic figures of intestinal epithelial cells of goldfish kept at different temperatures (Hyodo-Taguchi).

in these fish that a delay in the development and promotion of hepatic tumor nodules contributed to some extent to longevity at low temperature (Fig. 5) (6,7,8).

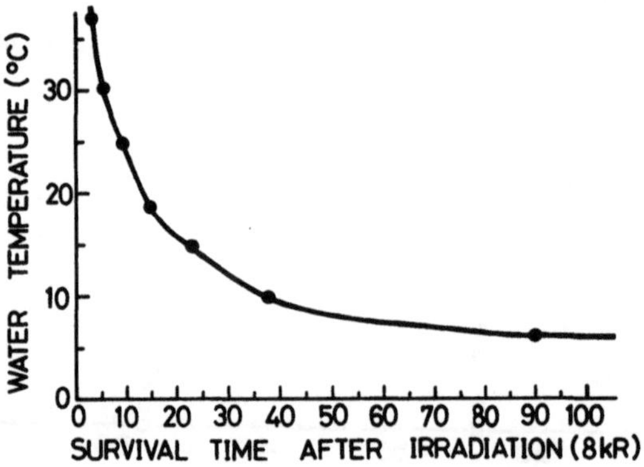

Fig. 3. Effects of temperature on rate of development of acute radiation injury in *Oryzias latipes*.

The behavior at different temperatures of cultured fish cells *in vitro* has also been studied by Shima, Etoh, Mano and Mitani. Details will be reported by Shima in his paper. These experimental results indicate that more can be learned from the use of fish and cultured fish cells to analyze the effects of temperature on the aging process of cells and organisms.

QUALITY AND QUANTITY OF FOOD

Comfort reported in 1963 that the restriction of food prolonged the life span of the female guppy (9). Similar experiments were repeated by him using fish of various ages, and the relationship between the growth rate and aging was discussed. Our experience using *Oryzias latipes* has been similar; however, no quantitative results have yet been obtained. The growth rate of fish is easy to control by controlling the food conditions, and fish can survive even if the growth rate is markedly modified. Therefore, the control of

TEMPERATURE	MEAN SURVIVAL TIME AFTER IRRADIATION	
	0 R	1000 R
NATURAL TEMPERATURE	725	320
10°C OR LESS	1042	431
20°C OR MORE	430	102

Fig. 4. Temperature effects on mortality of irradiated fish and non-irradiated fish.

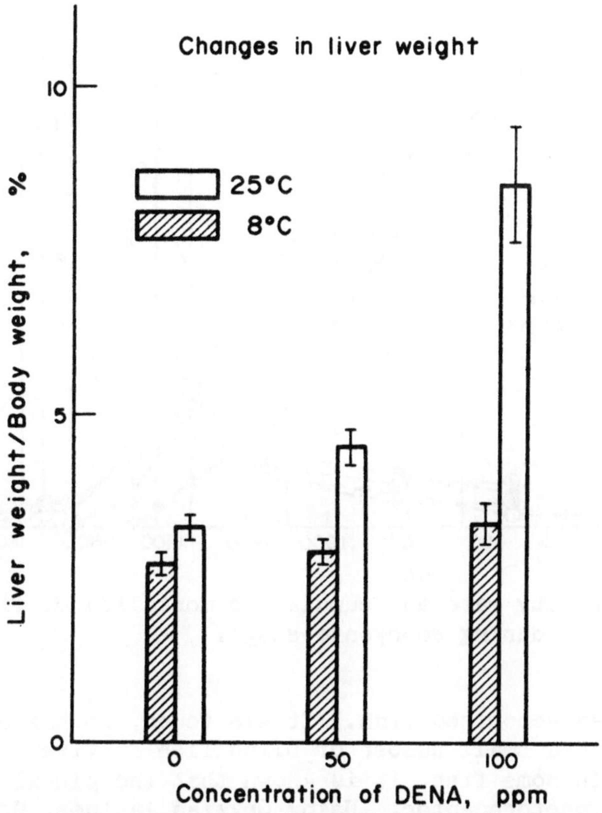

Fig. 5. The ratios of liver weight to body weight in DENA-treated fish kept at different temperatures. The weight indicates the development of the tumor.

longevity in fish is more easily accomplished than that of mammals. Recent developments in fish cultivation, particularly in Japan, have stimulated the scientific study of the nutrient value of feed. Many reports on the effects of the quantity and quality of food on growth, maturation, and the induction of various fish diseases, including tumors, have been published. Moreover, further fundamental studies of fish nutrition will be necessary before its relationship to the aging process of fish can be completely understood.

PHOTOPERIODICITY

If animals are exposed to short or long photoperiods over a considerable period, what happens to their aging rate? In an attempt to answer this question, Noumura and his co-workers are keeping mice exposed to artificial illumination for 20-, 24-, or 30-hour days. A similar type of experiment has been tried by our group with normal,

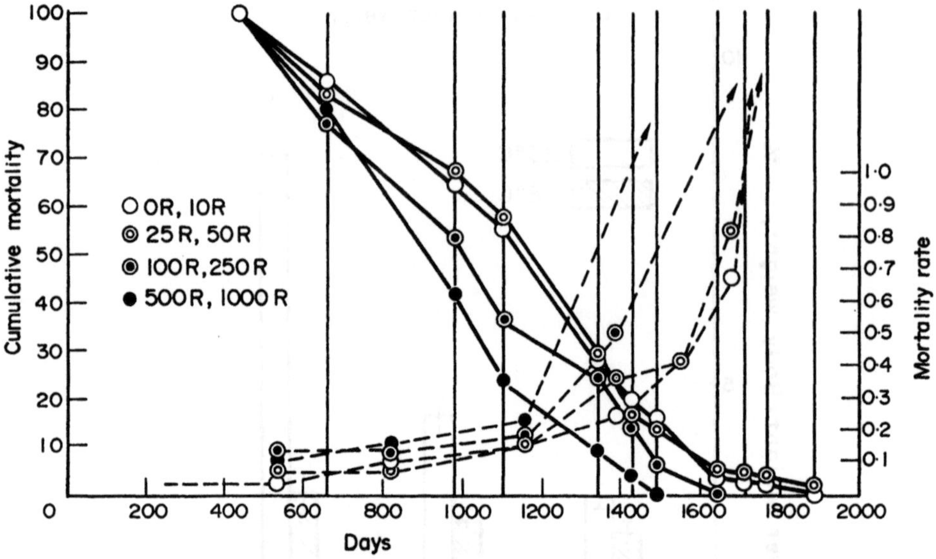

Fig. 6. Mortality rate and cumulative mortality of fish exposed to X-rays during embryonic stage.

blind, and pinealectomized fish. It was found, in the preliminary experiment, that a small number of blind fish survived longer than intact fish. In some fish, it is known that the pineal body functions as a photoreceptor. Using Oryzias latipes, Urasaki demonstrated in 1976 that photoperiods influence the pineal by way of the eyes (10). Positive effects of the photoperiods on the behavior and on the maturation of intact, but not pinealectomized, fish were

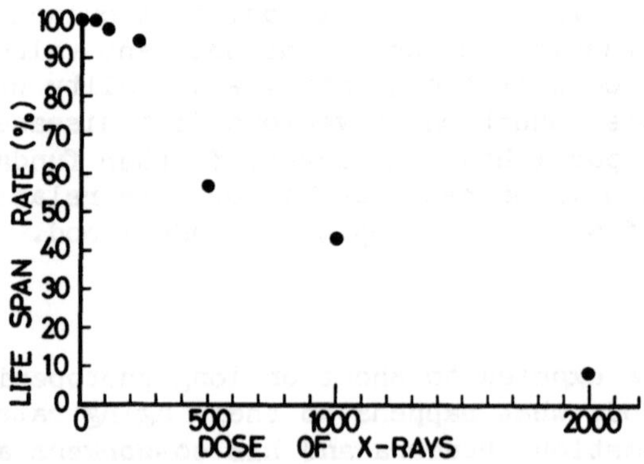

Fig. 7. Effect of X-irradiation of embryos on life span in Oryzias latipes.

Table 1. Important Histological Characteristics in Senile Fish

(1)	Degenerative changes (cerebrum)
(2)	Decrease in cell number (liver, kidney)
(3)	Enlargement of cells (liver, kidney)
(4)	Increase of conective tissue (testis)
(5)	Deposition of lipofuscin (cerebrum)
(6)	Degeneration of the thymus

recognized by a series of Urasaki's papers. The results on the effects of aging rate, however, are not yet conclusive.

RADIATION

The life-span-shortening effect of ionizing radiation has been well demonstrated in fish as well as in mammals (11). However, it is not yet certain that radiation does accelerate the non-specific aging process; nor that a low dose, or a low dose rate, of radiation exerts hormetic effects.

I have examined the effects of X- and γ-rays on the life span in Oryzias latipes, after establishing the life span table. Our results were reported at the symposium of the XIth International Congress of Gerontology. The conclusion we reached was that dose-dependent life-shortening effects of X-rays were demonstrated if these X-rays were given at high dose rates (11,12) (Figs. 6,7). However, under low-dose-rate conditions (less than 20 R/day), no significant effects on longevity were demonstrated.

Our histological studies of senile fish revealed various characteristics peculiar to them (Table 1). Most age-specific histo-cytologic changes in the liver, the spleen, the brain, and the testis occurred in irradiated fish. However, in some organs, the senile changes were not always felt to be stimulated by radiation (13). In addition, an examination of the effects of radiation on tumorigenesis is now in progress. Generally speaking, the nature of the radiation effects on fish is the same as that on mammals, so fish can be used as model animals (Table 2).

The data of the fish experiments show that radiation has clear life-shortening effects, but further quantitative study is necessary before we can conclude that radiation stimulates the non-specific aging processes.

Table 2. Summary of the Radiation Effects on Life Span in *Oryzias latipes*

(1) Life span shortening effects of radiation was clearly demonstrated at high dose-rate.
(2) At 320-35 R/day, accumulated dose for 50% mortality was 10-17 KR.
(3) At lower dose-rate, no clear effects were observed.
(4) Histological observation did not always demonstrate "radiation accelerates all non-specific aging processes".

MUTAGENIC, CARCINOGENIC, AND OTHER TRACE SUBSTANCES

The so-called "somatic mutation theory" as a mechanism for the aging process seems one of the most attractive. Therefore, the effects on tumorigenesis, mutagenesis, and lethality of compounds that specifically bind to DNA and interfere with DNA metabolism, such as actinomicin D, ethidium bromide, 5-bromodeoxyuridine (BUdR), and some alkylating agents and nitrosamine compounds, caffeine and urethane were examined in our laboratory. In addition, the effects of trace elements and trace metals, particularly $HgCl_2$ and CH_3HgCl in water, on mortality and mutagenicity were examined in our laboratory using *Oryzias latipes* by Sakaizumi. The effects of these substances were compared to those of ionizing radiation.

Some effects were measured by examining the chromosome aberration and DNA content distribution of cultured fish cells (Shima). We tried to demonstrate change in the template-primer activities of nuclear DNA to various types of DNA-polymerase by autoradiography, with sections of ethanol-fixed fish tissue treated with some drugs by a method similar to that reported by Price, Modak, and Makinodan (14). However, at the present time, no clear age-related changes have been demonstrated (15).

At any rate, aquatic organisms are very suitable for ascertaining the effects of Na and K, and their ion balance, (Ca, Mg, Zn, Fe, and some trace metals like Pb, Cd, and Hg) and of water-soluble mutagenic and carcinogenic substances on histological characteristics which are generally felt to indicate tumor formation and aging.

DISCUSSION

In order to properly study environmental effects on organisms, the organisms should be genetically homogeneous. Recently, at least eight pure inbred strains of Oryzias have been established by Hyodo-Taguchi. In addition, the very strange Amazon molly and Japanese silver tuna fish, which show gynogenetic reproduction, have been found, and genetically pure populations have been obtained. These fish have also been used as a model system of aging study by Setlow and our groups (16). Furthermore, the cultivaton in a germ-free environment of some fish has been successfully accomplished. Thus, the use of pathogen-free fish for gerontological research is also possible.

In order to obtain fundamental knowledge of the mechanism of the aging process in animals, comparative studies of the effects of environmental factors on aging process in different animals and their cells are essential. For instance, if the basic causes of biologial aging were related to somatic mutation, including chromosome aberration, or accumulation of errors in genetic information in the critical cells, ionizing radiation and some radiomimetic substances might accelerate the rate of aging process in all animals, even at cellular levels. If mesenchymal tissue changes were key causes of animal aging, the effects of temperature and of drugs interfering with collagen might be great on the aging rate in all animals in tissue, organ, or organism levels.

If the pineal body or homeostatic regulatory systems, such as hypothalamus, were the time keeper or biological clock of aging process in higher organisms, environmental factors which affect such systems, including photoperiod or administration of some exogenous hormonic substances, might change the rate of aging process only in vertebrate animals, and at whole animal levels. These effects might appear more markedly in higher species, in accord with the evolutionary development of the regulatory system. If more complicated factors, like psychological or social conditions play a more important role in human aging process, the effects might appear only in the more advanced societies.

I would like to re-emphasize the significance of using various animals, including poikilothermic species in which homeostatic mechanism is simple, and environmental factors act more directly, as a way to approach this complicated problem. In conclusion, I will add that in order to analyze environmental effects on aging, the reevaluation of interrelationship among aging phenomena occurring in different animal species is also important, as well as that in different levels of organization (Fig. 8).

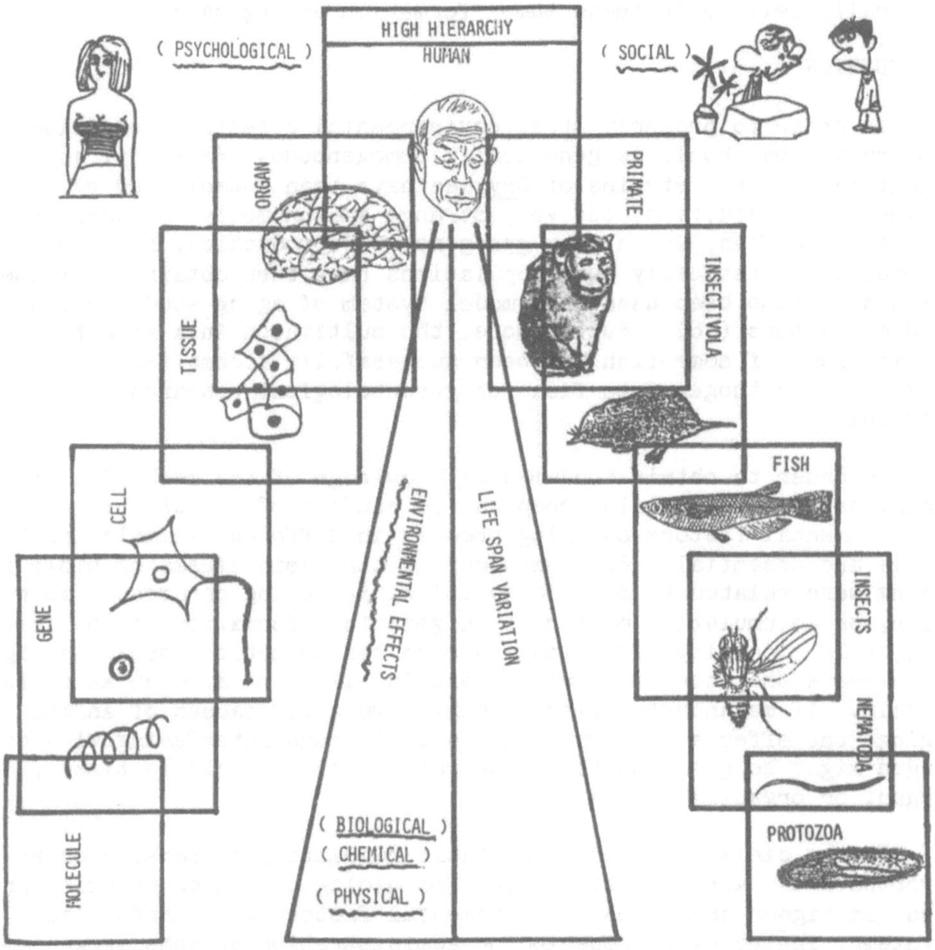

Fig. 8. Diagram showing approaches to analyze environmental effects on aging by reevaluation of interrelationships among aging phenomena occurring in different animal species and in different levels of organization.

REFERENCES

1. R. K. Liu and R. L. Walford, Observations on the life spans of several species of annual fishes and of the world's smallest fishes, Exp. Gerontol. 5:241 (1970).
2. R. K. Liu and R. L. Walford, The effect of lowered body temperature on life span and immune and non-immune processes, Gerontologia 18:363 (1972).

3. Y. Hyodo, Effect of X-irradiation on the intestinal epithelium of the goldfish Carassius auratus II. Influence of temperature on the development of histological changes in the intestine, Rad. Res. 24:133 (1965).
4. Y. Hyodo-Taguchi and N. Egami, Development of intestinal radiation injury and recovery at different temperatures in fish, in:"Comparative Cellular and Species Radiosensitivity," T. Suguhara and Y. P. Bond, eds., Igakushoin, Tokyo (1969).
5. N. Egami, Long-term observations of mortality of irradiated fish at different temperatures, Rad. Res. 59:132 (1974).
6. Y. Kyono and N. Egami, The effect of temperature during the diethylnitrosamine treatment on liver tumorigenesis in the fish, Oryzias latipes, Eur. J. Cancer 13:1191 (1977).
7. Y. Kyono, Temperature effects during and after the diethylnitrosamine treatment on liver tumorigenesis in the fish, Oryzias latipes, Eur. J. Cancer, 14:1089 (1978).
8. Y. Kyono, A. Shima, and N. Egami, Changes in the labeling index and DNA content of liver cells during liver tumorigenesis in the fish, Oryzias latipes, J. Natl. Cancer Inst., 63:71 (1979).
9. A. Comfort, Effect of delayed and resumed growth on the longevity of a fish (Lebistes reticulatus, Peters) in captivity, Gerontolgia 8:150 (1963).
10. H. Urasaki, The role of pineal and eyes in the photoperiodic effects on the gonad of the Medaka, Oryzias latipes, Chronobiologica 3:228 (1976).
11. N. Egami, Radiation effects on life span of the fish, Oryzias latipes, in:"Proc. XI Int. Congress Gerontology," 314 (1978).
12. N. Egami and H. Etoh, Effect of X-irradiation during embryonic stage on life span in the fish, Oryzias latipes, Expt. Gerontol. 8:219 (1973).
13. N. Egami, M. M. H. Ghoneum, A. Kikuta, and K. Ijiri, Effects of radiation on life span and lymphoid tissues in the fish, Oryzias latipes, in:"Abst. 2nd Radiation Biology Center Int. Symp.," 20.
14. G. B. Price, S. P. Modak, and T. Makinodan, Age-associated changes in the DNA of mouse tissue, Science 171:917 (1971).
15. M. Matsui, A. Shima, and N. Egami, Autoradiographic detection of the template-primer activities of DNA by exogenous DNA polymerase in fixed mouse tissues, J. Fac. Sci., Univ. Tokyo, IV, 13:399 (1976).
16. A. D. Woodhead, Ageing changes in the liver of two Poeciliid fishes, the guppy, Poecilia (Lebistes) reticulata and the Amazon molly, P. formosa, Expt. Gerontol. 13:37 (1978).

CENTRAL VS. PERIPHERAL AGING*

Richard G. Cutler

Gerontology Research Center
National Institute on Aging
National Institutes of Health
Baltimore City Hospitals
Baltimore, Maryland 21224

INTRODUCTION

The slow but progressive deterioration of man's health, followed by an increased onset frequency of diseases, results mostly from a complex spectrum of time-dependent changes collectively called aging (1). There is agreement that substantial prolongation of useful and enjoyable life span would require a uniform decrease in the rate of expression of most of these aging processes (2,3). However, there is much disagreement on the probability and advisability of slowing down man's aging rate, a process often considered to be incredibly complex (4,5).

At the present time, we know little about the biological nature of aging or about the genetic and biochemical complexity of processes which may be governing the aging rate. However, the hypothesis that specific processes may exist that govern the aging rate is fairly new and may, as we shall see later, be less complex than the aging process *per se* (5). In this regard, it must be determined whether the aging rate of man is controlled by a special set of genes. If so, we must also determine the number and informational complexity of these genes, and that of possible regulatory genes (6,7,8,9). Consideration of the evolutionary processes that gave rise to all living forms of life, and eventually to the unusually long period of longevity that man enjoys today (3,6,9,10), is likely to yield useful

*A similar lecture has also been presented for publication in "Biology of Aging," C. Borek and D. W. King, eds., Stratton Intercontinental Medical Book Corp., New York.

information toward this objective. Moreover, this endeavor requires a study of biology at its most general and fundamental level. The author believes that a clear understanding of all living processes, past and present, is not likely to be obtained without also an understanding of the basic nature of aging processes and how these processes are controlled (3,9). This paper presents highlights of such an evolutionary study of human longevity--and as part of this study, central vs. peripheral factors in aging are evaluated.

MAMMALIAN SPECIES HAVE DIFFERENT INNATE AGING RATES

There is little doubt that different mammalian species have substantial differences in their innate aging rates, even species that are genetically closely related. The major evidence supporting this concept is the different maximum life span potentials (MLP) found for different species. MLP is the life span of the last surviving member of a given population. Under conditions where the species' natural hazards have been largely removed and reasonable medical and sanitary conditions are observed (such as in modern zoos), this value approaches the innate biological ability of a species to survive. Obviously, the larger the initial young population observed, the more accurate the value obtained. For a number of primates and other animals, a reasonable MLP is known now that is probably no more than 20% underestimated (11,12,13). More importantly, from a comparative viewpoint, the different MLP's are probably even more accurate proportionally.

In Table 1, estimates of MLP's are given for some primate species. Man lives about 14 times longer than the shortest-lived of the primate species, the Phillipine tree shrew. Man appears to be the longest-lived of all living mammalian species, and probably of all mammalian species that ever lived.

Differences in ability to survive, or MLP, do not necessarily imply corresponding differences in aging rate. However, when rate of decline of physiological function is compared to MLP, an excellent correlation is observed. These studies have mainly been confined to mice, rats, guinea pigs, dogs, Rhesus monkeys, chimpanzees, and man (3,6,11). For example, the rate of loss of immune function in man and mouse is inversely proportional to MLP. This is also true for physical vigor, resistance to disease, and the rate of decline in mental function. Thus, MLP appears to be related to the innate ability of the animal to maintain its general mental and physical health. The different MLP's and the excellent correlation found with the rate of decline of common physiologic functions, mental abilities, and in the susceptibility to common diseases, strongly support the thesis that different aging rates exist which reflect a constitutive biological characteristic of an animal. It is emphasized, however, that very few comparative physiological and pathological studies have been carried out for the purpose of relating MLP, aging

Table 1. Maximum Life Span Potentials for Some Primates

Homo sapiens	man	113
Pan troglogytes	chimpanzee	55
Cebus capucinus	capucin	40
Galago senegalensis	galago	25
Saimiri sciureus	squirrel monkey	21
Tarsius syrichta	tarsier	12
Perodicticus potto	potto	12
Urogale everetti	Phillipine tree shrew	8

Taken from (11). MLP is in years.

rate, and onset frequency of disease, or the qualitative differences in these processes that may exist in different mammalian species. Clearly, much more comparative information is required.

WHY ANIMALS HAVE DIFFERENT MLP'S

If different mammalian species do have different innate capacities to maintain their physiology and mental health for a given period of time, then an evolutionary reason for it is likely to exist. An understanding of why animals have different MLP's would help clarify the concept of different aging rates and how these rates evolved mechanistically.

One possibility is that some type of biological limitation exists, unique to each species, preventing further increase in MLP regardless of how advantageous it might be to have a longer life span. Another possibility is that each species maintains its health for a characteristically optimum period of time because further increase would have no significant evolutionary selective advantage. This latter possibility appears at present to have more support. For example, mammalian species are essentially identical in their biological makeup, which is probably why mammals age qualitatively in a similar manner. It seems reasonable that similar metabolic and general physiological processes would give rise to similar aging processes. Also, an excellent correlation appears to exist between the intensity of a species' environmental hazards and its MLP--the life span observed when most of these environmental hazards are

Table 2. Correlation Between Mortality Rate in the Wild and Maximum Life Span Potential for Some Birds

Common name	Average annual adult mortality (fraction that is killed)	Maximum life span potential (yrs)
Blue tit	0.72	9
European robin	0.62	12
Lapwing	0.34	16
Common swift	0.18	21
Sooty shearwater	0.07	27
Herring gull	0.04	36
Royal albatross	0.03	45

Taken from (9).

removed. Typical data showing this correlation are shown in Table 2 for some birds and in Table 3 for some rodents. However, more data is needed to establish this correlation as a general phenomenon. If true, it could be hypothesized that animals in the wild seldom undergo significant senescence in their natural environment as a result of the balance of nature. Most animals would be killed by their natural predators or by accident before their performance is seriously reduced by their innate aging processes. Thus, there would be no evolutionary selective advantage for a mouse to be able to maintain optimum physical and mental health for 10 years if, on the average, 95% of the population could not survive beyond one year. Only animals at the top of the food chain, such as the elephant and man, appear to undergo senescence in the wild.

Not too many years ago, man's average life span (not MLP) was much shorter, and the problem of senescence was minor compared to other causes of death. In Table 4, the average life span of man is seen to be about 30 to 40 years under conditions of natural environmental hazards. Only after the age of 30 or 40 years did man's mental and physical health begin to show significant decline.

Table 3. Mortality Rate of Some Rodent Species in their Natural Ecological Environment

Species	Average mortality rate	Maximum life span potential	Maximum calorie consumption (MCC) (Kilocalories/g/MLP
Peromyscus maniculatus (deer mouse)	63-94% in 1 yr (rarely live over 2 yrs)	3040 days	703
Peromyscus leucopus (white-footed mouse)	rarely live over 2-3 yrs	3300 days	672
Mus musculus (field mouse)	99% in 1 yr (rarely live over 1 yr)	1200 days	250
Tamias striatus	50% in 1.5 yrs	12 yrs	561

Taken from (9).

The good correlation found between mortality rate and MLP indicates that MLP evolved to the point where it was no longer advantageous. The almost total absence of senescence in the population of wild animals in their natural environment is also consistent with the idea that sensescence has no evolutionary advantage, and is postponed to an age that insures its non-occurrence.

Would MLP always increase if the environmental hazards permitted it? Clearly, there are advantages to limited life span, such as enhancing turnover in the population, thus increasing the rate of evolutionary selective processes. However, for mammlian species, it appears that natural turnover rate in the population has been sufficient. The need to evolve a genetic program to terminate it is bypassed.

A great number of variables are involved in determining the resultant evironmental hazards of a species. One important parameter is the ability of the organism to learn from its environment in order to better adapt, protect, and feed itself. A rough correlation appears to exist between the amount of learned vs. instinctive behavior a given species demonstrates and its innate MLP (10,11,14). Apparently, longer lived mammalian species have been able to lower their environmental hazards by taking advantage of their ability to learn and reason. This implies, of course, that longer lived species in general have superior intelligence capabilities, which also appears to be true (11,14). Longer life spans could provide more time for an individual to achieve a certain degree of mental

Table 4. Average Mortality Rate of Present-Day Man in His Past and Present Environment

Time period	Average chronoage at 50% survival (yrs)	Maximum life span potential (yrs)
Würm (about 70,000-30,000 yrs ago)	29.4	69-77
Upper Paleolithic (about 30,000-12,000 yrs ago)	32.4	95
Mesolithic (about 12,000-10,000 yrs ago)	31.5	95
Neolithic Anatolian (about 10,000-8000 yrs ago)	38.2	95
Classic Greece (1100 B.C.-1 A.D.)	35	95
Classic Rome (753 B.C.-476 A.D.)	32	95
England (1276 A.D.)	48	95
England (1376-1400)	38	95
United States (1900-1902)	61.5	95
United States (1950)	70.0	95
United States (1970)	72.5	95

Taken from (9).

development and knowledge, and to pass this on to the young. Thus, a slower aging rate would be essential to take advantage of a superior cognitive ability. In this manner, the great differences in MLP and mental capacities that exist among the mammalian species can be explained by the conventional chance and necessity mechanisms of evolution. In this case, adaptive and learned behavior with increased MLP marks the evolutionary success of the mammalian species, and in particular for the primates.

THE BIOLOGICAL BASIS OF THE DIFFERENT MLP'S OF MAMMALIAN SPECIES

As was previously mentioned, differences in MLP do not seem to involve fundamental qualititative differences in biological makeup. Nevertheless, species that are remarkably similar at the biological level age at significantly different rates. The chimpanzee, having an MLP one-half that of man, appears to age twice as fast in all biological aspects, in spite of remarkable similarities to man at the biological level. The whole gamut of aging processes, such as changes in hearing, taste, smell, heart and kidney capacities, function of the immune system, mental function, as well as the onset frequency of age-dependent diseases, including cancer, would be expected to uniformly run at twice the rate in the chimpanzee as in man. It this proves true, then how is man able to maintain his mental and physical health so much longer? Further, can we enhance man's health for an even longer period of time by using means similar to those that have evolved in the past? This question represents a completely new approach in biomedical science: to discover the basis of general health maintenance and the origin of age-related dysfunctions of man.

Of course, some genetic differences must exist between species having different MLP's; but how much difference is there, and can we estimate an upper limit to the genetic complexity governing the aging rate of man? Two approaches have been used to make this estimate. The first was a biological comparison of the nucleic acids and proteins known in genetically closely related species having substantial differences in MLP. A study of about 50 major proteins of man and chimpanzee indicates that 99% of the amino acid sequences were identical, and many of the differences found were trivial in terms of biological function (15,16,17). Also, the nucleic acid sequence differences were found to be only about 1% between man and chimpanzee. In fact, man and chimpanzee are so similar at the genetic level that they are classified as sibling species (species that are remarkably similar in appearance) (15). Yet, man and chimpanzee are placed in different families on the basis of their obvious morphological and behavioral differences.

The second approach was to determine how quickly longevity can change, and to compare this value with how rapidly useful genetic alterations are known to occur. Two different methods were used to estimate this value (5,11). The first method compares the MLP between living species with the time when they had a common ancestor. For example, man and chimpanzee, with MLP's of about 100 and 50 years, respectively, had a common ancestor 15 x 10^6 years ago, the time the evolutionary lines of man and chimpanzee diverged. Thus, a minimum change of 50 years of MLP occurred with a time period of 15 x 10^6 years, or a change of 1.6 years MLP per 10^6 years of evolution. Tables 5, 6, and 7 show how this method was used to estimate the direction and speed MLP changed during the evolution of the primate species. The results show that MLP tended to always increase; the rate of increase of MLP increased as the higher-order primate species emerged; and the maximum rate of increase occurred during the emergence of the Hominidae-Pongidae families.

Table 5. **Estimates of the Evolutionary Rate of Increase in Maximum Life Span Potential within the Superfamilies of the Primates**

Order	Suborder	Superfamily	Mean MLP within a superfamily	MLP differences within a superfamily	Common divergence time (x 10^{-6} yrs) (Fossil dates)	Change in MLP per 10^6 yrs (Fossil)
	Prosimii	TUPAIOIDEA	6	1.5	65	0.02
		LORIDOIDEA	14	18	30	0.6
		LEMUROIDEA	19	24	30	0.8
Primates						
		CEBOIDEA	22	25	30	0.83
		CERCOPITHECOIDEA	30	27	25	1.1
	Anthropoidea	HOMINOIDEA	52	63	30	2.1

Taken from (11). MLP is in years.

Table 6. Estimates of the Evolutionary Rate of Increase in Maximum Life Span Potentials Between Closely Related Superfamilies of the Primates

Superfamily	Mean MLP of the two superfamilies	Difference in mean MLP between superfamilies	Common divergence time (x 10^{-6} yrs) (Fossil dates)	Increase in MLP (yrs) per 10^6 yrs (Fossil)
LORISOIDEA-TUPAIOIDEA	10.3	8	65	0.12
LEMUROIDEA-LORISOIDEA	16.8	5	40	0.13
CERCOPITHECOIDEA-CEBOIDEA	25.6	8	55	0.15
HOMINOIDEA-CERCOPITHECOIDEA	40.8	22	40	0.55

Taken from (11). MLP is in years.

Table 7. Estimates of the Evolutionary Rate of Increase in Maximum Life Span Potential between the Closely Related Families of Hominoidea

Family	Largest difference in MLP between families	Common Divergence time (x 10^{-6} yrs) (Fossil dates)	Increase in MLP (yrs) per 10^6 yrs (Fossil)
PONGIDAE-HYLOBATIDAE	18	30	0.6
HOMINIDAE-PONGIDAE	55	15	4.0

Taken from (11). MLP is in years.

The second method estimates the MLP of extinct fossil species using the empirical correlation found between MLP and brain and body weights for living species. This method was used by Cutler (5,11) and Sacher (13). The equation used is taken from Sacher's work in this area (18) and is:

$$\text{MLP} = (10.839)\,(\text{brain wt., g})^{0.636}\,(\text{body wt., g})^{-0.225}$$

The stongest rationale for using this equation to predict MLP for extinct species is that the prediction works equally well for living fossil species and for progressive species (11). Sacher did not support his findings using this rationale (13). Estimates of MLP using the brain and body weights for living fossils are shown in Table 8, and agree with known MLP's. The equation is also shown to predict MLP for mammals in general and primates, shown in Tables 9 and 10, respectively.

MLP was predicted for 59 ungulates, 32 carnivores, 24 primates, and 156 Hominidae fossil species. Knowing when the fossil species existed, a phylogenetic tree for the evolution of MLP was constructed. The results found were similar to that using the first method. Table 11 summarizes the ungulate and carnivore data, and Figure 1 illustrates that, although MLP generally increased, an increase in dispersion of MLP also occurred, reaching a maximum for present living species.

Table 8. Estimation of Maximum Life Span Potential for Living Fossil and Recent Mammals Living in a Mesozoic Niche

Common name	Cranial capacity (cm^3)	Body Wt (g)	MLP Pred.	MLP Obs.	Time of appearance ($x\ 10^{-6}$ yrs)
Short tailed shrew	0.347	17.4	2.9	3.3	14-0
Pygmy shrew	0.11	5.3	1.8	1.5	14-0
European shrew	0.2	10.3	2.3	1.5	14-0
long tailed shrew	0.12	5.7	1.9	1.5	14-0
tenrec	2.75	832	4.5	2	10-0
Madagascar hedgehog	1.51	248	4.1	3	10-0
streaked tenrec	0.83	110	3.3	3	5.5-0
Norwegian rat (wild)	1.59	200	4.4	3.4	5.5-0
field mouse	0.45	22.6	3.2	3.5	5.5-0
vole	0.66	23.7	4.1	2-3	3-0
vole	0.74	27.9	4.2	2-3	3-0

Taken from (12). MLP is in years.

Table 9. Prediction of Maximum Life Span Potential on the Basis of Body and Brain Weight for Some Mammalian Species

Common name	Cranial capacity (cm^3)	Body wt (g)	Maximum life span potential (MLP) Observed	Predicted
Pigmy shrew	0.11	5.3	1.5	1.8
Field mouse	0.45	22.6	3.5	3.2
Opossum	7.65	5000	7.0	5.8
Mongolian horse	587	260,000	46	38
Camel	570	450,000	30	33
Cow	423	465,000	30	27
Giraffe	680	529,000	34	35
Elephant (India)	5045	2,347,000	70	89
Mountain lion	154	54,000	19	23
Domestic dog	79	13,400	20	21

Taken from (9,12). MLP is in years.

The phylogenetic tree of MLP for the primate species is shown in Figure 2. The general increase in MLP is clearly evident, indicating maximum rate of increase along the ancestral-descendant-sequence leading to modern man. This latter observation is illustrated in Figure 3, showing the entire hominid ancestral-descendant-sequence lineage over the 60 x 10^6 years of primate evolution. More detailed data was obtained from the analysis of the 156 hominid species, and is shown in Figure 4, indicating an exponential rise of increased MLP and the sudden stop in the increase of MLP about 100,000 years ago. The rate of change in MLP over the past 2 million years is shown in Figure 5 for both MLP and the number of neurons for the hominid species. Richard Leakey's recent findings of a Homo habilis species existing 2 x 10^6 years ago are compatible with these conclusions (19).

The main conclusions of these studies are that: (1) increased longevity and not increased senescence evolved during the evolutionary history of mammals, and (2) the maximum rate of increased MLP for the primate species, which is about 14 years of MLP per 100,000 years, occurred along the hominid ancestral-descendant-sequence about 100,000 years ago.

Table 10. Prediction of Maximum Life Span Potential on the Basis of Body and Brain Weight for Some Primates

Common name	Cranial capacity (cm^3)	Body wt (g)	Maximum life span potential (MLP)	
			Observed	Predicted
Tree shrew	4.3	275	7	7.7
Marmoset	9.8	413	15	12
Squirrel monkey	24.8	630	21	20
Rhesus monkey	106	8719	29	27
Baboon	179	16,000	36	33
Gibbon	104	5500	32	30
Orangutan	420	69,000	50	41
Gorilla	550	140,000	40	42
Chimpanzee	410	49,000	45	43
Man	1446	65,000	95	92

Taken from (11). MLP is in years.

The increase in MLP is predicted to be the result of a uniform decrease in the aging rate of the entire spectrum of aging processes as we observe the spectrum of aging processes to exist in primate species living today. The basis of this argument is that, although different primates living today have different MLP's, they nevertheless appear to have qualitatively similar biological makeup, aging processes, and age-dependent diseases.

The next question is how fast adaptive point mutations can occur over a 100,000 year period. Three different methods were used to make this estimate (5,10,13). The first is based on Haldane's approximation that the maximum genomic load of harmful recessive mutations that can exist in germ cells limits the mutation rate that can occur to one substitution per genome per 300 generations. Using this, the mutation rate is calculated to be 44 adaptive amino acid substitutions per 40,000 genes per 100,000 years (where 40,000 genes are taken to be the average number of functional genes in a typical primate cell). Sacher arrived at a similar conclusion using Haldane's approximation, but made no calculations (13).

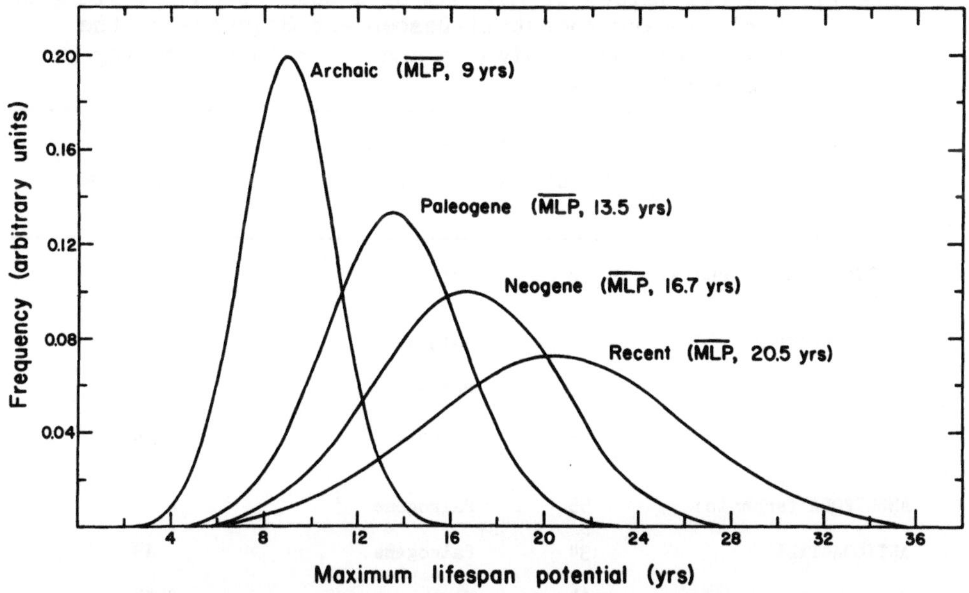

Fig. 1. Increase in mean MLP and dispersion of MLP in the archaic and progressive ungulates. Archaic species became extinct but progressive ones did not. Data represents analysis of about 10 species at each time era. Similar results were found for the carnivores. Taken from (12).

The second method is based on the DNA and protein sequence differences measured between the different primate species. These data are used to calculate the average change in nucleotide sequence of the DNA that actually did occur throughout the evolutionary history of the primates. From this data, an adaptive mutation rate is calculated at about 250 amino acid substitutions per 40,000 genes per 100,000 years for the hominid species 100,000 years ago.

The last method is based on a theoretical calculation to predict how rapidly adaptive mutations can occur. Using a spontaneous mutation rate of 10^{-9} per cell and a selective value parameter of 10^{-2}, the adaptive mutation rate calculated is 160 amino acid substitutions per 40,000 genes per 100,000 years.

Thus, all three methods used to estimate the number of adaptive mutations occurring during hominid evolution 100,000 years ago indicate that about 40 to 250 adaptive amino acid substitutions per genome occurred over a period of 100,000 years. This change has to account not only for the 14 years of uniform increase in the general maintenance of physical and mental health (a slowing down of aging rate by about 20%), but also for the morphological and cognitive changes that occurred during the recent evolution of man. Could this

Table 11. Average Values of Maximum Life Span Potential Along the Evolutionary Ancestral-Descendent Sequence of the Ungulates and Carnivores and Their Corresponding Archaic Species

Order	Average time of presence ($x\ 10^6$ yrs) and epoch		Average MLP
CONDYLARTHRA (archaic)	52	Paleogene	12
PERISSODACTYLA	44	Paleogene	16
	5	Neogene	29
	-	Recent	34
AMBLYPODA (archaic)	55	Paleogene	7
ARTIODACTYLA	34	Paleogene	13
	14	Neogene	18
	-	Recent	26
CREODONTA (archaic)	41	Paleogene	11
CARNIVORA	26	Paleogene	13
	17	Neogene	17
	-	Recent	20

Taken from (12). MLP is in years.

be true, or did some genetic parameter other than point mutation underlie this change? One important assumption made in these calculations is that the total number of functional genes is only 40,000 out of a potential maximum number of about 3.5×10^6, if all the genome is utilized. If more genetic information is utilized (over 40,000), then the possible number of adaptive mutations would increase proportionally.

Similar calculations and results to those described here have been made by other investigators (15,16,17,20,21,22,23,24). The general conclusion has been that it is difficult to account for the evolutionary changes that have occurred in mammals as being a result of point mutations in structural genes. Instead, the major genetic changes that best account for mammalian evolution are at the

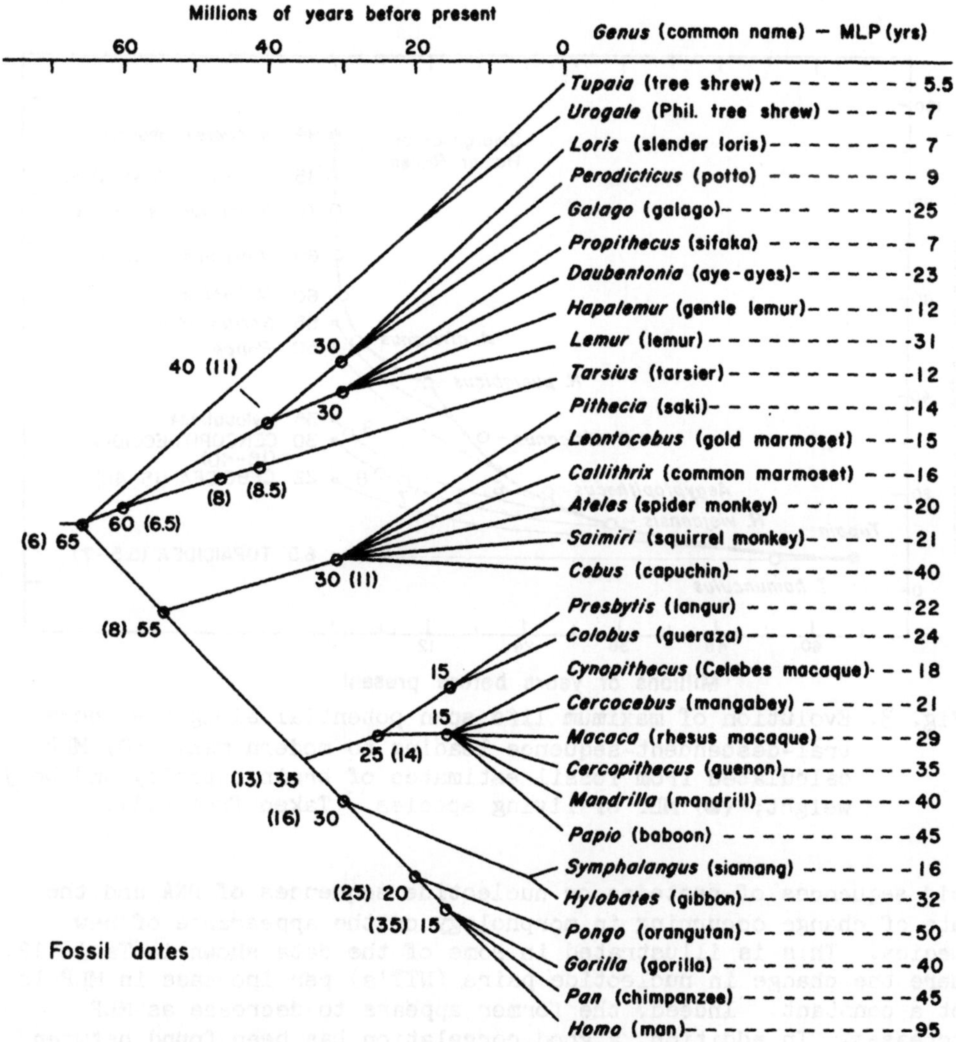

Fig. 2. Maximum life span potential phylogenetic tree for the primate species. Numbers in parenthesis are estimates of MLP of the species existing at that time. Neighboring numbers are millions of years according to geological dating. Taken from (11).

regulatory gene level (14,15,16). That is to say, mammalian evolution occurred as a result of changes in the expression of regulatory genes governing the same set of structural genes, either by a few point mutations or by chromosomal rearrangements.

There is major support for this new concept. It underlies the finding of little correlation between the rate of change in amino

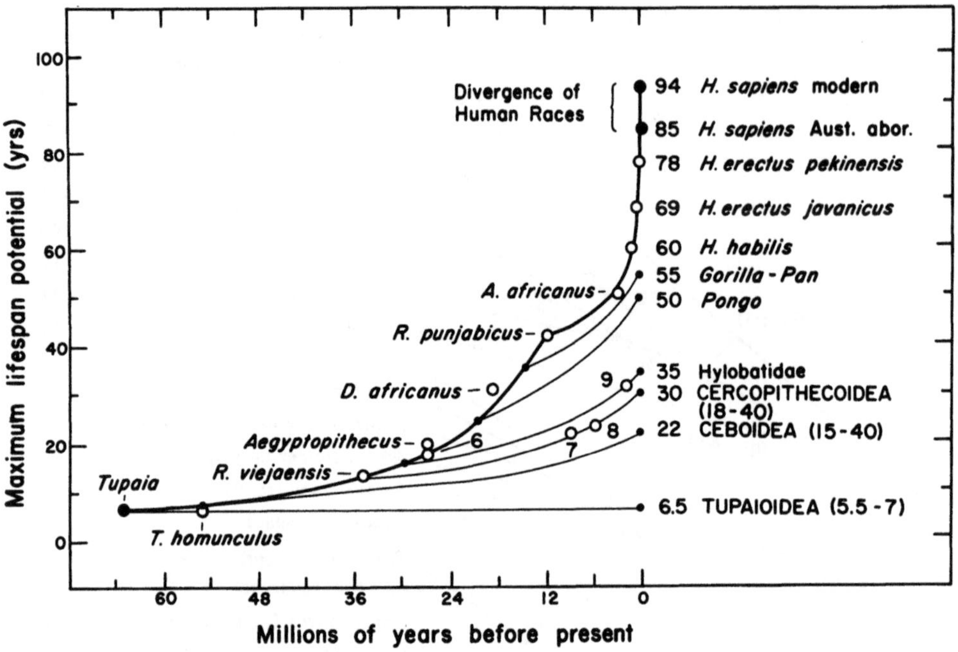

Fig. 3. Evolution of maximum life span potential along the ancestral-descendent-sequence leading to modern man. (O) MLP calculated from fossil estimates of brain capacity and body weight; (●) MLP of living species. Taken from (11).

acid sequences of proteins or nucleotide sequences of DNA and the rate of change occurring in morphology or the appearance of new species. This is illustrated in some of the data shown in Table 12, where the change in nucleotide pairs (NTP's) per increase in MLP is not a constant. Indeed, the former appears to decrease as MLP increases. In addition, a good correlation has been found between morphological change and the change in chromosomal morphology, which indicates that perhaps chromosomal rearrangement played an important role in governing timing and levels of gene expression during the differentiation and development of the organism. Also, adaptive studies with microorganisms and recently with Drosophila demonstrate that the type of genetic change involved, when the organism adapts to a new food source or to environmental condition, is almost always a regulatory change in existing genes, and not the appearance of new gene products. Finally, morphological differences occurring during the evolution of man and other primates have an underlying similarity.

Many of the changes in the morphology of primates with increasing MLP can be explained by a general retardation of development, a process called neoteny. Man is more fetal and child-like at all

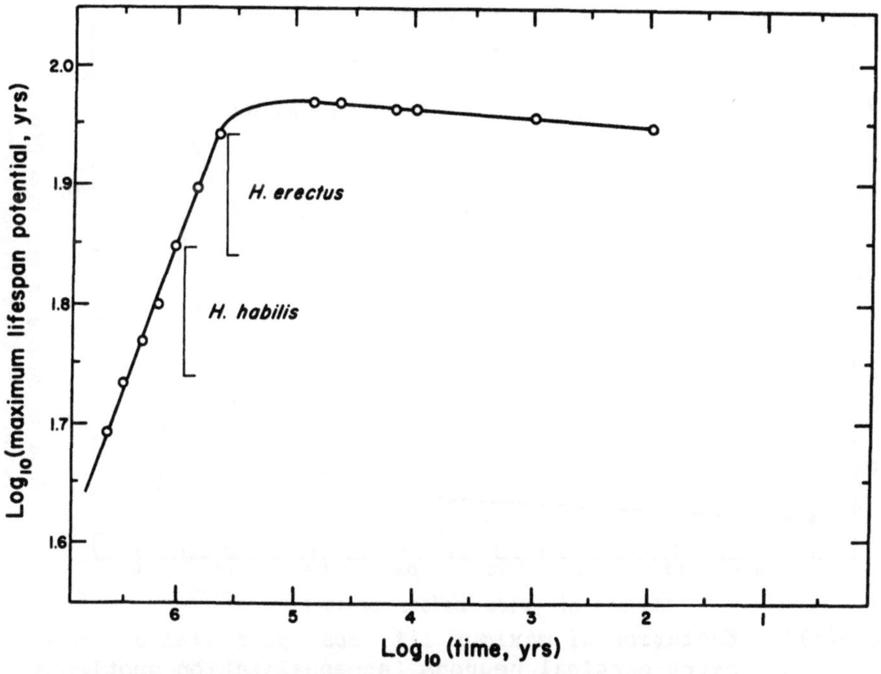

Fig. 4. Evolution of maximum life span potential for the hominid species calculated from a regressive analysis of 156 independent estimates of brain capacity and body weight. Open circles represent typical data indicating spread of data. Taken from (11).

stages of development than is the chimpanzee. Thus, different rates of development are also likely to be governed by regulatory genes and not by different types of structural genes (9,17,25,26).

To summarize, there is now substantial evidence indicating a surprisingly high rate of increase of MLP during the evolutionary appearance of man. Few point mutational changes occur during this period. Moreover, morphological changes cannot be accounted for easily by the accumulation of point mutational changes in structural genes. This concept is supported by the conservation of molecular and cellular biology, physiology and morphology among different species. The differences that are found can be explained as a result of timing and degree of expression of a common set of genes. The author has therefore suggested that the genetic differences between man and other primates that account for their innately different aging rates and mental capacities are not different types of structural genes but rather a common set of genes being expressed at different times and to different degrees (3,5,9,11). This common set of genes governing aging rate is postulated to be internally governed by

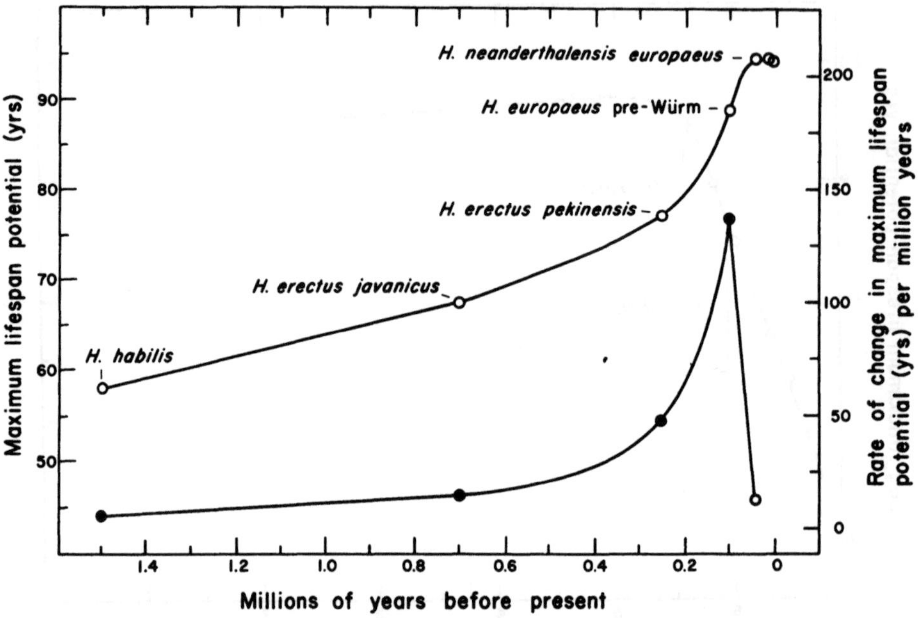

Fig. 5(a). Evolution of maximum life span potential and number of extra cortical neurons (encephalization quotient) during the recent emergence of the hominid species. (O) MLP; (●) rate of change of MLP. Taken from (11).

a common set of regulatory genes. These regulatory genes have undergone a few simple genetic modifications which have resulted in changes in the timing and level of expression of the genes they control and that determine the aging rate.

How many regulatory genes are involved in controlling aging rate, and to what extent and speed were these genes altered to give rise to man's rapid increase in MLP? If point mutational changes were the major source of change, and there is a random distribution of regulatory genes along the genome, then the estimate remains at about 40 to 250 amino acid substitutions per 14 years of increased MLP per 100,000 years. On the other hand, if chromosomal rearrangements are involved, we have no way at present to estimate how rapidly these changes can occur. Comparative analysis is now being undertaken at the chromosomal level between man and the chimpanzee, and the differences do not appear to be outstanding at this time (22). Nevertheless, we have to consider that, although the likelihood of changes at the point mutation level affecting the aging rate appear to be low, chromosomal rearrangement superimposed on these changes could substantially increase the complexity of the regulatory processes governing the aging rate of man.

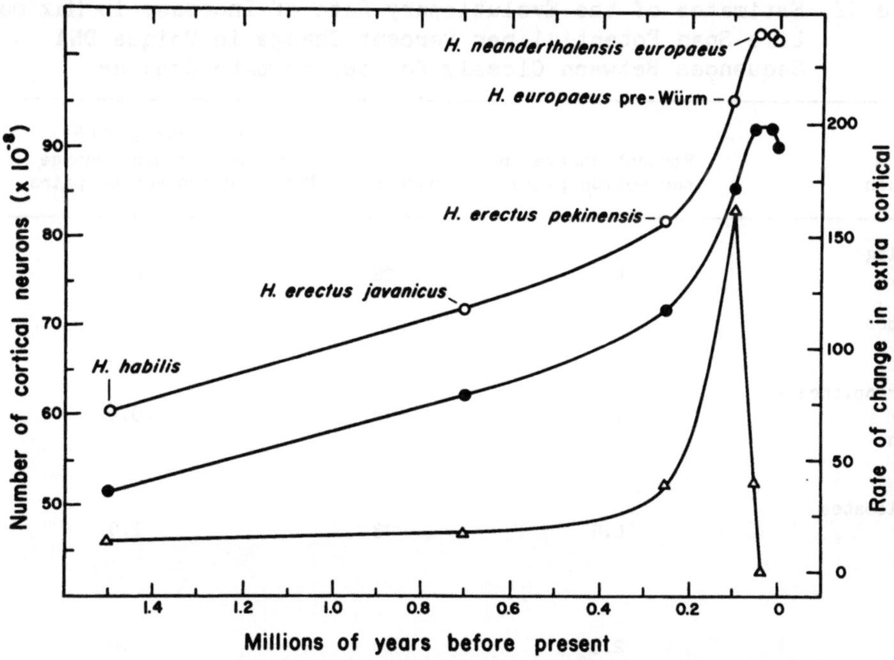

Fig. 5(b). Evolution of maximum life span potential and number of extra cortical neurons (encephalization quotient) during the recent emergence of the hominid species. (O) MLP; (●) number of cortical neurons; (Δ) rate of change of cortical neurons. Taken from (11).

GENERAL AND SPECIAL HYPOTHESES OF AGING AND LIFE MAINTENANCE

The data and ideas presented above can be summarized most clearly in a general hypothesis for all forms of life and a special hypothesis for the mammalian species (3,6,9). Both hypotheses are based on the notion that two opposing processes, aging and life maintenance, played major roles in the origin and evolution of all living systems.

Life maintenance processes are broadly defined as any characteristics or properties of a living system that act to increase the probability of its survival. Two major types of life maintenance processes exist. The first is related to the maintenance of the organism relative to external environment hazards. This includes morphological and the common house-keeping functions, plus special biological functions unique to a species. The second type of life maintenance process relates to internal environmental hazards, or to the intrinsic aging processes. This includes the finite functional life span of biological constituents making up the organism and the side-effects of metabolic reactions evolved to provide the life

Table 12. Estimates of the Evolutionary Rate of Increase in Maximum Life Span Potential per Percent Change in Unique DNA Sequences Between Closely Related Primate Genuses

Genus	Percent change in nucleotide pairs	Increase in MLP	Increase in MLP per percent change in nucleotide pairs
Galago → Cebus	54	26	0.5
Cercopitheous → Pan	11	10	0.9
Hylobates → Pan	6.5	13	2.0
Pan → Homo	2.5	50	20.0

Taken from (11). MLP is in years.

maintenance properties of the constituents. The side-effects of metabolic reactions, the harmful pleiotropic nature of metabolism and development, are considered by many to be the major aging processes. Special life-maintenance processes are postulated to exist solely to reduce these long-term detrimental effects.

The general hypothesis postulates that much of the morphology and biochemistry of cells and organisms today reflects the co-evolutionary history of these aging and life maintenance processes. Most of these two opposing processes emerged during the 3 to 4 billion year period leading to the evolution of the free-living eukaryotic cell. Some additional aging and life maintenance processes were added during the remaining evolutionary history of multicellular organisms, and were associated with their differentiation and developmental characteristics. From the appearance of mammalian species about 150 million years ago to the emergence of primate species 60 million years ago, few different aging and life maintenance processes evolved. Even fewer have evolved during the 15 to 4 million year period of hominid evolution. For these reasons, in addition to the remarkable biochemical similarities between the primate species, the recent increase in MLP is postulated not on the appearance of new structural genes or radically new biochemical pathways, but rather on a difference in the timing and degree of expression of a common set of life maintanance genes found in all primate species.

These conclusions, expressed in a general hypothesis for all life forms on the origin and evolution of aging and life maintenance processes, lead to a special unified hypothesis for the evolution of mammals, and in particular for the evolution of the primates. This special hypothesis unifies the aging and life maintenance processes of the mammalian species in seven major postulates, which are as follows:

1. All mammalian species express the same qualitative specturm of aging processes at the genotypic and phenotypic levels.

2. All mammalian species' aging processes are of a pleiotropic nature and are of two major types: (a) Continuously-Acting Aging Processes and (b) Developmentally-Linked Aging Processes.

3. All mammalian species express the same qualitative and time-dependent patterns of general physiological decline in function and increased sensitivity to disease as the result of these two common pleiotropic-acting aging processes.

4. All mammalian species express the same set of life maintenance processes or genes acting to control the rate of expression of the Continuously-Acting and Developmentally-Linked Aging Processes.

5. Differences in the time period in which each mammalian species is intrisically capable of maintaining its optimal physical and mental health (MLP) are a result of the timing and degree of expression of the common set of life maintenance processes.

6. The timing and degree of expression of this common set of life maintenance processes is controlled by a common set of regulatory genes that may constitute a small fraction of the functional genetic material of the cell.

7. Evolution of increased MLP was the result of changes, either by rearrangement within the genome and/or by point mutations of a common set of regulatory genes. These mechanisms are considered to be of a nature similar to those involved in the recent evolution of different morphological, developmental, and behavioral features of the primate species.

The ideas presented here as general and special hypotheses were first published in general form in 1972 (6) and later expanded (3,9). The hypotheses are unique so far as this author can determine, and should not be confused with the related and interesting

Table 13.

Accumulation of Damage or Dysfunctions that are or may be a Function of MLP

1. Chromosomal aberration frequency
2. Age pigments
3. Physiological functions
4. Mental or cognitive functions
5. Resistance to pathogenic diseases
6. Onset frequency of degenerative diseases
7. Physico-chemical alteration of chromatin (protein and DNA)*
8. Alteration of enzyme induction kinetics*
9. Ability of cells to maintain a given state of differentiation*
10. Accumulation of methionine sulfoxide residues in protein*

Repair or Protective Processes that are or may be a Function of MLP

1. DNA repair (UV, depurination, DNA-protein adducts)
2. Selective protein degradation*
3. Superoxide dismutase level*
4. Glutathionine peroxidase*
5. Catalase*
6. Vitamin E*
7. Vitamin C*
8. Activation of precarcinogen agents
9. Ratio of B/A lactate dehydrogenase
10. Metabolic rate
11. Encephalization index
12. Reduction of developmental rate
13. Neoteny
14. Free radical scavanger and antioxidant levels*
15. Rate of general nucleic acid and protein synthesis and degradation*
16. Fidelity of DNA and protein synthesis*
17. Interferon levels*
18. Methionine sulfoxide reductase*

*Under investigation in our laboratory
Taken from (3,6,8,9).

work of Sacher (13,18,27).

The most important role of the special hypothesis is to suggest meaningful experiments that might elucidate the biological nature of human aging and the processes determining the period during which optimum physical and mental health is maintained. A new experimental approach is suggested that would search for the "natural" differences governing aging rate by using a comparative analysis of species closely related genetically but having significant differences in their innate aging rate. A comparision of age-dependent changes, as well as other innate characteristics of the organism, as a function of MLP would give important insights as to which are important aging and life maintenance processes. Table 13 summarizes some data that is already known and areas where experiments are planned that relate to MLP.

DEDIFFERENTIATION AS THE PRIMARY SENESCENT PROCESS

A common idea in gerontology is that organismal aging is related to the time-dependent accumulation of some type of damage, be it cellular or extracellular (8,28,29). This damage is usually predicted to interfere with the proper function of the cell or lead to cell death. According to this idea, time-dependent accumulation of damage would be expected where the rate of accumulation is proportional to the characteristic aging rate of the species (8,30).

However, a completely different and more recent idea is that aging is primarily a result, not of accumulation of damage, at least primarily (31), but instead is the result of an inherent instability of organs or cells in terms of their ability to maintain their properly differentiated state, or the ability of the organism to maintain proper homeostatic processes. For example, the advent of sexual maturity brings a new set of hormones which could affect the long-term functional stability of many different cells, and not merely the immediate changes in the target tissues. This developmentally-linked type of aging process is of an epigenetic nature.

It is not necessary to observe any time-dependent accumulation of damage as the result of the Continuously-Acting or Developmentally-Linked Action Processes. Although it is possible that some type of accumulation of damage occurs, the author suggests a new concept in which a constant time-independent pool of defective or damaged cellular constituents exists within the cell or organism. A simple model follows, illustrating this idea, and is coupled with the hypothesis that the key primary aging process results from a slow dedifferentiation of cells.

Continuously-Acting and Developmentally-Linked Aging Processes are suggested to act by slowly destabilizing and altering the proper, differentiated states of cells following sexual maturation. Every type of differentiated cell is postulated to have a characteristic level, or pool, of agents that cause damage. This, in turn, produces a characteristic level (pool) of damaged cellular constituents. However, counteracting processes exist that reduce the level of these damaging agents and remove or repair the damaged cellular components. Thus, an equilibrium is maintained. The net rate of turnover, and the resultant "pool of damage," is determined by the cells' characteristic rates of input and removal of damage.

It is proposed that the degree and rate of turnover of this complex spectrum of damage within the cell determine the time-dependent probabilty that dedifferentiation or epigenetic-like cell alterations will occur.

Thus, cells from an organism which has a long MLP would be expected to have a higher differentiated stability state as the result of a lower constitutive pool of damage. This lower pool of damage would be the result of higher levels of protective and repair processes, as well as initially lower levels of production of damaging agents.

Aging is produced by Developmentally-Linked Aging Processes by a similar mechanism. It is proportional to the length of time cells are exposed to the developmentally-related harmful agents, as well as to the amounts of these substances to which cells are exposed. The agents would not result in an accumulation of damage, but would simply increase the time-dependent probability that a dedifferentiation-like cellular alteration would occur.

Aging would not necessarily be a result of a time-dependent loss of repair or protective processes. Each cell would have an innate and characteristic probability of dedifferentiating on the basis of its constitutive levels of damage. Different cell types within an organism would be expected to have different probabilities of dedifferentiation. Of course, the original state of dedifferentiation would direct the probability of what types of dedifferentiation events would most likely occur.

The idea of a correlation existing between MLP and the constitutive level of damage within a cell leads to the question of how this level is controlled. A feedback relationship probably exists between the levels of damage within a cell and the level of repair and protective processes that are expressed. Thus, the sensitivity of such a feedback loop may determine the species' innate levels of Continuously-Acting Anti-Aging Processes and would therefore be a key regulatory process governing aging rate.

What evidence supports the innate loss of ability of cells to maintain their proper post-maturational state of differentiation as a primary aging process? There is at present very little positive data (33), and perhaps the most convincing aspect of the dedifferentiation hypothesis is that it can satisfactorily explain, as a causative process, many of the different physiological problems and diseases associated with aging. For example, the slow loss of a particular physiological function could be the result of a higher fraction of the cells in a tissue not producing the optimum spectrum of enzyme levels, hormone receptors, structural proteins, hormones, and so forth. A detailed search for something radically wrong with the cells making up the tissue, such as an accumulation of defective proteins, reduced protein synthesis capacity, or defective structures in the genetic apparatus of the cell, would be fruitless. Yet, significant loss of proper function is evident.

More damaging to the organism could be the synthesis of a protein with high biological activity from a certain cell type that should not normally be synthesizing that protein. For example, suppose a liver cell began to synthesize small amounts of a hormone that inhibited proper homeostatic regulation of thyroid or immune function.

Strong evidence for such dedifferentiation processes occurring more frequently as a function of increased physiological age is found on analysis of the proteins present in many types of tumors (34-37). A common finding is a complex appearance of gene derepression, where often a tumor of an adult synthesizes proteins normally found in fetal development, such as alpha-fetal protein, or when non-endocrine cancerous tissue synthesizes hormones. In this sense, the age-dependent increase in at least some types of cancers may represent a special case of the general much broader age-dependent dedifferentiation process apparently occurring in all cells with time (38). A slight change in a cell's differentiated state would not be noticed, particularly in post-mitotic tissue. However, if the change in differentiation represents a reverse back to a dividing state, then the process of simple uncontrolled growth would amplify this type of dedifferentiation until it is readily detected and results in the early death of the organism.

Any protein synthesized by a cell that was not present when general immunocompetence occurred in early life could be antigenic. Thus, dedifferentiation could be the basis for many of the autoimmune diseases associated with increased age (39,40). Furthermore, the well known age-dependent changes in hair growth, density and appearance of wild coarse hair, blemishes such as age-spots and moles in skin, the decrease of response time of cells to hormones or other types of stimuli, the loss of hormone receptor sites and the appearance of abnormal protein in the brain (41,42), all can be accounted for by a slight alteration in the cells' differentiated state, and without proposing that the cell operates improperly because of a high accumulation of some type of damage or basic impairment to cell life-maintenance functions.

It is also known that viruses and/or virus-related genetic material is endogenous in the normal genome of cells by a vertical transfer mechanism (through germ cells) (43,44). The role of such viral-related genetic information is not known--but it may be related to cancer and slow-type virus diseases (45,46). The age-dependent loss of a cell's ability to maintain repression of these genes by random dedifferentiation events could also be an important component of the aging process (47,48).

We have recently investigated the dedifferentiation aging model in our laboratory by searching for the age-dependent expression of genes in cells where these genes are not expected to be expressed (38). Specifically, the possible expression of α and β globin genes and the endogenous mouse leukemia virus genes (MuLV) as a function of increased age in liver and brain of mouse was investigated. The assay system utilized a highly radioactive synthesized probe called complementary DNA (cDNA), produced by a purified preparation of globin mRNA or MuLV RNA and reverse transcriptase enzyme. The cDNA probe was mixed with RNA preparations obtained from liver and brain at different ages and examined for the presence of cDNA-RNA hybrid complexes. The presence of a cDNA-RNA hybrid would show that RNA complementary to that specific cDNA probe was present in the RNA preparation. The results, shown in Table 14, reveal an age-dependent two-fold increase in the levels of α and β globin in liver and brain. Results shown in Table 15 for the MuLV show a two-fold increase in the amount of MuLV-related RNA, which is related to an increased fraction of RNA complementary to the entire virus genome found present. More experimentation along these lines should be undertaken to evaluate the role dedifferentiation might play in aging.

EXTENSION OF HUMAN MENTAL AND PHYSICAL HEALTH--POSSIBILITY AND ADVISABILITY

Most persons prefer good health, with mental health as the most prized possession (49). But would people prefer a short healthy life span or a long healthy one? Recent surveys on this question clearly indicate that, although many social, economical and theological problems would surface upon any substantial extension of human mental and physical health, most of the people of the United States at least favor the opportunity of having a choice (50-54).

The most serious difficulty in discussing this subject is that of evaluating whether a significant extension of human health is a real possibility in the near future (55-57). The subject is brought up here because the unified hypothesis of aging and life maintenance processes as presented in this chapter suggests that, although a reasonable understanding of the vast complexity of the biological nature of the aging process may lie in the distant future, some significant control of the aging rate may be possible in the near future. For example, processes which govern aging rate are likely to be far less difficult to investigate than aging processes. If the unified hypothesis presented here proves correct, then we should be prepared for a substantial increase in our knowledge in the near future about these specific life maintanance processes and how their effectiveness to slow aging may be enhanced. Progress in this area would almost be impossible to stop, for it could come not only from laboratories primarily interested in the biological nature of aging, but also from cancer and environmental toxicology groups.

One interesting idea that may result in our first significant reduction of innate aging rate is based on the notion that levels of repair and protective processes are governed by a cell's characteristic level, or pool, of damaged cellular constituents. It may prove

Table 14. Amount of Globin Sequences in Brain and Liver as a Function of Age[a]

	6-month old animal		20-month old animal		27-month old animal	
	Nucleus	Cytoplasm	Nucleus	Cytoplasm	Nucleus	Cytoplasm
Brain						
$\frac{\text{globin RNA (g)}}{\text{total RNA (g)}} \times 10^6$	5.3	11.3	11.2	14.4	12.0	20.6
$\frac{\text{globin RNA}}{\text{cell}}$	15	282	32	360	34	515
Liver						
$\frac{\text{globin RNA (g)}}{\text{total RNA (g)}} \times 10^6$	3.8	1.9	7.5	4.7	9.5	8.6
$\frac{\text{globin RNA}}{\text{cell}}$	12	111	23	274	30	502

[a]Taken from Ono and Cutler (38).

Table 15. Amount of Murine Leukemia Virus-Related RNA in Brain and Liver Nuclei as a Function of Age[a]

	6 month animal	27 month animal
Brain		
$\frac{\text{virus RNA}}{\text{total RNA}} \times 10^5$	5	9
percent genome transcribed	42	70
Liver		
$\frac{\text{virus RNA}}{\text{total RNA}} \times 10^5$	9	16
percent genome transcribed	50	74

[a]Taken from Ono and Cutler (38).

possible to induce higher levels of a complex spectrum of repair and protective processes within a cell, without knowing what they are or the details of how they are controlled, by simply compelling a cell to incorporate a complex spectrum of damaged cellular components (9).

In terms of Developmentally-Linked Aging Processes, means to induce a slower rate of development, or to selectively remove or inhibit hormone secretions after their useful period is over, may also prove practicable in the near future.

Thus, I believe the possibility of developing life-extension technology, such that the aging rate is slowed down by a factor of two or so, should be taken seriously. Consequently, consideration as to whether life-extension would be advisable should begin now (56,57). Too frequently in the past, such possibilities were thought unrealistic and were readily discarded (53). Hence, life span extension has not been sufficiently considered either in terms of its possible benefits or problems. Resolute decisions in this area are essential for proper distribution of funds supporting research that is more oriented toward the development of life-extension technology.

If significant life extension is a real possibility in the near future, say over the next 50 years, what about advisability? People seem more capable of picking out the problems rather than the benefits. Some obvious problem areas are (1) population growth control,

(2) economic institutions, such as the Social Security System, which now depends on existing MLP, (3) the fair distribution of life extension technology to the poor and rich, and (4) the conflict extended life span might cause for different ethnic and religious groups.

And what about the benefits? At the individual level, a longer period of good physical and mental health is usually associated with a correspondingly greater enjoyment of life, but this, of course, could be highly debated. However, one could have less fear that many of the enjoyments of life would pass him by simply because there was not enough time. Moreover, a postponement of death and the suffering that frequently accompanies it would be welcome.

Less obvious are social and economic benefits for the entire human race. If we reflect on why increased longevity of man evolved in the first place and how this played a key role in his evolutionary success, I believe the benefits for man will become more obvious. It is disappointing to find even in recent and popular publications on the evolutionary history of man a complete lack of coverage on the role longevity may play in the evolutionary success of man. We learn of the importance of bipedalism, of the importance of the thumb and fingers, of the ability to talk, of the spoken and written language and, of course, of man's other remarkable mental abilities. But could man have possibly survived without a corresponding extension of his years of good physical and mental health? I doubt it very much.

Further extension of life span may produce more of the same type of benefits that occurred in the past. If so, there would be more time for learning, resulting perhaps in a higher qualitative increase in our knowledge, not only about the universe, but also of ourselves. With more time to explore and discover, with greater understanding of life and the control over it, would not this lead to a better world? In terms of economics, would not increased productivity, as well as creativity, offset an increase in the length of time an individual might spend in the senescent period of life?

This last question bears importantly on just how life extension might be achieved. If life is extended in a way similar to how it evolved in the past, then an increased period of health would bring a proportional increase in the period of senescence. Would this be acceptable?

It is unrealistic to believe that some type of treatment may be developed to maintain health up to, say, 100 years, and then for the organism suddenly to grow older overnight and die, thus eliminating the senescent phase of life. Such an idea is frequently stated as an interpretation of a further squaring of the percent survival curve (53,58). But, as noted before, this idea simply conveys the incorrect concept that the declining slope of the survival curve is related to the rate of aging.

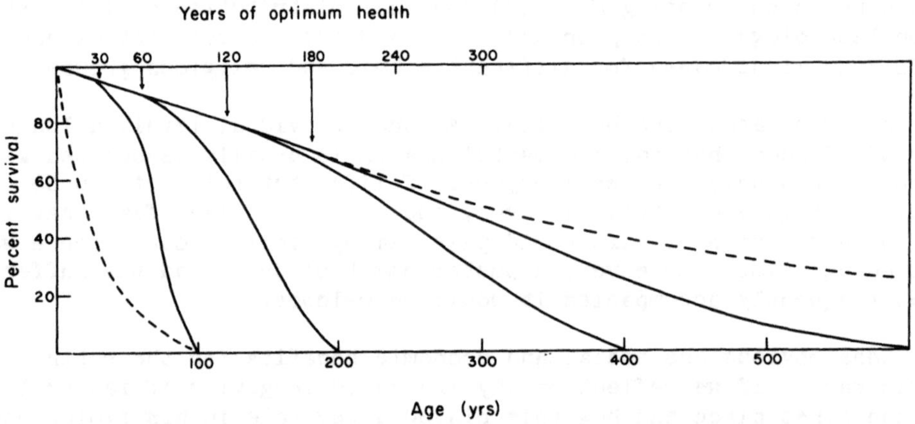

Fig. 6. Percent survival curves for man in the past, present and possible future. Dotted lines represent the two exponential decline curves where smallest fraction of senescent individuals occurs, first curve with MLP of about 100 years about 10,000 years ago and second curve, with infinite MLP. For the various curves shown, number of years of optimum health is taken to be when the curve breaks for the theoretical maximum level of percent survival where aging rate of zero or MLP is infinite.

What happens instead as the curve becomes squared is that the percent of senescent individuals increases. For example, let us go back several thousand years, where man, as a Homo sapien with a MLP of 100, had an average life span (50% mean) of 30 years. This is shown in Figure 6 for percent survival and Figure 7 for the corresponding rate of mortality curve. The exponential decline in percent survival, or a constant rate of death with time, determined how long man lived under the natural environmental hazards that led to his evolution. An increased probability of death with time, where death becomes more related to senescence, was an exception.

As man becomes able to diminish his environmental hazards, but unable to reduce his innate aging rate correspondingly, the 50% mean survival increased, as well as did the percent senescent individuals in the population (see Figs. 6,7). This trend continued to what we have today, where average life span has reached about 75 years in the developed nations, and MLP has remained constant. Further significant squaring of the curve in the future is unlikely. Even if it does occur, it would only further increase the high level (about 50%) of people over 35 years of age that we now have in the population.

However, one result not frequently considered is that, given the present intensity of environmental hazards and medical care, a

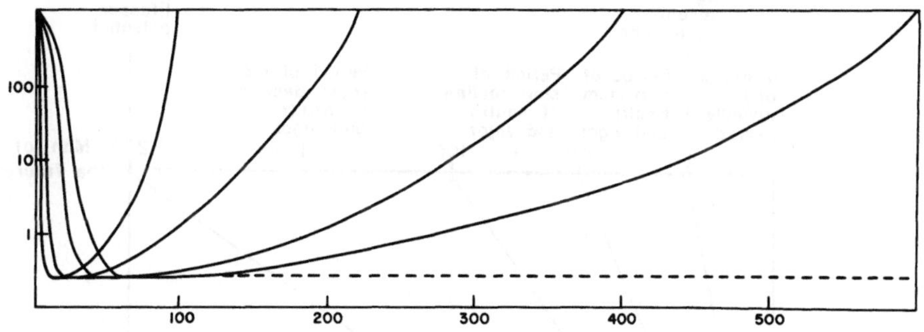

Fig. 7. Rate of mortality for man in the past, present and possible future. Curves correlate to the present survival curves in Fig. 6, including the dotted lines where probability of death is independent of physiological age.

reduction in aging rate or an increase in MLP would reduce, not increase, the percent of senescent individuals in the population. Examples of how an increase in MLP would affect future percent survival curves are shown in Figures 6 and 7 for 200, 400, 600 and infinite MLP's. In effect, increasing MLP would bring the cycle back to normal, to a balance between probability of death and innate capacity to maintain health--the way it originally was several thousand years ago. Thus, if MLP begins to increase again, an individual would have more of a chance of being killed before he reached a given level of senescence. For example, if the aging process can be stopped so that the probability of death does not exceed that for a 30-year-old man today in the U.S., then MLP would be about 1246 years and 50% mean survival would be 374 years. Of course, if environmental hazards began to reduce in proportion to increased MLP, then the percent of senescent individuals in the population would remain constant.

The population problem may also not become as serious as is frequently believed. Increased MLP does not imply a correspondingly increased reproduction rate. Couples today could have up to 20 children, but instead they usually have 2 or 3. Even further birth control measures are being undertaken in some nations today. As long as the rate of birth is balanced by the rate of death, any population would be stable, regardless of the longevity of its members. A more immediate problem is the initial size to which the population would increase before such an equilibrium came into play. Estimates of this equilibrium value, if MLP were doubled today and maintained for 100 years, appear to be small compared to the normal population growth that is expected under no change in MLP.

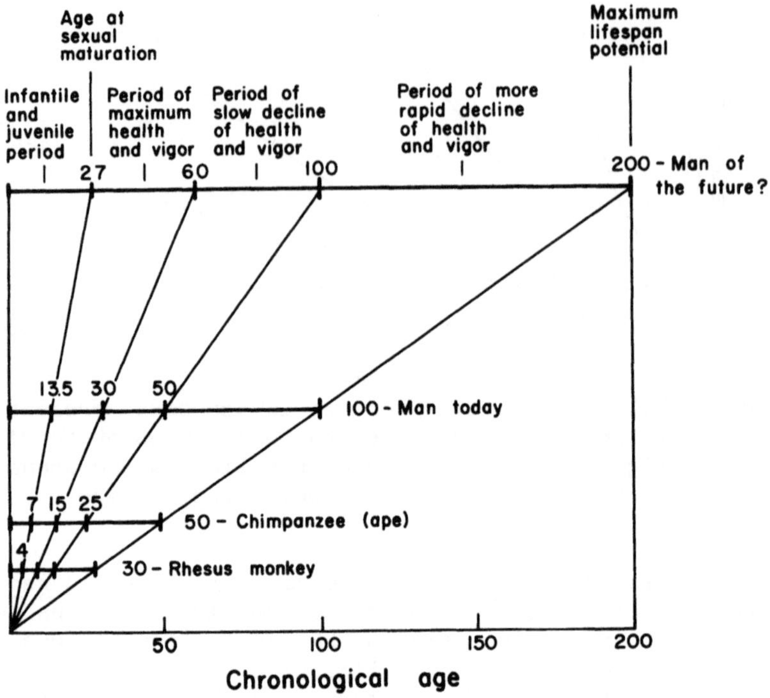

Fig. 8. Stages of development of the primate species relative to one another and the projection of these stages to man with a maximum life span potential of 200 years. Taken from (9).

Life extension up to a MLP of 200 or more years, if achieved by similar processes as those that have recently evolved, would likely require a uniform prolongation of the stages of development. Figure 8 shows the different developmental periods of life span in Rhesus, chimpanzee, and man; and from these values an extrapolation is made as to what the extended time-period of these various phases of life span would be for man with a MLP of 200 years. In the example, the period of maximum health and vigor increases from 16.5 years to 33 years, and the period of rapid decline in vigor and health increases from 50 years to 100 years. It appears that more years of senescence would be gained than years of youth. However, it should be clear from our previous discussion and Figures 6 and 7 that, in spite of an increased period of senescence, the percent of the population in such a phase of life would decrease.

Another remarkable change occurring during the recent evolutionary history of man is his increase in brain size with the accompanying increase in mental ability (59,60). Figure 9 illustrates the correlation of brain weight to MLP during recent hominid evolution. If such a trend continued, a brain size increase from about 1450 g to 5000 g would evolve for a corresponding increase of MLP from 100 to

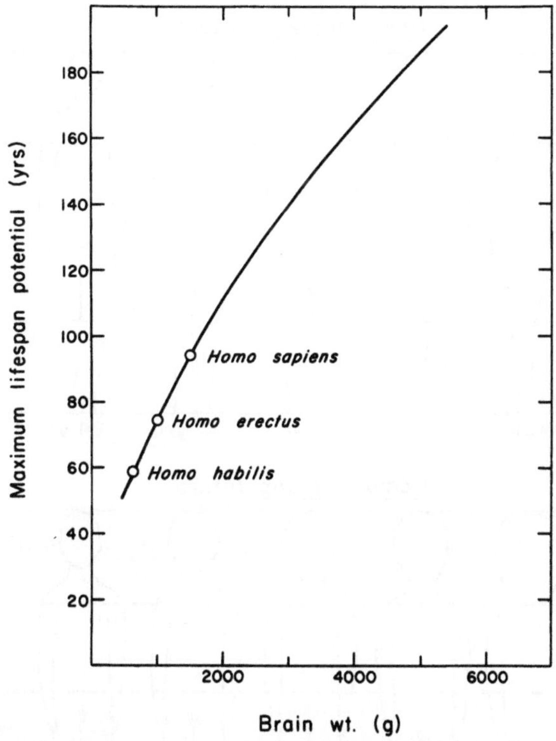

Fig. 9. Evolutionary trend of increased brain size in relation to increase in MLP for man in his recent evolutionary past and a projection for the future. Equation for this projection is:

$$\text{MLP (yrs)} = 1.607\ (\text{Brain wt., g})^{.5579}$$

200 years. Whether such an increase also would result in higher mental functions, remains to be determined (61,62), but recent comparative studies on neuron networks between man and chimpanzee show few qualitative differences. It may very well be that higher brain functions, as evident in man, result from a relatively small amount of genetic information, where there is much redundancy in its design. This would be consistent with such a high evolutionary rate of development of the brain, along with an increased MLP.

An interesting hypothesis on the mechanism of how the morphological functions of man evolved, known as neoteny, is that certain stages of early development were retarded, as compared to similar stages of development in the apes (63-66). In this sense, adult man has many fetal characteristics that are found only in the infant developmental stages of man's hominid ancestors, as well as some of the living ape species (67,68). This idea suggests that the general

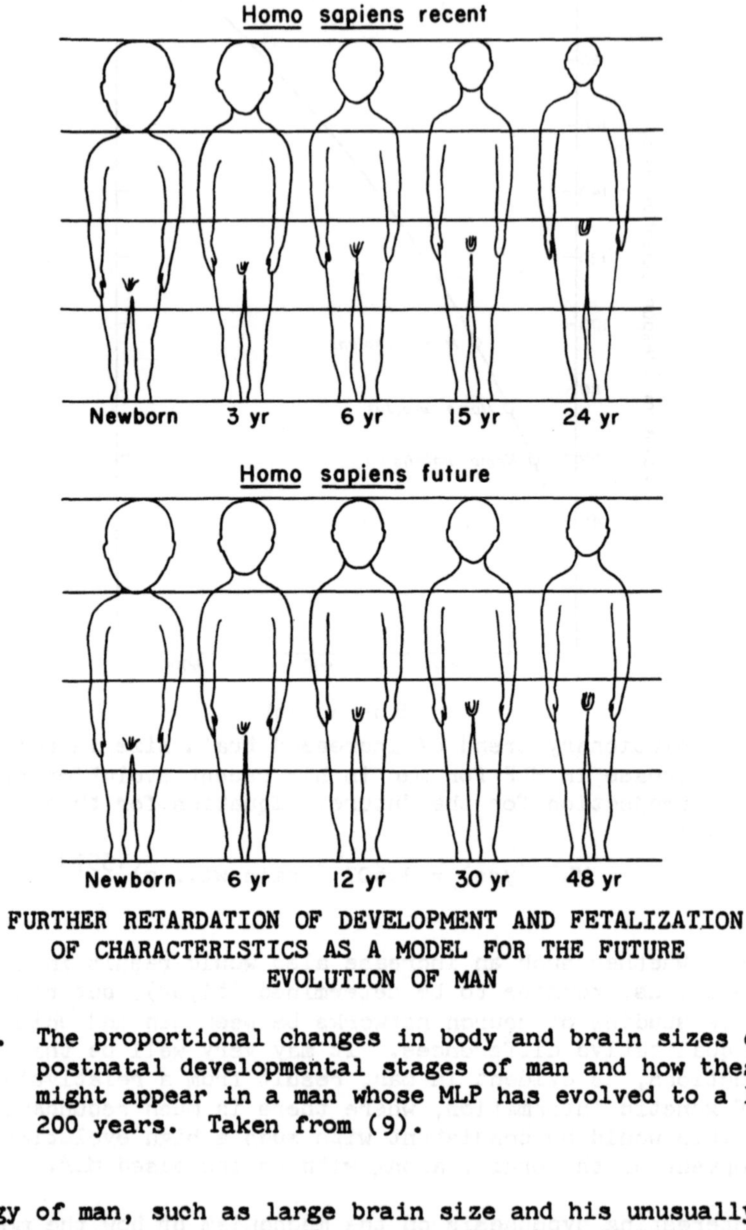

Fig. 10. The proportional changes in body and brain sizes during postnatal developmental stages of man and how these stages might appear in a man whose MLP has evolved to a level of 200 years. Taken from (9).

morphology of man, such as large brain size and his unusually slow pattern of development, evolved as a result of small alterations in the regulatory processes governing developmental rate (69).

The general morphological appearance of postnatal developmental stages of man today, and what it may be in the future if continued along similar lines, is shown in Figure 10. Table 16 summarizes some of the major developmental and physical characteristics of man with a

Table 16. Model of Continued Evolution of Human Longevity[a]

MLP, yrs	92	150	200
Brain capacity, cm^3	1446	3396	5688
EQ	7.5	15.2	22.6
$N_c \times 10^{-8}$	91	168	240
Body wt, g	65	81	97
SMR, c/g/d	23	21.8	20.8
MCC, Kc/g	780	1198	1523
ASM, yr	14-17	22-27	30-37
% Br wt/Body wt, g/g	2.2	4.2	5.8

[a]The assumption is made that these parameters continued to evolve along the same equation as they have during the past 2.5 million years of hominid evolution.

MLP of 100 and 200 years.

Just as man thought his earth to be the center of the universe, so he has also thought his body to be nearly perfect and improvement to be impossible. We are now closer to challenging this idea directly by inquiring about what biological processes determine the innate duration of health, how these processes might be improved, and what might be the consequences if significant life extension occurs. If the potential benefits of extended physical and mental health are realized, man may be nearing a quantum jump in his evolution--a self-evolutionary process that is perhaps as natural as his evolutionary past, and as inescapable.

REFERENCES

1. C. E. Finch and L. Hayflick, eds., "Handook of the Biology of Aging," Van Nostrand Reinhold, New York (1977).
2. P. S. Timiras, ed., "Developmental Physiology and Aging," Macmillan Co., New York (1972).
3. R. G. Cutler, in:"Interdisciplinary Topics in Gerontology," Vol. 9, R. G. Cutler, ed., Karger, Basel (1976).
4. P. Weiss, in:"Perspectives in Experimental Gerontology," Charles C. Thomas, Springfield, Illinois (1966).
5. R. G. Cutler, Proc. Natl. Acad. Sci. USA 72:4664 (1975).
6. R. G. Cutler, in:"Advances in Gerontological Research, Vol. 4," B. L. Strehler, ed., Academic Press, New York (1972).
7. R. G. Cutler, Mech. Ageing Dev. 2:381 (1974).

8. R. G. Cutler, in:"Genetic Effects on Aging," D. Bergsma, D. E. Harrison, and N. W. Paul, eds., Alan R. Liss, New York (1978).
9. R. G. Cutler, in:"The Biology of Aging," J. A. Behnke, C. E. Finch, and G. B. Moment, eds., Plenum Press, New York (1978).
10. K. M. Weiss, J. Human Evol. (in press).
11. R. G. Cutler, J. Human Evol. 5:169 (1976).
12. R. G. Cutler, Gerontology 25:69 (1979).
13. G. A. Sacher, in:"Primate Functional Morphology and Evolution," R. Tuttle, ed., Mouton, The Hague (1975).
14. H. J. Jerison, "Evolution of the Brain and Intelligence," Academic Press, New York (1973).
15. M. C. King and A. C. Wison, Science 188:107 (1975).
16. F. J. Ayala, "Molecular Evolution," Sinauer Pub., Sunderland, Mass. (1976).
17. G. B. Kolata, Science 189:446 (1975).
18. G. A. Sacher, in:"Ciba Foundation Colloquium on Aging," Vol. 5 (1959).
19. R. E. Leakey and R. Lewin, "Origins," E. P. Dutton (1977).
20. A. C. Wilson, L. R. Maxson, and V. M. Sarich, Proc. Natl. Acad. Sci. USA 71:2843 (1974).
21. A. C. Wilson, V. M. Sarich, and L. R. Maxson, Proc. Natl. Acad. Sci. USA 71:3028 (1974).
22. A. C. Wilson, S. S. Carlson, and T. J. White, Ann. Rev. Biochem. 46:573 (1977).
23. G. L. Bush, S. M. Case, A. C. Wilson, and J. L. Patton, Proc. Natl. Acad. Sci. USA 74:3942 (1977).
24. J. F. MacDonald, G. K. Chambers, J. David, and F. J. Ayala, Proc. Natl. Acad. Sci. USA 74:4562 (1977).
25. D. Pilbeam and S. J. Gould, Science 186:892 (1974).
26. S. J. Gould, "Ontogeny and Phylogeny," Belknap Press of Harvard University Press, Cambridge, Mass. (1977).
27. G. A. Sacher, Exp. Geront. 3:265 (1968).
28. R. G. Cutler, in:"Aging, Carcinogenesis and Radiation Biology," K. C. Smith, ed., Plenum Press, New York (1976).
29. J. P. Ogrodnik, J. H. Wulf, and R. G. Cutler, Exp. Geront. 10:119 (1975).
30. R. G. Cutler, Exp. Geront. 10:37 (1975).
31. C. E. Finch, Quart. Rev. Biol. 51:49 (1976).
32. U. Reiss and D. Gershon, Eur. J. Biochem. 63:617 (1976).
33. H. Ursprung, "The Stability of the Differentiated State," Springer-Verlag, New York (1968).
34. C. L. Markert, Cancer Res. 28:1908 (1968).
35. A. D. Braun, "The Biology of Cancer," Addison-Wesley, Reading, Mass. (1974).
36. J. H. Goggin and N. G. Anderson, Adv. Cancer Res. 19:105 (1974).
37. J. Uriel, in:"Cancer, A Comprehensive Treatise," F. Becke, ed., Plenum Press, New York (1975).
38. T. Ono and R. G. Cutler, Proc. Natl. Acad. Sci. USA 75:4431 (1978).
39. R. L. Walford, Gerontologia 21:184 (1975).

40. R. L. Walford, "The Immunologic Theory of Aging," Williams and Wilkins, Baltimore (1969).
41. K. Nandy, in:"The Aging Brain," K. Nandy and I. Sherwin, eds., Plenum Press, New York (1976).
42. R. D. Terry, in:"A New Look at Biological Aging," J. A. Behnke, C. E. Finch, and G. B. Moment, eds., Plenum Press, New York (1978).
43. R. J. Huebner and G. J. Todaro, Proc. Natl. Acad. Sci. USA 64:1087 (1969).
44. H. M. Temin, Science 192:1075 (1976).
45. J. Uriel, Cancer Res. 36:4269 (1976).
46. M. R. Ahuja and R. Anders, in:"Recent Advances in Cancer: Cell Biology, Molecular Biology, and Tumor Virology, Vol. 1," R. C. Galli, ed. (1977).
47. E. J. Field and A. Peat, Gerontologia 17:129 (1971).
48. E. J. Field and B. K. Shelton, Gerontologia 19:211 (1973).
49. G. J. Gruman, Trans. Amer. Phil. Soc. New Series, Part 9:56 (1966).
50. B. L. Strehler, Fed. Proc. 34:5 (1975).
51. P. G. Goldschmidt and I. H. Jillson, "A Comprehensive Study of the Ethical, Legal, and Social Implications of Advances in Biomedical and Behavioral Research and Technology," Policy Research Inc., Baltimore, Md.
52. B. L. Neugarten and R. J. Havighurst, "Extending the Human Life Span: Social Policy and Social Ethics," Committee on Human Development, University of Chicago, Chicago (1977).
53. B. L. Neugarten and R. J. Havighurst, "Social Policy, Social Ethics and the Aging Society," Committee on Human Development, University of Chicago, Chicago (1977).
54. H. Gerjuoy, in:"Frontiers in Aging: Life Extension," F. M. Lassman, ed., International J. Aging and Human Development, in press.
55. Life-Span Conference: The Center for the Study of Democratic Institutions/The Fund for the Republic, Inc., Santa Barbara, CA (1970).
56. R. G. Cutler and R. A. Kalish, Gerontologist 17:141 (1977).
57. R. G. Cutler, in:"Frontiers in Aging: Life Extension," R. M. Lassman, ed., International J. Aging and Human Development, in press.
58. L. Hayflick, Nat. Hist. 86:22 (1977).
59. P. V. Tobias, "The Brain in Hominid Evolution," Columbia University Press, New York (1971).
60. R. E. Leakey and R. Lewin, "Origins," E. P. Dutton, New York (1977).
61. B. Rensch, Amer. Naturalist XC:81 (1956).
62. L. Van Halen, Amer. J. Phys. Anthrop. 40:417 (1974).
63. A. H. Schulz, Proc. Amer. Phil Soc. 94:428 (1950).
64. S. J. Gould, Nat. Hist. 85:22 (1976).
65. S. J. Gould, Nat. Hist. 85:18 (1976).

66. S. J. Gould, "Ontongeny and Phylogeny," Harvard University Press, Cambridge, Mass. (1977).
67. A. H. Schultz, Quart. Rev. Biol. 1:465 (1926).
68. G. F. R. S. DeBeer, "Embryos and Ancestors," Oxford University Press, London (1971).
69. S. J. Gould, "Ever Since Darwin," W. W. Norton & Co., New York (1977).

LONGEVITY POTENTIAL, PHYLOGENETIC AND ECOLOGICAL CONSTRAINTS IN MAMMALS

François Bourlière

INSERM Gerontology Research Unit
Paris, France

The dependence of mammalian life span on some constitutional variables, adult body weight, brain body weight, specific metabolic rate and deep body temperature, has been repeatedly discussed by Sacher (1,2). Furthermore, having found, in his 1976 paper, a relationship between the rate of entropy production and the duration of life when body weight is constant, Sacher goes so far as to conclude that "everything we know about the neurological concomitants of mammalian longevity--sensory, intellectual, and motor--supports the intuition that the length of life of a species is closely related to its intelligence and, indeed, that longevity is a major teleonomic purpose and manifestation of animal intelligence."

Such a view is hard to substantiate when one considers the numerous data on mammalian longevity recently made available in the literature (3,4,5,6,7). The maximum recorded life span of a number of small animals is given in Table 1, together with the adult body weight, and the capability of the species to undergo hibernation (H) or periods of daily torpor (T).

The extreme longevity potential of bats (Chiroptera) stands out at once, despite the fact that the behavioral performances of this mammalian order are not particularly sophisticated, and in spite of a brain/body weight ratio not very different from that of the short-lived and non-heterothermic small rodents. It is also to be noted that within a given taxonomic category--whether it be Marsupialia, Insectivora, Chiroptera, Primates, or Rodentia--all the species sharing a similar body weight which are also able to lower their body temperature when environmental conditions become unfavorable, are at the same time those which enjoy the greater longevity potential. This is quite obvious when one compares murids and heteromyids among the Rodentia.

Table 1. Adult Body Weight (g), Maximum Recorded Life Span (years), Ability to Hibernate or Estivate (H) and to Enter Daily Torpor (T), Among Small Mammals

	Adult body weight	Maximum longevity	Hibernation or Torpor
Marsupialia			
Planigale sp.	5	1	
Sminthopsis crassicaudata	10-15	3	T
Acrobates pygmaeus	12-14	4	T
Cercartetus caudatus	15-25	>5.5	T
Antechinus stuartii	24-49	>3	T
Petaurus norfolcensis	90-130	12	
Dasycercus cristicaudata	120-170	>5	T
Caluromys derbianus	190-220	>5	
Caluromysiops irrupta	ca 200	>7.5	
Dasyuorides byrnei	ca 200	>5	
Macrotis lagotis	300-1600	>7	T ?
Dasyurus viverrinus	680-1130	7	
Potorous tridactylus	1360-1810	>9.5	
Insectivora			
Suncus etruscus	1.25-2.3	>2	
Sorex araneus	6-10	1.5	
Crocidura russula	6-10	4	
Neomys fodieus	10-22	1.5	
Blarina brevicauda	14-22	2.5	
Chiroptera			
Pipistrellus pipistrellus	3.8-6.5	11	H.T
Myotis mystacinus	4-8	18	H.T
Rhinolophus hipposideros	4-9	> 18	H.T
Myotis daubentoni	6-12	18	H.T
Plecotus auritus	6-12	13	H.T
Barbastella barbastellus	6-13	18	H.T
Myotis nattereri	7-12	17	H.T
Plecotus austriacus	7-14	12	H.T
Rhinolophus ferrum-equinum	13-34	> 22	H.T

Another constitutional variable that must be taken into consideration is the reproductive potential of species. Those with a high reproductive rate (large litter-size and several litters per year), like rodents of the microtine or murine type, have a low longevity potential. In contrast to these "r-strategists," the "K-strategists," such as bats and primates with a low reproductive potential, have a much longer life span (8,9).

"Intelligence" as such has, therefore, quite probably very little to do with the longevity potential of mammals. Those species which

Table 1. (Continuation). Adult Body Weight (g), Maximum Recorded Life Span (years), Ability to Hibernate or Estivate (H) and to Enter Daily Torpor (T), Among Small Mammals

	Adult body weight	Maximum longevity	Hibernation or Torpor
Chiroptera (continued)			
Myotis myotis	20-45	18	H.T
Desmodus rotundus	33-47	12.5	
Eidolon helvum	250-310	21.5	
Primates			
Microcebus murinus	45-170	>11	H.T
Galago demidovii	50-90	10	H.T
Cebuella pygmaea	110-160	10	
Galago senegalensis	150-300	>10	
Callithrix jacchus	260-320	12.5	T
Microcebus coquereli	300-400	15.5	H.T
Cheirogaleus major	340-600	11	H.T
Saguinus fuscicollis	370-436	> 7	T ?
Leontopithecus rosalia	430-654	10	
Perodictitus potto	600-1600	11	
Calimico goeldi	645-680	10	
Miopithecus talapoin	800-900	28	
Galago crassicaudatus	1000-1800	14	
Rodentia			
Micromys minutus	7-10	4	
Perognathus longimembris	7-19	>8	T
Perognathus fallax	14-17	>8	T
Mus musculus	14-25	3.5	
Peromyscus leucopus	14-30	>8	T
Microtus arvalis	16-51	>1.5	
Apodemus sylvaticus	16-30	>4	
Peromyscus maniculatus	17-35	8	T
Apodemus flavicollis	18-40	5	
Microtus agrestis	20-47	>1.5	
Muscardinus avellanarius	23-43	6	H
Rattus rattus	150-250	4.5	
Rattus norvegicus	240-360	3	

are endowed with the longest life span appear to be basically those most capable of efficiently adapting to environmental changes, both at the individual and at the population levels. Such a high degree of adaptability can actually be achieved in two different (and not forcibly exclusive) ways, through adaptive behaviors (i.e., "intelligence," according to Sacher) as well as through physiological mechanisms like heterothermy which enable an organism to temporarily withstand adverse environmental conditions.

A relationship between an extended longevity potential and a high degree of physiological and/or behavioral adaptability to changing environmental conditions might also help to explain why, in a toxonomic category like bats, long-lived species are more frequently ecountered in temperate than in tropical areas. The more adaptable, thus, the potentially more longevous species would in our view have a better chance to be selected by the extreme seasonality or the impredictability of climatic conditions in northern latitudes.

REFERENCES

1. G. A. Sacher, Relations of lifespan to brain weight and body weight in mammals, in:"The Lifespan of Animals," G. E. W. Wolstenholme and M. O'Connor, eds., Churchill, London (1959).
2. G. A. Sacher, Evaluation of the entropy and information terms governing mammalian longevity, Interdis. Top. Gerontol. Basel 9:69 (1976).
3. L. R. Collins, "Monotremes and Marsupials. A Reference for Zoological Institutions," Smithsonian Institution, Washington (1973).
4. G. B. Corbet and H. N. Southern, eds., "The Handbook of British Mammals, Second Edition," Blackwell, Oxford (1977).
5. Th. Haltenorth and H. Diller, "Bestimmungsbuch. Saugetiere Afrikas und Madagascars," BLV Verlagsgesellschaft, Munchen (1977).
6. P. Hershkovitz, "Living New World Monkeys (Platyrrhini). Volume I," University of Chicago Press, Chicago (1977).
7. J. Niethammer and F. Krapp, "Handbuch der Saugetiere Europas, Band I," Akademische Verlagsgesellschaft, Wiesbaden (1978).
8. F. Bouliere, Lifespans of mammalian and bird populations in nature, in:"The Lifespan of Animals," G. E. W. Wolstenholme and M. O'Connor, eds., Churchill, London (1959).
9. F. B. Golley, K. Petruscewicz, and L. Ryszkokwski, "Small Mammals: Their Productivity and Population Dynamics," Cambridge University Press, Cambridge (1975).

POPULATION DOUBLING NUMBERS IN CELLS WITH GENETIC DISORDERS

Osamu Nikaido, Sadayuki Ban* and Tsutomu Sugahara

Radiation Biology Center and Department of Experimental Radiology, Faculty of Medicine*, Kyoto University
Kyoto 606, Japan

INTRODUCTION

The limited life spans of fibroblasts derived from human embryonic lungs were first reported by Hayflick (1). Then, the correlation between doubling potentials of cells and maximal life spans of donor animals (2) as well as the inverted correlation between doubling potentials of human fibroblasts and ages of donors were established (3). Thus, it has been thought that cells age as donors age, or cells *in vitro* at least mimic parts of various processes of *in vivo* aging, although the mechanisms of cellular aging are not yet known.

Comparative evolutionary studies on the relationship between the extent of unscheduled DNA synthesis (UDS) induced in the cells by exposure to ultraviolet light (UV), and maximal life spans in various placental animals from which the cells were derived, offered the hypothesis that the ability of cells to repair DNA damage induced by various environmental agents determines the life spans in animals (4). On the other hand, cells obtained from patients with a genetic disease, Hutchinson-Gilford progeria, were reported to be defective in repairing single strand breaks formed in cellular DNA by gamma-irradiation (5,6) and to have low doubling potentials in culture (7). A contradictory result was also reported, however, for the same disease (8). Nevertheless, these results have called the attention of many investigators to the role of DNA repair in cellular aging.

Ontogenetic analyses are necessary to elucidate the role of a cell's ability to repair DNA damage in its aging process. Results of the alterations in this cellular reparability throughout *in vitro* life spans, as obtained by many workers, are controversial (9,10,11).

For example, it was recently reported that the extent of UDS in mouse embryonic fibroblasts gradually decreased as _in vitro_ age increased (12). A similar decrease in the extend of UDS as cells proceed through their life spans has never been reported for human cells. This decrease is seen in human cells only at very late passages (13).

By applying the repair hypothesis to _in vitro_ aging, one can suggest that the limited life spans of cultured human cells result from the accumulation of DNA damage introduced by various environmental agents present in culture conditions. At the moment, it is unknown what sorts of and to what extent DNA damage accumulates in cells during their life spans. The biological characterization and identification of these damages is necessary before it will be possible to establish causal relationship between "cellular reparability" and cellular aging.

Cells obtained from patients with recessive genetic diseases, such as xeroderma pigmentosum (XP) and ataxia telangiectasia (AT), are known to be sensitive to UV and X-rays, respectively (14). It is well known that the sensitivity of these cells to various agents is due to their deficient ability to repair specific types of DNA damage (15,16). One might expect early cessation of growth potentials in such repair deficient mutants if the damage accumulated during culture, in ambient conditions, contained at least some damage the cells could not repair. Therefore, evaluation of doubling potentials of cells obtained from patients with XP, AT, and Werner's syndrome (WS), showing "premature" aging, and from healthy donors of various ages, was carried out.

For the assessment of "cellular reparability" to UV-damaged DNA, host-cell reactivation (HCR), using herpes simplex virus irradiated with UV, was applied to various cells as well as to cells at various _in vitro_ ages (17,18). This technique was employed because the UDS induced in cells following treatment with UV, which is usually applied to detect the DNA repair, might not show actual completion of DNA repair. Rather, it might show only insertion of exogenous radioactive bases into the sites of damage. Virus production in host cells, on the other hand, implies complete repair of UV-induced damage in viral DNA.

MATERIALS AND METHODS

Cells, Culture Method and Medium

Fetal lung and heart tissues at five months gestational age were provided by the courtesy of the Human Embryo Center for Teratological Studies, Faculty of Medicine, Kyoto University. Skin biopsies taken from healthy donors of various ages were obtained through Kansai Electric Co. Hospital by courtesy of Dr. Y. Isobe. Skin biopsy specimens of patients with conditions known to produce defective DNA repair were provided by the courtesy of Professor Takebe, Radiation Biology Center, Kyoto University, and those of Werner's syndrome were offered by Kyoto University Hospital, Chiba University Hospital, Tenri Hospital, and Obama Municipal Hospital.

Fibroblasts propagated from tissues or biopsy fragments by a method being published elsewhere (19) were cultured in TD-40 culture bottle at a concentration of 10^6 cells per 10 ml of Eagle's MEM medium (Nissui Seiyaku Co , Tokyo) supplemented with 10% calf serum (Flow Laboratories, Stanmore). The same batches of calf serum were used throughout this experiment. Three bottles of cells were successively cultured. Cells were fed every 2 days with fresh medium and subcultured at the 4th to 7th day, prior to reaching to near confluency. After harvesting the cells with 0.1% trypsin (Difco Laboratories, Detroit) and 0.01% EDTA (Waken Pharmacy Co., Osaka) in phosphate buffer saline, an aliquot of 10^6 cells was inoculated into a TD-40 culture bottle. The cessation of growth of a cell population was recognized when lower cell yields than inoculum cell number (10^6 cells) were obtained twice in successive subcultures. The number of population doublings (PDN) attained by cells was calculated by the method being published elsewhere (19).

The Virus and its Assay

Herpes simplex virus, type I, a large plaque variant of the +GC Miyama strain (20), having a titer of 1.7×10^7 pfu/ml against human aminon Fl cell line, was used for all virus experiments. After diluting viral suspensions with phosphate buffer saline to the appropriate concentration, various doses of UV were given with germicidal lamps (10 watt x 2, Toshiba GL-10) at a dose rate of 1.7 to 1.8 J/m^2/sec., and monitored at each exposure by Topcon radiometer (Tokyo Kogaku Co. Ltd., Tokyo). 0.5 ml of UV-irradiated viral suspension was delivered to freshly confluent cells in plastic dishes (6 cm in diameter), which had been previously washed once with phosphate buffer saline and incubated for 90 min. at 37°C. Virus adsorption was stopped by adding 4.5 ml of complete medium containing 0.25% human gammaglobulin (human immunoglogulin, Midorijuji Co., Osaka). Plaques were scored on the 3rd day of incubation, and survival curves for successful UV-irradiated herpes simplex virus infection of various cell strains were depicted as the function of UV doses. The survival curves were usually composed of two components (17). D_0 values were obtained from the first component.

RESULTS

Repair of UV-Damaged Virus DNA by Various Host Cells

When cell progression had reached 20% of usual life spans, various cells were assayed for the UV-survival of herpes simplex

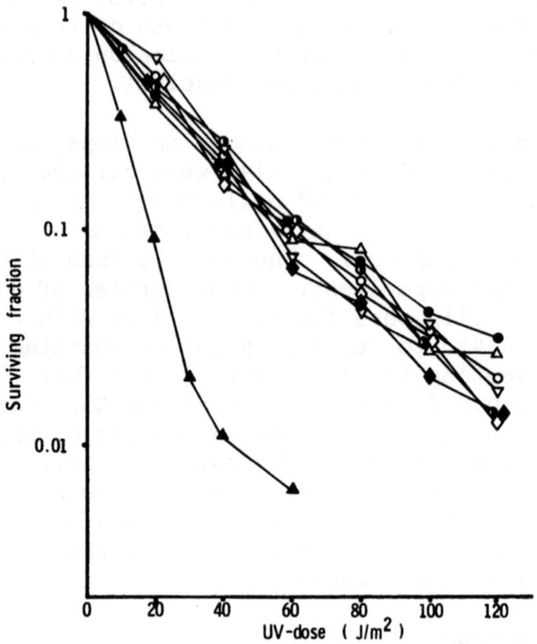

Fig. 1. Host-cell reactivation of UV-irradiated herpes simplex virus in cells derived from healthy donors. △ 1.5-year-old female; ▽ 33-year-old female; ◇ 65-year-old female, from patient with genetic disorders; ◆ AT1SE, 9-year-old male; ▲ XP6NA, 6-year-old female; ● WS10B, 47-year-old male, and from fetus; ○ lung; and ◐ heart.

viruses. Cells obtained from healthy donors, patients with ataxia telangiectasia and those with Werner's syndrome were most efficient in HCR of UV-irradiated viruses, while cells from xeroderma pigmentosum patients were most reduced in HCR. D_0 values in J/m^2 for the first component of the survival curves were 25 for normal cells and 8 for XP cells, as shown in Figure 1.

It is noteworthy that the lung and heart fibroblasts obtained from a single fetus showed the same D_0 values in HCR of UV-irradiated viruses, though they had distinctly different doubling potentials, as shown later. Age-dependent changes of D_0 values were not observed in three cell strains obtained from healthy donors of various ages.

Relationship Between in Vitro Ages and HCR

Cells cultured for various lengths of time were assayed for HCR of UV-irradiated herpes simplex viruses. The D_0 values of the

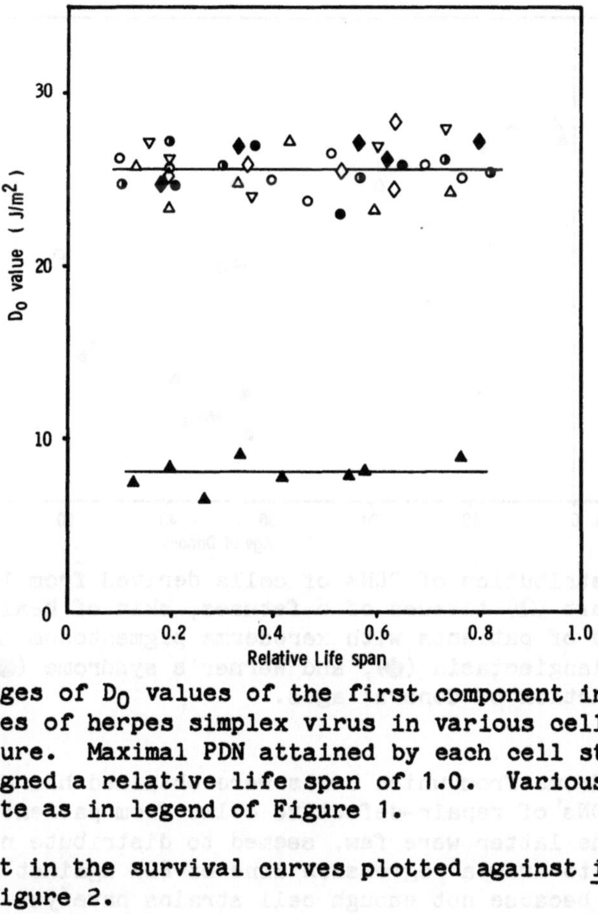

Fig. 2. Changes of D_0 values of the first component in UV-survival curves of herpes simplex virus in various cells during culture. Maximal PDN attained by each cell strain was assigned a relative life span of 1.0. Various symbols denote as in legend of Figure 1.

first component in the survival curves plotted against in vitro ages are shown in Figure 2.

As shown in this figure, no marked changes in D_0 values were observed in each cell population throughout 80% of its life span, though low D_0 values were observed in XP cells. It is remarkable that different D_0 values were not observed among cells derived from fetal lung and heart having different PDNs, and that WS cells having lower PDNs as proved in Figure 3 showed the same magnitude of D_0 values as normal cells. This is in agreement with the results obtained from UDS experiment after UV exposure (21).

Distribution of PDNs in Cells Obtained from Various Donors

Cells derived from donors of various ages and patients with genetic disorders were assayed in terms of their PDNs. Figure 3 shows the relationship between PDNs in various cells and ages of donors. Donors with a history of diabetes mellitus and cortisone medication were carefully excluded from this experiment, with the exception of those with Werner's syndrome. All patients with

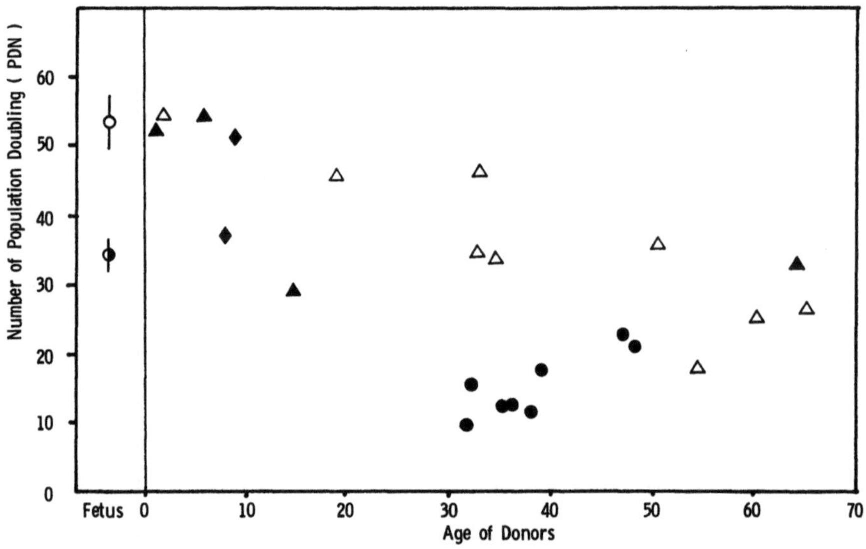

Fig. 3. Distribution of PDNs of cells derived from lung (○) and heart (◑) tissues of 6 fetuses, skin of healthy donors (△), and of patients with xeroderma pigmentosum (▲), ataxia telangiectasia (◆), and Werner's syndrome (●), as a function of donors' ages.

Werner's syndrome from which cells were obtained had a history of diabetes. PDNs of repair-defective cells from patients with XP and AT, though the latter were few, seemed to distribute normally. It is not possible to draw a regression line of PDN against donors' ages in this figure, because not enough cell strains have yet been examined. However, an apparent tendency in reduction of PDNs as donors' ages increased may exist among various cells, with the exception of WS cells. PDNs of WS cells fell well below the range of PDNs for normal cells.

DISCUSSION

The aim of the present study was, first, to statistically confirm the results on the doubling potentials of XP cells previously reported by Goldstein (22), and then to extend the experiment further by testing other repair-defective cell strains. Because the number of population doublings attained by human cells was known to spread within a wide range (3,23), either repeat cultures of a cell strain or an increase in the number of cell strains in culture was necessary to obtain statistically significant results. Our results were in good agreement with those previously reported (22). XP cells, known to be defective in the first step of excision repair to UV damage in DNA (24), showed a low D_0 value in the first component of UV survival curve of herpes simplex virus. However, their number of population doublings fell well within the normal range. On the other hand, the number of population doublings of AT cells, which were defective in gamma-endonuclease (16), also fell within the range of PDNs attained by normal cells. These results might suggest that defects in both UV- and gamma-specific endonucleases in cells do not shorten their life spans and that the damages accumlated in cellular DNA during culture does not require both endonucleases for their repair, even if the accumulation of damage in cellular DNA is a causal event in cellular aging.

A striking correlation between the extent of UDS in cells derived from various placental animals, following irradiation with UV as a model agent, and maximal life spans of donor animals suggested to us the important role of DNA repair in aging. The present results, however, do not readily establish this correlation in cases of human cells, because XP cells defective in HCR for UV-irradiated viruses had age-matched population doubling numbers comparable to those of normal cells. Furthermore, it is known that cellular sensitivities to UV do not differ largely among cells derived from various animals (25), so cells showing low extent of excision repair might have other compensatory repair mechanisms. Therefore, it is also conceivable that repair mechanisms other than excision repair play important roles in cellular aging.

It was recently reported that non-cycling cells in WI-38 cell population at very late passages had a reduction in the extent of UDS to UV-induced DNA damages (13). Non-cycling cells, defined as cells unable to enter the S period for a long time, accumulated in cell populations with increasing <u>in vitro</u> age (26) and with increasing donor age (27). The accumulation rates of non-cycling cells per unit time were higher in both WS and heart cells having low PDNs than in their counterparts, age-matched normal cells and lung cells, respectively (Nikaido, unpublished). Despite the growing subpopulations of non-cycling cells, the reparability of whole cell population to repair UV-damaged DNA, assayed by HCR in the present study, remained unchanged among the various cell strains, with the exception of XP cells and cells at various passages up to 80% of their life spans. One way to explain these results is that non-cycling cells, as well as cycling cells, are susceptible to virus production. It is also possible that only the residual cycling cells in a population participate in the production of viruses, which masks the lack of susceptibility of non-cycling cells to viruses. Thus, the increasing heterogeneity in a cell population as it ages may disturb biological characteristics such as DNA repair and DNA synthesis in cells. Analyses and purification of subpopulations showing different characteristics in aging cells may increase our knowledge of the mechanisms of cellular aging. An experiment on this is now in progress.

ACKNOWLEDGEMENTS

The authors wish to express their gratitude to Dr. S. Arase for introducing to us the virus experiment, and to Drs. H. Imura, O. Nagatani, M. Nishikawa, and Y. Tanabe for providing us with specimens obtained from patients with Werner's syndrome. We also wish to acknowledge Professor H. Takebe for his helpful discussions and for providing us with various biopsy specimens. This research was supported in part by a Grant-in-Aid for Cancer Research from the Ministry of Education, Science and Culture, Japan.

REFERENCES

1. L. Hayflick and P. S. Moorhead, The serial cultivation of human diploid cell strains, Exp. Cell Res. 25:585 (1961).
2. L. Hayflick, The longevity of cultured human cells, J. Amer. Geriat. Soc. 22:1 (1974).
3. G. M. Martin, C. A. Sprague, and C. J. Epstein, Replicative life span of cultivated human cells, effect of donor's age, tissue and genotype, Lab. Invest. 23:86 (1970).
4. R. W. Hart and R. B. Setlow, Correlation between deoxyribonucleic acid excision-repair and life span in a number of mammalian species, Proc. Natl. Acad. Sci. USA 71:2169 (1974).
5. J. Epstein, J. R. Williams, and J. B. Little, Deficient DNA repair in human progeroid cells, Proc. Nat. Acad. Sci. USA 70:977 (1973).
6. J. Epstein, J. R. Williams, and J. B. Little, Rate of DNA repair in progeria and normal human fibroblasts, Biochem. Biophys. Res. Comm. 59:850 (1974).
7. S. Goldstein, Lifespan of cultured cells in progeria, Lancet 1:424 (1969).
8. J. D. Regan and R. B. Setlow, DNA repair in human progeroid cells, Biochem. Biophys. Res. Comm. 59:858 (1974).
9. R. B. Painter, J. M. Clarkson, and B. R. Young, Ultraviolet induced repair replication in aging diploid human cells (WI-38), Radiation Res. 56:560 (1973).
10. J. M. Clarkson and R. B. Painter, Repair of X-ray damage in aging WI-38 cells, Mutat. Res. 23:107 (1974).
11. P. D. Bowman, R. L. Meek, and C. W. Daniel, Decreased unscheduled DNA synthesis in nondividing aged WI-38 cells, Mech. Age. Dev. 5:251 (1976).
12. V. Paffenholts, Correlation between DNA repair of embryonic fibroblasts and different life span of 3 inbred mouse strains, Mech. Ageing Dev. 7:131 (1978).
13. R. W. Hart and R. B. Setlow, DNA repair in late passage human cells, Mech. Ageing Dev. 5:67 (1976).
14. J. E. Cleaver, DNA repair and radiation sensitivity in human (xeroderma pigmentosum) cells, Int. J. Radiat. Biol. 18:557 (1970).

15. R. B. Setlow, J. D. Regan, J. German, and W. L. Carrier, Evidence that xeroderma pigmentosum cells do not perform the first step in the repair of ultraviolet damages in their DNA, Proc. Nat. Acad. Sci. 64:1035 (1969).
16. M. C. Paterson, B. P. Smith, P. H. M. Lohman, A. K. Anderson, and L. Fishman, Defective excision repair of X-ray-damaged DNA in human (ataxia telangiectasia) fibroblasts, Nature 260:444 (1976).
17. C. D. Lytle, Host-cell reactivation in mammalian cells. I. Survival of ultraviolet-irradiated herpes simplex virus in different cell lines, Int. J. Radiat. Biol. 19:329 (1971).
18. H. Takebe, S. Nii, M. I. Ishii, and H. Utsumi, Comparative studies of host cell reactivation of Xeroderma pigmentosum, normal human and some other mammalian cells, Mutat. Res. 25:383 (1974).
19. S. Ban, O. Nikaido, and T. Sugahara, Acute and late effects of a single exposure of ionizing radition on cultured human diploid cell populations, Radiat. Res. in press.
20. O. Niwa and S. Nii, Applicability of microbiological technique to selection of HCR- mutants of mammalian cells, Biken J. 15:39 (1972).
21. Y. Fujiwara, T. Higashikawa, and M. Tatsumi, A retarded rate of DNA replication and normal level of DNA repair in Werner's syndrome fibroblasts in culture, J. Cell. Physiol. 92:365 (1977).
22. S. Goldstein, The role of DNA repair in aging of cultured fibroblasts from xeroderma pigmentosum and normals, Proc. Soc. Exp. Biol. Med. 137:730 (1971).
23. R. Holliday, L. I. Huschtscha, G. M. Tarrant, and T. B. L. Kirkwood, Testing the commitment theory of cellular aging, Science 198:366 (1977).
24. K. Tanaka, M. Sekiguchi, and Y. Okada, Restoration of ultraviolet-induced unscheduled DNA synthesis of xeroderma pigmentosum cells by the concomitant treatment with Bacteriophage T4 endonuclease V and HVJ (Sendai virus), Proc. Nat. Acad. Sci. USA 72:4071 (1975).
25. A. M. Rauth, Effects of ultraviolet light on mammalian cells in culture, in:"Current Topics in Radiation Research," Vol. 6, M. Evert and A. Howard, eds., North-Holland, Amsterdam (1970).
26. V. J. Cristofalo and B. B. Sharf, Cellular senescence and DNA synthesis. Thymidine incorporation as a measure of population age in human diploid cells, Exptl. Cell Res. 76:419 (1973).
27. E. Schneider and Y. Mitsui, The relationship between in vitro cellular aging and in vivo human age, Proc. Nat. Acad. Sci. USA 73:3584 (1976).

SUBJECT INDEX

MIX
Papier aus verantwortungsvollen Quellen
Paper from responsible sources
FSC® C105338

If you have any concerns about our products,
you can contact us on
ProductSafety@springernature.com

In case Publisher is established outside the EU,
the EU authorized representative is:
Springer Nature Customer Service Center GmbH
Europaplatz 3, 69115 Heidelberg, Germany

Printed by Libri Plureos GmbH
in Hamburg, Germany